2014 YEAR BOOK OF PATHOLOGY AND LABORATORY MEDICINE®

The 2014 Year Book Series

Year Book of Endocrinology®: Drs Schott, Apovian, Clarke, Eugster, Khaodhiar, Meikle, Oetgen, Petersenn, Toth, and Willenberg

Year Book of Hand and Upper Limb Surgery®: Drs Yao, Adams, and Rizzo

Year Book of Medicine®: Drs Barker, DeVault, Garrick, Gold, Khardori, Lawton, LeRoith, and Pearson

Year Book of Neonatal and Perinatal Medicine®: Drs Fanaroff, Benitz, Donn, Neu, Papile, and Van Marter

Year Book of Ophthalmology®: Drs Rapuano, Fudemberg, Gupta, Hammersmith, Milman, Nagra, Nelson, Penne, Pyfer, Sergott, Shields, and Talekar

Year Book of Orthopedics®: Drs Morrey, Huddleston, Rose, Swiontkowski, and Trigg

Year Book of Pathology and Laboratory Medicine®: Drs Raab and Bissell

Year Book of Pediatrics®: Dr Cabana

Year Book of Plastic and Aesthetic Surgery™: Drs Miller, Gutowski, and Smith

Year Book of Pulmonary Disease®: Drs Barker, Jones, Maurer, Spradley, Tanoue, and Willsie

Year Book of Surgery®: Drs Behrns, Daly, Fahey, Hines, Howe, Huber, Klodell, Mozingo, and Pruett

Year Book of Urology®: Drs Andriole and Coplen

Year Book of Vascular Surgery®: Drs Gillespie, Bush, Passman, Starnes, and Watkins

2014

The Year Book of PATHOLOGY AND LABORATORY MEDICINE®

Editor-in-Chief

Stephen S. Raab, MD

Professor of Pathology, University of Washington, Seattle, Washington, and Memorial University of Newfoundland/Eastern Health Authority, St John's, Newfoundland, Canada

Editor-in-Chief, Laboratory Medicine

Michael G. Bissell, MD, PhD, MPH

Professor Emeritus, Department of Pathology, The Ohio State University, Columbus, Ohio

Editor

Maxwell L. Smith, MD

Assistant Professor, Department of Laboratory Medicine and Pathology, Mayo Clinic, Scottsdale, Arizona

ELSEVIER
MOSBY

ELSEVIER
MOSBY

VP Global Medical Reference: Mary E. Gatsch
Publisher: Adrianne Brigido
Supervisor, Electronic Year Books: Donna M. Skelton
Electronic Article Manager: Mike Sheets
Illustrations and Permissions Coordinator: Dawn Vohsen

2014 EDITION

Printed in the United States of America
Composition by TNQ Books and Journals Pvt Ltd, India
Printing/binding by Sheridan Books, Inc.

Editorial Office:
Elsevier
Suite 1800
1600 John F. Kennedy Blvd.
Philadelphia, PA 19103-2899

International Standard Serial Number: 1077-9108
International Standard Book Number: 978-0-323-26481-5

Contributing Editors

Mary C. O'Keefe, MD
Anatomic and Clinical Pathology Resident, University of Colorado Anschutz Medical Campus, Aurora, Colorado

Damon R. Olson, MD
Anatomic and Clinical Pathology Resident, University of Colorado Anschutz Medical Campus, Aurora, Colorado

Miriam D. Post, MD
Assistant Professor, Department of Pathology, University of Colorado School of Medicine, Aurora, Colorado

Megan E. Quinn, MD
Anatomic and Clinical Pathology Resident, University of Colorado Anschutz Medical Campus, Aurora, Colorado

Abby M. Richmond, MD
Anatomic and Clinical Pathology Resident, University of Colorado Anschutz Medical Campus, Aurora, Colorado

M. Sherif Said, MD, PhD, FCAP
Associate Professor of Pathology, University of Colorado Denver; Associate Director of Pathology, Denver Health, Denver, Colorado

Heather Signorelli, DO
Pathology Resident at University of Colorado Health Sciences Center, Denver, Colorado

Table of Contents

Journals Represented

Journals represented in this YEAR BOOK are listed below.

Acta Pathologica, Microbiologica, et Immunologica Scandinavica
American Journal of Clinical Pathology
American Journal of Infection Control
American Journal of Kidney Diseases
American Journal of Surgical Pathology
American Journal of Transplantation
Annals of Diagnostic Pathology
Archives of Disease in Childhood
Archives of Pathology and Laboratory Medicine
BMC Nephrology
Cancer
Cancer Investigation
Ceskoslovenská Patologie
Clinical Chemistry
Clinical Endocrinology
Clinical Infectious Diseases
Clinical Toxicology
Critical Care Medicine
Cytopathology
Diagnostic Cytopathology
Digestive and Liver Disease
Endocrine Pathology
European Respiratory Journal
Experimental and Molecular Pathology
Gynecologic Oncology
Head and Neck
Hepatology
Histopathology
Human Pathology
International Journal of Gynecological Cancer
International Journal of Gynecology and Pathology
International Journal of Pediatric Otorhinolaryngology
Journal of Clinical Microbiology
Journal of Clinical Pathology
Journal of Heart and Lung Transplantation
Journal of Immunology
Journal of Infectious Diseases
Journal of Molecular Diagnostics
Journal of the American Medical Association
Kidney International
Lancet Oncology
Laryngoscope
Liver International
Modern Pathology
Nephrology Dialysis Transplantation
New England Journal of Medicine
Pathology Research and Practice

Public Library of Science One
Respiratory Medicine
Science
Thrombosis Research
Transfusion
Transplantation
Virchows Archiv

Standard Abbreviations

The following terms are abbreviated in this edition: acquired immunodeficiency syndrome (AIDS), cardiopulmonary resuscitation (CPR), central nervous system (CNS), cerebrospinal fluid (CSF), computed tomography (CT), deoxyribonucleic acid (DNA), electrocardiography (ECG), health maintenance organization (HMO), human immunodeficiency virus (HIV), intensive care unit (ICU), intramuscular (IM), intravenous (IV), magnetic resonance (MR) imaging (MRI), ribonucleic acid (RNA), ultrasound (US), and ultraviolet (UV).

Note

The Year Book of Pathology and Laboratory Medicine is a literature survey service providing abstracts of articles published in the professional literature. Every effort is made to assure the accuracy of the information presented in these pages. Neither the editors nor the publisher of the Year Book of Pathology and Laboratory Medicine can be responsible for errors in the original materials. The editors' comments are their own opinions. Mention of specific products within this publication does not constitute endorsement.

To facilitate the use of the Year Book of Pathology and Laboratory Medicine as a reference tool, all illustrations and tables included in this publication are now identified as they appear in the original article. This change is meant to help the reader recognize that any illustration or table appearing in the Year Book of Pathology and Laboratory Medicine may be only one of many in the original article. For this reason, figure and table numbers will often appear to be out of sequence within the Year Book of Pathology and Laboratory Medicine.

PART I

ANATOMIC PATHOLOGY

1 Outcomes Analysis

Consensus Statement on Effective Communication of Urgent Diagnoses and Significant, Unexpected Diagnoses in Surgical Pathology and Cytopathology From the College of American Pathologists and Association of Directors of Anatomic and Surgical Pathology

Nakhleh RE, Myers JL, Allen TC, et al (Mayo Clinic Florida, Jacksonville; Univ of Michigan Med Ctr, Ann Arbor; Univ of Texas Health Science Ctr, Tyler; et al)

Arch Pathol Lab Med 136:148-154, 2012

Context.—Recognizing the difficulty in applying the concept of critical values to anatomic pathology diagnoses, the College of American Pathologists and the Association of Directors of Anatomic and Surgical Pathology have chosen to reevaluate the concept of *critical diagnoses*.

Objective.—To promote effective communication of urgent and significant, unexpected diagnoses in surgical pathology and cytology.

Design.—A comprehensive literature search was conducted and reviewed by an expert panel.

Results.—A policy of effective communication of important results in surgical pathology and cytology is desirable to enhance patient safety and to address multiple regulatory requirements.

Conclusions.—Each institution should create its own policy regarding urgent diagnoses and significant, unexpected diagnoses in anatomic pathology. This policy should be separate from critical results or panic-value policies in clinical pathology, with the expectation of a different time frame for communication. *Urgent diagnosis* is defined as a medical condition that, in most cases, should be addressed as soon as possible. *Significant, unexpected diagnosis* is defined as a medical condition that is clinically unusual or unforeseen and should be addressed at some point in the patient's course. Further details of this statement are provided.

► There has been little study of the hand-off between anatomic pathologists and clinicians in the providing of a diagnosis. The medical legal literature indicates that a failure in this hand-off may have catastrophic consequences. This article presents a consensus statement for effective communication regarding those diagnoses that are considered urgent and significant/unexpected. Examples of these diagnoses are provided in the article's reference section.

S. Raab, MD

The Ideal Laboratory Information System

Sepulveda JL, Young DS (Columbia Univ, NY; Univ of Pennsylvania, Philadelphia)

Arch Pathol Lab Med 137:1129-1140, 2013

Context.—Laboratory information systems (LIS) are critical components of the operation of clinical laboratories. However, the functionalities of LIS have lagged significantly behind the capacities of current hardware and software technologies, while the complexity of the information produced by clinical laboratories has been increasing over time and will soon undergo rapid expansion with the use of new, high-throughput and high-dimensionality laboratory tests. In the broadest sense, LIS are essential to manage the flow of information between health care providers, patients, and laboratories and should be designed to optimize not only laboratory operations but also personalized clinical care.

Objective.—To list suggestions for designing LIS with the goal of optimizing the operation of clinical laboratories while improving clinical care by intelligent management of laboratory information.

Data Sources.—Literature review, interviews with laboratory users, and personal experience and opinion.

Conclusions.—Laboratory information systems can improve laboratory operations and improve patient care. Specific suggestions for improving the function of LIS are listed under the following sections: (1) Information Security, (2) Test Ordering, (3) Specimen Collection, Accessioning, and Processing, (4) Analytic Phase, (5) Result Entry and Validation, (6) Result Reporting, (7) Notification Management, (8) Data Mining and

TABLE 3.—Desirable Functionalities of an Order Appropriateness Expert System

The system displays previous relevant test results (graphically, if required) and pending related orders, with an opportunity for the provider to cancel the order after being made aware of such information.
The system has built-in and customizable medical necessity review and acceptance or rejection criteria, including criteria for maximum frequency of appropriate ordering for different situations, eg, by patient location, clinic, specialist, diagnosis.
The system merges or cancels redundant orders falling within preestablished criteria (institutionally or nationally developed). For example, if 2 providers order thyroidstimulating hormone tests in the same week, the orders are merged and both providers will receive the results. If a provider orders a hemoglobin A1c test a month after a result is available in the system, the order is cancelled and the provider is notified to call the laboratory if an override is needed.
The system uses available clinical and laboratory inputs to determine appropriateness. For example, if patient sex is female and ordered test is prostate-specific antigen, the order is flagged for cancelling. If patient is receiving rapamycin and cyclosporine treatment, and only cyclosporine is ordered, the system asks the provider if rapamycin measurements are also desired.
The system has the ability to cancel flagged orders with hard stops to prevent inappropriate work-around of the rules, while providing a mechanism for the ordering provider to justify an exception, eg, by asking the provider to call the laboratory for rule overriding. Certain order types, eg, associated with research protocols, should be exempted from appropriateness protocols by policy.
The expert order appropriateness system should be able to halt orders that are not associated with a proper diagnostic code (such as ICD-9 or ICD-10).

Abbreviation: ICD, International Classification of Diseases.

Crosssectional Reports, (9) Method Validation, (10) Quality Management, (11) Administrative and Financial Issues, and (12) Other Operational Issues (Table 3).

▶ In this report, Sepulveda and Young provide an outline of the limitations of our current laboratory information system (LIS) and components that are needed for a more optimal system. Fig 1 in the original article shows a modular approach to building a LIS that would create more than just an information reporting and billing tool. A modular approach would allow for laboratories to use the components that they need for specific areas and would allow for upgrades and changes that could be tailored to specific laboratory needs. This type of system would permit laboratories to build quality assurance and improvement components within the system. Table 3 describes examples of these built-in quality procedures. These types of systems would be transformative in allowing pathologists and other laboratory personnel to work to provide an optimal diagnosis instead of working to avoid a making a mistake. For further reading, see reference list.[1,2]

S. Raab, MD

References

1. Fraser CG. Improved monitoring of differences in serial laboratory results. *Clin Chem.* 2011;57:1635-1637.
2. Hoffman MA, Williams MS. Electronic medical records and personalized medicine. *Hum Genet.* 2011;130:33-39.

Frozen Section Diagnosis: Is There Discordance Between What Pathologists Say and What Surgeons Hear?

Roy S, Parwani AV, Dhir R, et al (Univ of Pittsburgh Med Ctr, PA)
Am J Clin Pathol 140:363-369, 2013

Objectives.—Communication in various medical settings is subject to misinterpretation. The frozen section (FS) diagnosis in patient care is dependent on successful communication between pathologists and surgeons. However, very few studies looking at FS errors analyzed postanalytic communication issues.

Methods.—A total of 300 consecutive cases, in which an FS was performed and corresponding surgical note was available, were studied. The FS diagnosis and surgeon's interpretation were recorded for all cases. Discrepancies were classified as major (clinical impact) or minor (no clinical impact).

Results.—We found 8 (2.7%) miscommunications, all with only minor clinical impact. These were attributed mainly to the surgeon's misinterpretation of a deferred diagnosis. Also contributing to miscommunication was the pathologist's use of nonspecific terminology such as "favor" or "scattered."

Conclusions.—We found that the rate of miscommunicated FS diagnoses was low at our institution during the period of our study. However, the rate of miscommunication was similar to the much more widely recognized problem of sampling error.

▶ In the patient safety literature, root cause analysis indicates that a major cause of medical error is in a failed hand-off between health care providers. A solution to this problem is the read-back activity, in which the receiver reports back to the sender what the sender just said. The methods of this study are not rigorous, as Roy and coauthors do not record what the pathologists actually said and only what they wrote down. Understanding the complexity of the pathologist-surgeon discussion is not even attempted. Likewise, what the surgeons actually thought was being said also is not recorded. It is unclear if the authors recommend read-backs in light of their data, showing only a low number of miscommunications; such a return communication is not listed in their typical frozen section event workflow. As catastrophic miscommunications are relatively infrequent in intraoperative consultation services, the sample size of this study may have been too low to detect any major error. For further reading, see the reference list.[1,2]

S. Raab, MD

References

1. Powsner SM, Costa J, Homer RJ. Clinicians are from Mars and pathologists are from Venus. *Arch Pathol Lab Med.* 2000;124:1040-1046.
2. Talmon G, Miller R, Horn A, et al. How well do we communicate? A comparison of intraoperative diagnoses and operative notes [abstract poster no. 45]. *Arch Pathol Lab Med.* 2012;136:1095.

Clinician compliance with laboratory regulations requiring submission of relevant clinical data: A one year retrospective analysis

Layfield LJ, Factor RE, Jarboe EA (Univ of Utah School of Medicine and ARUP Laboratories, Salt Lake City)

Pathol Res Pract 208:668-671, 2012

Background.—The College of American Pathologists (CAP) recognizes the need for clinical data in the interpretation of specimens submitted for histopathologic evaluation. Anecdotal evidence indicates that clinician compliance with requests for clinical history is variable.

Design.—Quality assurance data from August 1, 2010 to September 31, 2011 were searched for all cases listing no clinical history. Four consecutive weeks of surgical pathology request forms were also reviewed for the presence or absence of clinical history and its accuracy.

Results.—21,700 cases were accessioned in the study period and 1293 (5.9%) requisitions contained no clinical history. The four-week review documented that 143 of 1698 (8.4%) requisitions had no clinical history and 12 cases contained incorrect history (0.7%).

Conclusions.—Between 5.9% and 8.4% of requisitions contain no clinical history. In 0.2% of cases, clinical history was incorrect. Compliance with the CAP policy for clinical history appears poor.

▶ Providing clinical information on a surgical pathology requisition form is a hand-off from the clinical practitioner to laboratory personnel. The importance of this hand-off in surgical pathology has not been evaluated rigorously,[1,2] and most commentary on the value of this hand-off is based on anecdotal opinion. For example, we know that the hand-off point is a step prone to error if critical information is not provided or incorrect information is provided. Practicing pathologists are easily able to relate instances in which the incorrect or no information affected the quality of diagnosis. However, in most instances, the failure to provide clinical information or the providing of incorrect information presumably does not affect patient care. In addition, the laboratory decrease in efficiency resulting from the extra work in obtaining this information is unknown. Layfield and coauthors simply present data to show the frequency of which clinical information is lacking or defective. Ideally, we need studies showing the importance of these hand-offs and how this information is incorporated into pathologist and other laboratory personnel cognitive processes. Pathologists need to study what they need specifically for diagnostic purposes, or the quality of clinical data currently provided (eg, ?mass – r/o pathology) may be no better than no information.

S. Raab, MD

References

1. Nakhleh RE, Zarbo RJ. Surgical pathology specimen identification and accessioning: a College of American Pathologists Q-Probes Study of 1 004 115 cases from 417 institutions. *Arch Pathol Lab Med.* 1996;120:227-233.
2. Joint Commission. *1998–1999, Comprehensive Accreditation Manual for Pathology and Laboratory Services.* 1998. Oakbrook Terrace, IL: Joint Commission on Accreditation of Healthcare Organizations; 1998.

Equivocal or Ambiguous Terminologies in Pathology: Focus of Continuous Quality Improvement?

Idowu MO, Wiles A, Wan W, et al (Virginia Commonwealth Univ Health System, Richmond)

Am J Surg Pathol 37:1722-1727, 2013

Ambiguous terminologies introduce uncertainty into pathology reports and may be misinterpreted by clinicians. Although absolute diagnostic certainty in all cases is not attainable, nevertheless, unbridled use of equivocal or ambiguous terminologies may lead to additional, sometimes unnecessary, tests and/or procedures directly or indirectly leading to increase in health care costs, as well as patient and clinician dissatisfaction. We evaluated the degree of certainty attributed to the commonly used ambiguous terminologies ("consistent with", "compatible with", "indicative of", "favor", "suggestive of", "suspicious for", "not excluded", "cannot exclude," "not ruled out", "not definite for," "not specific for," "indeterminate," "not identified") used in pathology reports by groups of attending physicians and their respective trainees using an online survey. There is no statistical difference in the interpretation of each terminology between attending pathologists and pathology trainees. There is also no significant difference between pathology and other attending groups for majority of the terminologies. However, there are significant differences between at least 2 of the 4 attending physician categories in the following pathology terminologies: "consistent with" (overall $P = 0.01$), "compatible with" ($P = 0.02$), "not excluded" ($P = 0.008$), and "cannot exclude" ($P = 0.01$). The pairwise comparisons among the 4 specialties show that there is significant difference in the interpretation of the degree of certainty between pathology and medicine in terms of "not excluded" ($P = 0.007$) and "cannot exclude" ($P = 0.03$). Focused peer review or monitoring of pathology reports with ambiguous terminologies may reduce their use and represent a worthwhile and achievable goal.

▶ The pathologist uses a report as a method of hand-off or communication to the clinical team. Clearly, equivocal and or ambiguous terminology expresses pathologist uncertainty and the inability to be precise. Although the goal to reduce this type of terminology is laudable, a fundamental problem is that pathologists struggle with the application of diagnostic criteria and assessment of sample quality. Perhaps equivocal and/or ambiguous terminology would be decreased if we dealt directly with these issues. In addition, we should ask the clinicians the best means by which they would like pathologists to express uncertainty instead of having them guess. For further reading, see the reference list.[1,2]

S. Raab, MD

References

1. O'Brien BJ. Words or numbers? The evaluation of probability expressions in general practice. *J R Coll Gen Pract.* 1989;39:98-100.
2. Nakao MA, Axelrod S. Numbers are better than words. Verbal specifications of frequency have no place in medicine. *Am J Med.* 1983;74:1061-1065.

Accounting for the Professional Work of Pathologists Performing Autopsies

Sinard JH, for the Autopsy Committee of the College of American Pathologists (Yale Univ School of Medicine, New Haven, CT)

Arch Pathol Lab Med 137:228-232, 2013

Context.—With an increasing trend toward fee-code-based methods of measuring the clinical professional productivity of pathologists, those pathologists whose clinical activities include the performance of autopsies have been disadvantaged by the lack of generally accepted workload equivalents for autopsy performance and supervision.

Objective.—To develop recommended benchmarks to account for this important and often overlooked professional activity.

Design.—Based on the professional experience of members of the Autopsy Committee of the College of American Pathologists, a survey of autopsy pathologists, and the limited additional material available in the literature, we developed recommended workload equivalents for the professional work associated with performing an autopsy, which we elected to express as multiples of established Current Procedural Terminology codes.

Results.—As represented in Table 3, we recommend that the professional work associated with a full adult autopsy be equivalent to 5.5 × 88309-26. Additional professional credit of 1.5 × 88309-26 should be added for evaluation of the brain and for a detailed clinical-pathologic discussion. The corresponding value for a fetal/neonatal autopsy is 4.0 × 88309-26.

Conclusion.—Although we recognize that autopsy practices vary significantly from institution to institution, it is hoped that our proposed guidelines will be a valuable starting point that individual practices can then adapt, taking into account the specifics of their practice environment (Table 3).

▶ Sinard and the Autopsy Committee of the College of American Pathologists attempted to develop recommended workload equivalents for autopsy performance and supervision using multiples of established Current Procedural Terminology (CPT) codes (Table 3). Because autopsies are not performed in a standard manner among North American institutions, standardizing the workload equivalents is challenging. Presumably, linking autopsy workload to pre-existing CPT codes also has a reimbursement connotation. I find the proposal of Sinard et al intriguing in that the technical performance is weighted far more than the detailed clinical-pathologic discussion, which is defined as an in-depth discussion of the findings at autopsy correlated with the clinical

TABLE 3.—Autopsy Committee Suggested Values for Measuring the Professional Activity Associated With the Performance of Autopsies[a]

Adult autopsy	
Full autopsy (without brain):	88309-26 × 5.5
Additional (add-on):	
Adult brain	88309-26 × 1.5
Detailed clinical-pathologic discussion[b]	88309-26 × 1.5
Fetal/neonatal autopsy	
Full autopsy (without brain):	88309-26 × 4.0
Additional (add-on):	
Fetal brain	88309-26 × 0.5
Placenta (if done with autopsy)	88307-26 × 1.0 for third trimester 88305-26 × 1.0 prior to third trimester
Detailed clinical-pathologic discussion[b]	88309-26 × 1.5

[a]The final multiplier for a given case is the sum of the base multiplier for that case type and any appropriate add-on multipliers. These values do not include any technical component that may be performed by the pathologist.

[b]For purposes of these recommendations, a detailed clinical-pathologic discussion is defined as an in-depth discussion of the findings at autopsy, correlated with the clinical history, presentation, and clinical course; an explicit statement as to the most likely underlying cause and sequence of events leading to the death; and a researched and referenced discussion of the major disease process(es) present in the patient.

history, presentation, and clinical course; an explicit statement as to the most likely underlying cause and sequence of events leading to the death; and a researched and referenced discussion of the major disease process(es) present in the patient. As the clinicians and patients rely on this discussion, which truly is the quality assurance of a time of patient care, I would think that this discussion should be weighted higher. For further reading, see the reference list.[1,2]

S. Raab, MD

References

1. Hemphill RR, Heavrin BS, Lesnick J, et al. Those who can, do and they teach too: faculty clinical productivity and teaching. *West J Emerg Med.* 2011;12:254-257.
2. Hynes WM, MacMillan DH. Establishing a compensation model in an academic pathology department. *Am J Clin Pathol.* 2005;124:S8-S15.

Template-based synoptic reports improve the quality of pathology reports of prostatectomy specimens

Aumann K, Amann D, Gumpp V, et al (Univ Med Ctr Freiburg, Germany)

Histopathology 60:634-644, 2012

Aims.—Traditionally, pathology reports have been textual, with a high degree of variability. In part, they miss some of the information needed, e.g. for therapy decisions. To meet all requirements, it would be helpful to have a tool providing reminders of the necessary data and facilitating the transfer of these data into a pathology information system (PIS). Here, we describe a TNM-adapted toolset including a PIS-integrated structured template that contributes to improving pathology reports of prostatectomy specimens.

Methods and Results.—All prostatectomy reports between January 2002 and August 2010 ($n = 1049$) were classified into descriptive reports (DRs) ($n = 411$), structured reports (SRs) arranged according to tumour spread, lymph node status, and surgical margin status ($n = 333$), and template-based synoptic reports (TBSRs) ($n = 305$). The report types were compared with regard to the content of 11 organ-specific essential data (ED) items crucial for exact TNM classification, therapy decisions, or prognostication. All 11 ED items were included in 2.7% of DRs, 43.5% of SRs and 97.2% of TBSRs, with a statistically highly significant difference ($P < 0.001$).

Conclusions.—SRs, and particularly TBSRs, are advantageous as compared with DRs regarding the content of ED and the clarity of the data layout. The use of TBSRs leads to a reduction in failed data transfer and therefore to an increase in the quality of pathology reports (Table 1).

► Aumann and colleagues report that template-based synoptic reports (TBSR) improve the standardization and quality of the clinical communication of prostatectomy specimen essential data. Table 1 defines these essential data points and highlights the close clinical connection between pathology and clinical

TABLE 1.—Data Recommended for Inclusion in Histopathology Reports of Prostatectomy Specimens [Essential Data (ED)] With Assessed Values, Including Descriptions for Calculating the Essential Data Score (EDS) (the Total Number of Essential Data Reported); if the ED Were Not Evaluable, the Case Was Excluded From the Calculation

ED	Value	Description
Intraprostatic tumour spread	Not evaluable	Resection in many parts or larger tissue probes were removed
	0	Not acquired or incomplete (without percentage if only one lobe is involved)
	1	Tumour confined within one lobe (in percentage) or involves both lobes
Capsule	Not evaluable	Prostatectomy without the complete capsule
	0	Not acquired
	1	Capsule intact or penetrated
Seminal vesicle	Not evaluable	Prostatectomy without seminal vesicles
	0	Tumour infiltration of seminal vesicle not acquired
	1	Infiltration status of seminal vesicle documented
Histological tumour type	Not evaluable	Not definable
	0	Not acquired or incomplete (e.g. 'carcinoma')
	1	Complete histological tumour type according to the WHO classification (e.g. 'adenocarcinoma')
Gleason score	Not evaluable	Preoperative hormonal or radiation therapy
	0	Not acquired
	1	Grading according to Gleason score
Surgical margin status	Not evaluable	Resection in many parts or larger tissue probes were removed
	0	Not acquired or positive resection margins without exact specification of involved margins
	1	Negative or positive resection margins with exact specification of involved margins
Lymph node status	Not evaluable	Resection without lymph nodes
	0	Not acquired
	1	Information about lymph node status
TNM	Not evaluable	Resection in many parts or larger tissue probes were removed
	0	TNM classification not or partly acquired
	1	TNM classification completely acquired
Perineural invasion	0	Not acquired
	1	Pn0/1 or verbal
Lymph vessel invasion	0	Not acquired
	1	L0/1 or verbal
Blood vessel invasion	0	Not acquired
	1	V0/1 or verbal

WHO, World Health Organization.

care. The use of TBSRs generally is not debated in the pathology field, although individual data fields may be questioned depending on the actual clinical need. For some laboratory information systems, the incorporation of TBSRs may be challenging but necessary for quality improvement.[1,2]

S. Raab, MD

References

1. Epstein JI, Srigley J, Grignon D, et al. Recommendations for the reporting of prostate carcinoma: association of Directors of Anatomic and Surgical Pathology. *Am J Clin Pathol.* 2008;129:24-30.
2. Harnden P, Berney D, Shelley M. Dataset for histopathology reports for prostatic carcinoma, 2nd edition. http://www.rcpath.org/resources/pdf/g084datasetprostaticcarcinomaoct09.pdf. Accessed June 29, 2010.

Utility of whole slide imaging and virtual microscopy in prostate pathology

Camparo P, Egevad L, Algaba F, et al (Cabinet de Pathologie Amiens, France; Karolinska Institutet, Stockholm, Sweden; Fundacio Puigvert-Univ Autonomous, Barcelona, Spain; et al)

APMIS 120:298-304, 2012

Whole slide imaging (WSI) has been used in conjunction with virtual microscopy (VM) for training or proficiency testing purposes, multicentre research, remote frozen section diagnosis and to seek specialist second opinion in a number of organ systems. The feasibility of using WSI/VM for routine surgical pathology reporting has also been explored. In this review, we discuss the utility and limitations of WSI/VM technology in the histological assessment of specimens from the prostate. Features of WSI/VM that are particularly well suited to assessment of prostate pathology include the ability to examine images at different magnifications as well as to view histology and immunohistochemistry side-by-side on the screen. Use of WSI/VM would also solve the difficulty in obtaining multiple identical copies of small lesions in prostate biopsies for teaching and proficiency testing. It would also permit annotation of the virtual slides, and has been used in a study of inter-observer variation of Gleason grading to facilitate precise identification of the foci on which grading decisions had been based. However, the large number of sections examined from each set of prostate biopsies would greatly increase time required for scanning as well as the size of the digital file, and would also be an issue if digital archiving of prostate biopsies is contemplated. Z-scanning of glass slides, a process that increases scanning time and file size would be required to permit focusing a virtual slide up and down to assess subtle nuclear features such as nucleolar prominence. The common use of large blocks to process prostatectomy specimens would also be an issue, as few currently available scanners can scan such blocks. A major component of proficiency testing of prostate biopsy assessment involves screening of the cores to detect small atypical foci. However, screening virtual slides of wavy fragmented prostate cores using a computer mouse aided by an overview image is very different from screening glass slides using a microscope stage. Hence, it may be more appropriate in this setting to mark the lesional area and focus only on the interpretation component of competency testing. Other issues limiting the use of digital pathology in prostate pathology include the cost of high quality slide scanners for WSI and high resolution monitors for VM as well as the requirement for fast Internet connection as even a subtle delay in presentation of images on the screen may be very disturbing for a pathologist used to the rapid viewing of glass slides under a microscope. However, these problems are likely to be overcome by technological advances in the future.

▶ In this review article, Camparo et al outline the strengths and weaknesses of whole-slide digital imaging (WSI) in the field of prostate pathology. Currently, WSI may be used in education, external quality assurance schemes, and secondary case review. Camparo et al indicated that the slow processes in image acquisition (digitization and visualization) and the large number of slides that would need to be digitized in prostate pathology limited the use of WSI, especially in primary diagnostic care. However, if these barriers were overcome, would prostate pathologists actually switch out their microscopes for WSI technology? This question touches more on current pathology culture than on anything else. The argument to switch from light microscopy to WSI most likely will depend on quality metrics, such as safety, efficiency, effectiveness, patient centeredness, patient equity, and timeliness of care delivery. In many systems, efficiency drives system changes, as these systems are accustomed to evaluating costs of care delivery. Pathologists have the ability to drive this system change by examining other quality metrics. For further reading, see reference list.[1,2]

S. Raab, MD

References

1. Fine JL, Grzybicki DM, Silowash R, et al. Evaluation of whole slide image immunohistochemistry interpretation in challenging prostate needle biopsies. *Hum Pathol.* 2008;39:564-572.
2. Chargari C, Comperat E, Magné N, et al. Prostate needle biopsy examination by means of virtual microscopy. *Pathol Res Pract.* 2011;207:366-369.

Approach to Intraoperative Consultation for Donor Liver Biopsies

Melin C, Miick R, Young NA, et al (Univ of Rochester, NY; Einstein Med Ctr—Philadelphia, PA)

Arch Pathol Lab Med 137:270-274, 2013

Context.—As demand for organs to treat end-stage liver disease increases, donor livers once deemed only marginally suitable for donation are being considered for transplantation. Pathologists are increasingly being asked to evaluate these livers for acceptability. This article provides guidelines for frozen section evaluation of livers for transplantation.

Objective.—This article concentrates on the histopathologic features of transplant suitability with appropriate clinicopathologic correlation for the practicing pathologist. Recommendations for proper handling and sampling of tissue are discussed. Relative and absolute contraindications as well as artifacts and benign conditions are emphasized.

Data Sources.—Sources include a compilation of the authors' experiences in academic and community liver transplantation centers. In addition, relevant medical literature was reviewed, as well as Web sites specializing in organ transplantation, such as Transplant Pathology Internet Services and the Organ Procurement and Transplantation Network.

Conclusions.—Malignancy and extensive necrosis in the liver are absolute contraindications to transplantation. Evaluation of macrosteatosis, fibrosis, hepatitis, and necrosis depends on the severity of disease and correlation with the clinical situation. Donor age of greater than 60 years does not preclude transplantation. Artifacts and benign conditions need

TABLE 1.—Acceptable and Unacceptable Criteria for Liver Transplantation Based on Frozen Section Histology

Finding	Acceptable for Transplantation	Unacceptable for Transplantation
Steatosis—macrovesicular	<30% hepatocytes involved	≥30% hepatocytes involved
Steatosis—microvesicular	Any type	N/A
Viral hepatitis	In positive recipients: Grade <2 Batts and Ludwig Grade <5 mHAI (Ishak/Knodell)	In all recipients: Grade ≥2 Batts & Ludwig Grade ≥5 mHAI (Ishak/Knodell)
Fibrosis	Stage <2 Batts and Ludwig or mHAI (Ishak/Knodell)	Stage ≥2 Batts and Ludwig or mHAI (Ishak/Knodell)
Granulomas	"Burned-out" or fibrotic/calcified granulomas	Active granulomas, caseating or noncaseating
Nonspecific portal inflammation	Mild	>Mild (particularly if the viral hepatitis status of the donor is unknown)
Necrosis	<10% of liver area	≥10% of liver area
Malignancy	No	Yes

Abbreviations: mHAI, modified hepatic activity index; N/A, not applicable.

to be understood to prevent wastage of precious organs and to ensure that an appropriate organ is provided for the recipient (Table 1).

▶ Melin and colleagues provide an important review for practicing pathologists who evaluate intraoperative consultations of donor liver biopsies. Table 1 lists the acceptable and unacceptable criteria for liver transplantation based on the liver biopsy histology. The challenges for the practicing pathologist lie in recognizing the appropriate diagnosis in borderline cases. For example, determining the difference between 25% and 35% macrosteatosis often is difficult even without the artifacts described by Melin et al. One wishes for a large slide or image bank demonstrating how an expert would diagnose borderline cases of macrosteatosis rather than a descriptive explanation. Sadly, these methods of helping the practicing pathologist generally are absent. For further reading, see the reference list.[1,2]

S. Raab, MD

References

1. Imber CJ, St Peter SD, Lopez I, et al. Current practice regarding the use of fatty livers: a trans-Atlantic survey. *Liver Transpl.* 2002;8:545-549.
2. Loinaz C, González EM. Marginal donors in liver transplantation. *Hepatogastroenterology.* 2000;47:256-263.

Outside Case Review of Surgical Pathology for Referred Patients: The Impact on Patient Care

Swapp RE, Aubry MC, Salomão DR, et al (Mayo Clinic, Rochester, MI)
Arch Pathol Lab Med 137:233-240, 2013

Context.—Original surgical pathology materials from external sources are reviewed by our pathologists for referred patients before their clinical evaluation and treatment.

Objective.—To identify the rate of major disagreements with diagnoses from external institutions and to characterize the nature and impact of discordant diagnoses on patient care.

Design.—We identified and reviewed all surgical pathology cases, except for medical liver, medical renal, and cardiac pathology cases, for the period between January 1, 2005, and December 31, 2010, to determine the overall frequency of major disagreements, defined as any change in diagnosis having a substantial impact on patient management.

Results.—Our review of 71 811 cases initially examined between 2005 and 2010 identified 457 major disagreements (0.6%). The most frequent areas of disagreement were gastrointestinal (80 cases; 17.5%), lymph node (73; 16.0%), bone/soft tissue (47; 10.3%), and genitourinary (43; 9.4%). For a subset of 166 cases reviewed between July 1, 2009, and December 31, 2010, follow-up data were available for 140 (84.3%). Treatment was affected by a changed diagnosis in 126 cases (90.0%), and prognosis was affected in 129 cases (92.1%). For 86 (51.8%) of the 166 cases, additional tissue was obtained. Revised diagnoses concurred with follow-up tissue diagnosis in 84.9% (73 cases), whereas they differed from follow-up tissue diagnosis in 15.1% (13 cases).

Conclusions.—Our findings demonstrate the value of outside case review of pathology materials for referred patients, and suggest that it decreases the likelihood of diagnostic errors and provides better protection for patients.

▶ Every year, a handful of academic institutions publish their data on the findings of secondary review of external cases involving referred-in patients. Swapp and colleagues reported that the Mayo Clinic found a secondary review discrepancy frequency of 6.0%, with a major discrepancy frequency of 0.6%. These data are similar to those published in a series reporting multiple years of these types of studies. The conclusions of these studies indicate that this secondary review is a beneficial practice and serves as a form of error prevention. In reality, the underlying practices that lead to these errors are not directly addressed. A large portion of these discrepancies is based on failures of diagnostic precision, which has causes involving our current apprenticeship education and training systems, lack of agreement in diagnostic criteria and patterns, and pathology cultures that are not trained in quality improvement. Although some practitioners recommend the benefits of subspecialty practice, the lack of precision among expert subspecialists still is an issue. The fundamental changes in eliminating errors in precision will need global collaboration and teamwork, components that only are just being learned in other areas of medicine.[1]

S. Raab, MD

Reference

1. Raab SS, Grzybicki DM. Quality in cancer diagnosis. *CA Cancer J Clin.* 2010;60: 139-165.

Cervical Histopathology Variability Among Laboratories: A Population-Based Statewide Investigation

Gage JC, for The New Mexico HPV Pap Registry Steering Committee (Natl Cancer Inst, Bethesda, MD; et al)

Am J Clin Pathol 139:330-335, 2013

To inform the proposed systematic adjudicative staining of cervical intraepithelial neoplasia grade 2 (CIN2) and equivocal diagnoses, we characterized diagnostic heterogeneity across 15 laboratories. Laboratory-specific distributions of 37,486 biopsy specimen diagnoses were compared after adjusting for preceding cytology. In a subset of preceding cytology specimens, HPV16 genotyping was considered an indicator of lesion severity. Distributions of normal and CIN1 diagnoses varied widely, with laboratories favoring either normal (5.5%-57.7%) or CIN1 diagnoses (23.3%-86.7%; $P < .001$ for normal:CIN1 variability). Excluding extreme values, 6.2% to 14.4% of diagnoses were CIN2 ($P < .001$). For CIN2 diagnoses, HPV16 positivity in the preceding cytology varied between 39.0% in the largest laboratory and 57.4% in others ($P < .001$), suggesting differential interpretation, not population differences, as a cause of variability. In conclusion, the frequency of diagnoses requiring special staining ($p16^{INK4a}$ immunostaining) to adjudicate equivocal CIN2 will be sizable and vary between laboratories, especially if extended to a fraction of CIN1 lesions.

▶ The article by Gage et al illustrates the remarkable diagnostic variability among New Mexico laboratories in cervical cancer screening pathology services. Fig 1 in the original article is emblematic and shows the percentage of distribution of cervical biopsy specimen diagnoses by laboratory, standardized by preceding cytology and to laboratory L because it processed the greatest number of biopsy specimens. It is interesting that this difference has not been shown to relate to differences in missed cervical cancers. However, the article illustrates how we apply different ancillary tests as a method to improve the reproducibility of diagnoses. The ability for the pathology field to improve diagnostic precision based on reassessment of diagnostic criteria and patterns is not clear and perhaps has never seriously been examined as a viable solution. For further reading, see reference list.[1,2]

S. Raab, MD

References

1. Ismail SM, Colclough AB, Dinnen JS, et al. Observer variation in histopathological diagnosis and grading of cervical intraepithelial neoplasia. *BMJ*. 1989;298: 707-710.
2. Stoler MH, Schiffman M. Interobserver reproducibility of cervical cytologic and histologic interpretations: realistic estimates from the ASCUS-LSIL Triage Study. *JAMA*. 2001;285:1500-1505.

2 Breast

Assessing the Potential Cost-Effectiveness of Retesting IHC0, IHC1+, or FISH-Negative Early Stage Breast Cancer Patients for HER2 Status

Garrison LP Jr, Lalla D, Brammer M, et al (VeriTech Corporation, Mercer Island, WA; Genentech, Inc, South San Francisco, CA; et al)

Cancer 119:3113-3122, 2013

Background.—Fluorescence in situ hybridization (FISH) and immunohistochemistry (IHC) tests are commonly used to assess human epidermal growth factor 2 (HER2) status of tumors in patients with breast cancer. This analysis evaluates the likely cost-effectiveness of expanded retesting to assess HER2 tumor status in women with early stage breast cancer.

Methods.—We developed a decision-analytic model to estimate the incremental cost-effectiveness ratio (ICER) of expanded reflex testing from a US payer perspective. Expanded reflex testing is defined as retesting tumor specimens from patients whose tumors are IHC0, IHC1+, or FISH-negative on their first test. In the base case, we assumed that 80% of patient tumors are initially IHC-tested and 20% are FISH-tested. Testing outcomes for IHC and FISH with and without retesting were based on published meta-analyses. The cost of tests and treatment and the long-term health outcomes were obtained from the literature.

Results.—In the base case, we estimated that 2.27% of women who received expanded reflex testing would be HER2-positive and receive trastuzumab treatment: the projected ICER was $36,721 per life year or $39,745 per quality-adjusted life year (QALY). This varied between $47,100 per QALY and $35,500 per QALY if we assumed that 1%-8% of patients retested were then HER2+, respectively. The results of deterministic and probabilistic sensitivity analysis were robust. This strategy would result in 4700 (2000-17,000) patients being eligible to receive trastuzumab treatment annually.

Conclusions.—Retesting patients who are IHC0, IHC1+, or FISH-negative is projected to be a cost-effective clinical strategy (Fig 1).

► Garrison et al cite 2 references that suggest a significant level of discordance between unequivocal immunohistochemistry (IHC) and fluorescence in situ hybridization (FISH) human epidermal growth factor 2 results in women with breast cancer. The authors also report that randomized trials suggest potential clinical benefit for treatment with trastuzumab in women whose tumors are IHC positive and FISH negative. Consequently, Garrison et al propose expanded reflex testing as shown in Fig 1. This proposal would markedly affect laboratory practice.

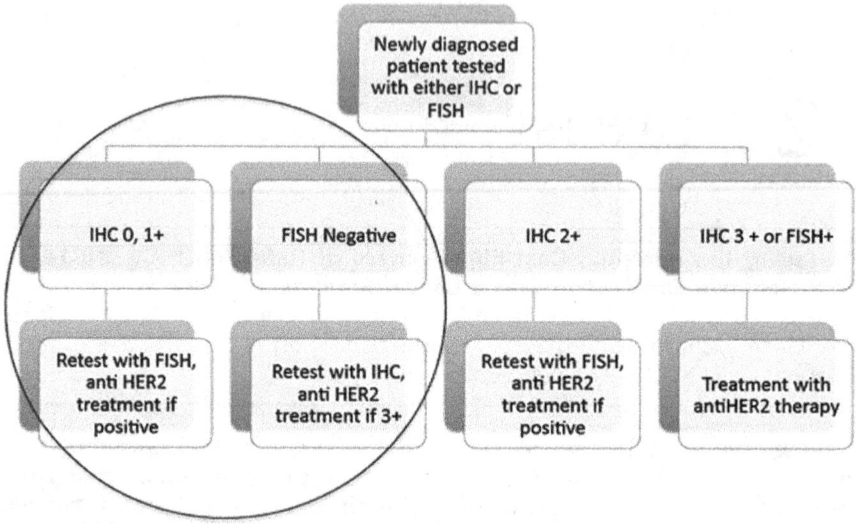

FIGURE 1.—Proposed expansion (circled) to the reflex testing algorithm. (Reprinted from Garrison Jr LP, Lalla D, Brammer M, et al. Assessing the potential cost-effectiveness of retesting IHC0, IHC1+, or FISH-negative early stage breast cancer patients for HER2 status. *Cancer.* 2013;119:3113-3122, Copyright 2013, American Cancer Society. This material is reproduced with permission of Wiley-Liss, Inc., a subsidiary of John Wiley & Sons, Inc., www.interscience.wiley.com.)

This practice is based on the "believe the positive" result approach. For additional reading, please see the reference list.[1,2]

S. Raab, MD

References

1. Grimm EE, Schmidt RA, Swanson PE, et al. Achieving 95% cross-methodological concordance in HER2 testing: causes and implications of discordant cases. *Am J Clin Pathol.* 2010;134:284-292.
2. Cuadros M, Villegas R. Systematic review of HER2 breast cancer testing. *Appl Immunohistochem Mol Morphol.* 2009;17:1-7.

Are Physician Recommendations for *BRCA1/2* Testing in Patients With Breast Cancer Appropriate? A Population-Based Study

McCarthy AM, Bristol M, Fredricks T, et al (Univ of Pennsylvania Perelman School of Medicine, Philadelphia)
Cancer 119:3596-3603, 2013

Background.—To the best of the authors' knowledge, few population-based studies to date have examined the use of *BRCA1/2* testing or patterns of physician recommendations for genetic testing among women diagnosed with breast cancer. The objective of the current study was to evaluate the rates and predictors of physician recommendation for *BRCA1/2* testing among patients with breast cancer.

Methods.—Women aged 18 years to 64 years who were diagnosed with invasive breast cancer in 2007 were identified from the Pennsylvania Cancer Registry and mailed a survey regarding their family history of cancer, physician treatment recommendations, and *BRCA1/2* testing. Of the 4009 women who were sent surveys, 2258 responded (56%). Based on age at diagnosis and family history, women were categorized as being at high, moderate, or low risk of *BRCA1/2* mutations.

Results.—Nearly 25% of the participants were classified as being at high risk of carrying a *BRCA1/2* mutation based on their age at the time of breast cancer diagnosis and family history of breast and/or ovarian cancer. Physician recommendations for *BRCA1/2* testing were found to be strongly associated with risk of carrying a mutation, with 53% of high-risk women reporting a testing recommendation compared with 9% of low-risk women. In addition, physician recommendations were strongly correlated with the use of testing in all risk groups. Among high-risk women, the lack of a recommendation for *BRCA1/2* testing was more common among older, low-income, and employed women.

Conclusions.—Although *BRCA1/2* testing recommendations appear to be appropriately correlated with mutation risk, a significant percentage of patients with breast cancer who meet criteria for *BRCA1/2* testing may not receive a recommendation for such testing from their health care providers.

▶ Clinical guidelines suggest that patients with breast cancer should consider genetic testing if they have the following criteria: early-onset disease (< 45 years), bilateral breast cancer, triple-negative cancer, Ashkenazi Jewish ancestry, or a strong family history of breast or ovarian cancer. Apart from the ancestry and family history criteria, pathology laboratories generally produce or have knowledge of the other criteria data and play an important role in providing this information to clinicians and patients. McCarthy et al suggest that a significant number of women with breast cancer who have the appropriate criteria to recommend *BRCA1/2* testing may not be receiving a recommendation. Pathology laboratories could potentially bridge this gap by developing strategies to inform providers (and patients) with genetic testing recommendations for individual patients. This practice could extend far beyond *BRCA1/2* genetic testing. For additional reading, please see the reference list.[1,2]

S. Raab, MD

References

1. Daly MB, Axilbund JE, Buys S, et al. National Comprehensive Cancer Network (NCCN) Clinical Practice Guidelines in Oncology. Genetic/Familial High-Risk Assessment: Breast and Ovarian. Version 1.2012. www.nccn.org/professionals/physician_gls/pdf/genetics_screening.pdf. Accessed January 2, 2014.
2. Ropka ME, Wenzel J, Phillips EK, et al. Uptake rates for breast cancer genetic testing: a systematic review. *Cancer Epidemiol Biomarkers Prev.* 2006;15:840-855.

Borderline Atypical Ductal Hyperplasia/Low-grade Ductal Carcinoma In Situ on Breast Needle Core Biopsy Should Be Managed Conservatively

VandenBussche CJ, Khouri N, Sbaity E, et al (The Johns Hopkins Med Institutions, Baltimore, MD)

Am J Surg Pathol 37:913-923, 2013

The differential diagnosis of low–nuclear grade intraductal epithelial proliferations of the breast includes atypical ductal hyperplasia (ADH) and ductal carcinoma in situ (DCIS). This distinction can be difficult on core needle biopsy (CNB) but can have significant clinical ramifications. We examined the clinical course of patients diagnosed on CNB with borderline ADH/DCIS lesions [marked ADH (MADH)] at our institution. A total of 74 patients were diagnosed with MADH on CNB and underwent an excisional biopsy (EB). The majority of these CNBs reviewed at outside hospitals had been classified as DCIS. Twenty patients (27%) had benign findings or lobular neoplasia in their EB, 18 (24%) had ADH, 33 (45%) had DCIS, and 3 (4%) had DCIS and invasive ductal carcinoma (IDC). Among the 38 patients who were not diagnosed with DCIS or IDC on EB, no patient underwent further surgery or radiation postoperatively. Thirty-seven of these 38 patients had no recurrences, whereas 1 patient developed a "recurrence" that on our review was likely residual localized MADH. The mean follow-up for these patients was 54 months. Of the 36 patients diagnosed with DCIS or IDC on EB, <20% required mastectomy. On review, MADH involving an intermediate-sized duct on CNB and the amount of residual lesion on imaging was significantly associated with DCIS or IDC on EB. Conversely, MADH involving columnar cell lesions and the presence of calcification on CNB were significantly associated with benign pathology on EB. In conclusion, our study provides preliminary data that justify a conservative approach to borderline ADH/DCIS lesions on CNB: that is, diagnose as MADH and treat by conservative excision.

▶ VandenBussche et al argue that marked atypical ductal hyperplasia (MADH) is not a diagnostic category but is a working diagnosis. However, the authors recommend a specific follow-up strategy for this working diagnosis, which essentially makes the category diagnostic in principle. The authors give 3 main types of lesions, with relatively specific histologic features that are classified as MADH and indicate that a conservative approach assists in the classification. Assuming that diagnostic criteria cannot be used to separate ADH and ductal carcinoma in situ on some core needle biopsy samples, and that more tissue is necessary, the authors stress that an excisional biopsy may be the follow-up strategy of choice. The challenge for the practicing pathologist is determining the scenarios in which to make the working MADH diagnosis (ie, the types of cases that are difficult). These types of categories often start out as great ideas but then blossom into categories in which overuse is problematic. For further reading, see reference list.[1,2]

S. Raab, MD

References

1. Page DL, Dupont WD, Rogers LW, et al. Atypical hyperplastic lesions of the female breast. A long-term follow-up study. *Cancer.* 1985;55:2698-2708.
2. Johnson NB, Collins LC. Update on percutaneous needle biopsy of nonmalignant breast lesions. *Adv Anat Pathol.* 2009;16:183-195.

Molecular alterations in metaplastic breast carcinoma

Cooper CL, Karim RZ, Selinger C, et al (Royal Prince Alfred Hosp, Camperdown, New South Wales, Australia; et al)
J Clin Pathol 66:522-528, 2013

Metaplastic carcinoma of the breast is a rare and heterogeneous subtype of breast carcinoma with a generally poor outcome, and few therapeutic options once disease recurs or progresses. Metaplastic carcinomas of the breast are usually of a larger size at diagnosis, with less frequent nodal metastasis compared with invasive ductal carcinoma no special type, and lack hormone and HER2 receptor expression. Recent research has revealed some potentially actionable genetic changes in a subset of these rare tumours. However, ongoing efforts to further characterise the genetic basis and the molecular alterations underlying the distinctive morphological and clinical characteristics of these tumours are needed in order to identify new targets for treatment. This review will describe the theories of pathogenesis of metaplastic breast carcinoma, and highlight genetic changes and potential therapeutic targets in this generally poor prognosis malignancy.

► In this review article, Cooper et al described the characteristics of metaplastic carcinomas of the breast, which have a poorer prognosis than matched triple negative carcinomas. The poor prognosis may be secondary to inherent biology and the initial presentation at a higher stage. Cooper et al detail the molecular features of metaplastic carcinomas, which may provide the potential to develop treatment strategies. For further reading, see reference list.[1,2]

S. Raab, MD

References

1. Luini A, Aguilar M, Gatti G, et al. Metaplastic carcinoma of the breast, an unusual disease with worse prognosis: the experience of the European Institute of Oncology and review of the literature. *Breast Cancer Res Treat.* 2007;101: 349-353.
2. Tomaskovic-Crook E, Thompson EW, Thiery JP. Epithelial to mesenchymal transition and breast cancer. *Breast Cancer Res.* 2009;11:213.

Primary Squamous Cell Carcinoma of the Breast: Predictors of Locoregional Recurrence and Overall Survival

Nayak A, Wu Y, Gilcrease MZ (Univ of Texas MD Anderson Cancer Ctr, Houston)

Am J Surg Pathol 37:867-873, 2013

Studies evaluating the biological behavior of primary squamous cell carcinoma (SCC) of the breast have yielded inconsistent results, perhaps in part because most studies have not taken into consideration specific histologic subtypes. We identified 21 cases of primary SCC of the breast diagnosed between the years 1985 and 2010 and analyzed the association between particular histologic features and disease outcome. Most tumors (17/21) were moderately or poorly differentiated, and most had a high nuclear grade (15/21). Five-year locoregional recurrence-free survival (LRRFS) for all patients was 54% ± 12%, and 5-year overall survival (OS) was 51% ± 13%. The only statistically significant feature associated with LRRFS was the presence of a spindle cell component in the tumor. Patients with >10% spindle cell component had decreased LRRFS (log rank; $P = 0.006$). The only statistically significant features associated with OS were patient age and tumor keratinization. Patients more than 60 years of age had decreased OS (log rank; $P = 0.035$), and patients with tumors having at least focal keratinization had improved OS (log rank; $P = 0.027$). Lymph node status, mitotic rate, tumor necrosis, cystic degeneration, clear cell change, and the presence of a pleomorphic component or associated ductal carcinoma in situ were not associated with either LRRFS or OS. In summary, primary SCC of the breast tends to be aggressive, particularly in patients more than 60 years of age and those with tumors having >10% spindle cell component. The presence of at least focal keratinization, however, is associated with significantly improved OS.

▶ Primary squamous cell carcinoma of the breast is a rare entry. Nayak et al indicate that the histologic features of a spindle cell component (poorer prognosis) and keratinization (better prognosis) are important to document in the pathology report. For additional reading, see the reference list.[1,2]

S. Raab, MD

References

1. Behranwala KA, Nasiri N, Abdullah N, et al. Squamous cell carcinoma of the breast: clinico-pathologic implications and outcome. *Eur J Surg Oncol.* 2003;29: 386-389.
2. Aparicio I, Martínez A, Hernández G, et al. Squamous cell carcinoma of the breast. *Eur J Obstet Gynecol Reprod Biol.* 2008;137:222-226.

Ductal carcinoma in situ associated with triple negative invasive breast cancer: evidence for a precursor–product relationship

Thike AA, Iqbal J, Cheok PY, et al (Singapore General Hosp)

J Clin Pathol 66:665-670, 2013

Aims.—We evaluated pathological features of the ductal carcinoma in situ component of 241 triple negative invasive breast cancers.

Results.—We found that 151 (62.6%) in situ lesions were of high nuclear grade, and 236 (97.9%) were triple negative (oestrogen receptor, progesterone receptor, cerbB2 negative). Immunohistochemistry for cytokeratin (CK)5/6, CK14, CK17, epidermal growth factor receptor (EGFR), CD117, 34βE12, p63 and smooth muscle actin (SMA) revealed positive staining in 5 (2.1%), 60 (24.9%), 69 (28.6%), 37 (15.4%), 69 (28.6%), 137 (56.8%), 3 (1.2%) and 22 (9.1%) in situ ductal components respectively, with fair to substantial agreement of staining results (positive versus negative) between in situ and corresponding invasive elements for CK5/6, CK14, CK17, EGFR, CD117 and 34βE12; but none to fair agreement for p63 and SMA respectively. When the tri-panel of CK14, EGFR and 34βE12 was used to define the basal phenotype, 68% revealed basal-like expression of both in situ and invasive components of the same case.

Conclusions.—Our data support the notion that triple negative ductal carcinoma in situ is the precursor of the corresponding invasive counterpart, and that basal-like expression is maintained in the majority of invasive cancers associated with basal-like in situ disease. Future studies that prospectively evaluate morphological and biological characteristics of invasive cancers that develop from triple negative and basal-like ductal carcinoma in situ lesions will assist in validating these findings (Table 5).

▶ This article by Thike et al examines the pathologic and immunohistochemical features of ductal carcinoma in situ in triple negative breast cancers (estrogen receptor, progesterone receptor, and cerbB2 negative; Table 5). The goal is to better understand the relationship of in situ and invasive components. This could have a future impact on how to immunohistochemically evaluate and describe pure in situ disease. For additional reading, see reference list.[1,2]

S. Raab, MD

TABLE 5.—Tri-panel (CK14, EGFR, 34βE12) Immunohistochemical Reactivity in Concurrent Ductal Carcinoma In Situ and the Invasive Component in Triple Negative Breast Cancer (N=241)

	Invasive Component		
	Tri-panel Negative	Tri-panel Positive	p Value
DCIS component			
Tri-panel negative (%)	31 (13.0)	6 (14.9)	<0.001
Tri-panel positive (%)	10 (4.1)	164 (68.0)	

DCIS, ductal carcinoma in situ.

References

1. Leong AS, Sormunen RT, Vinyuvat S, et al. Biologic markers in ductal carcinoma in situ and concurrent infiltrating carcinoma. A comparison of eight contemporary grading systems. *Am J Clin Pathol.* 2001;115:709-718.
2. Lampejo OT, Barnes DM, Smith P, et al. Evaluation of infiltrating ductal carcinomas with a DCIS component: correlation of the histologic type of the in situ component with grade of the infiltrating component. *Semin Diagn Pathol.* 1994;11: 215-222.

Pitfalls in outcome prediction of breast cancer

Rakha EA (Nottingham Univ Hosps NHS Trust and Univ of Nottingham, UK)

J Clin Pathol 66:458-464, 2013

Breast cancer represents a heterogeneous group of diseases with varied presentation, morphological and biological features, behaviour, and response to therapy. Management of breast cancer relies on availability of robust predictive and prognostic factors to support decision making. Identifying and validating the prognostic and predictive value of a given marker is based on studying its association with clinical outcome with or without consideration for therapy, respectively. In the field of cancer research, clinical outcome is determined by assessing certain time-dependent events: "endpoints" such as tumour progression, recurrence and patient mortality. Guidelines for reporting tumour markers have been published and there is a perception that outcome determination in breast cancer is well documented. However, reviewing the literature has highlighted the varied use of definitions used in clinical outcome measures and there are pitfalls in outcome analysis. This may have contributed to the discrepancies in the literature and to the inconsistent conclusions seen in published studies assessing the same markers. Identification of these pitfalls is expected to improve prognostic and predictive marker assessment. Here issues related to outcome determination in breast cancer including definitions and pitfalls and some critical views are presented (Table 1).

► In this review article, Rakha describes the pitfalls in outcome analysis of breast cancer studies. A take-home message is that distant recurrence-free interval and breast cancer–specific survival are the ideal outcome endpoints for the prognostic and predictive value of primary tumor characteristics. Table 1 provides excellent information regarding outcome endpoints.

S. Raab, MD

TABLE 1.—Definitions of outcome endpoints used in studies assessing morphological and molecular prognostic and predictive marker characteristics of breast cancer. These definitions include time-dependent events measured from the time of definitive surgery, assignment in a clinical trial or from the start of treatment in the neoadjuvant setting

Outcome endpoints	Events included	Events not included	Suitability
Overall survival	Death from any cause including cancer- and non-cancer-related, treatment-related and unknown cause	Patients lost to follow-up or alive at the last follow-up date are censored	Therapeutic clinical trials. In prognostication studies when the cause of death cannot be determined
Breast cancer specific survival	Death from breast cancer or death with breast cancer provided that other non-breast cancer-related causes are excluded	Death from other causes or from unknown causes. Lost to follow-up or alive at the end of follow-up are censored	Most reliable outcome endpoint in prognostication studies. It can be used in clinical trials whenever applicable (ie, testing long-term outcome of specific treatment)
Disease free survival*	All breast cancer events including locoregional and distant recurrences, second primary breast cancers, contralateral breast cancers and death from any cause. Some studies may include in situ carcinomas and second primary non-breast cancers	Patients lost to follow-up or alive at the last follow-up date are censored	Therapeutic and preventive trials. Not recommended in prognostication studies
Recurrence free survival	All breast cancer recurrences including locoregional and distant recurrences and death	Second primary cancers and in situ carcinomas	Therapeutic and preventive trials, less relevant in prognostication studies
Recurrence free interval	All breast cancer recurrences including locoregional and distant recurrences	Second primary cancer, in situ carcinomas and deaths	Therapeutic trials and prognostication studies
Local recurrence free interval	Recurrence in the ipsilateral breast, chest wall or mastectomy scar	Recurrences in other sites and deaths	Studies assessing efficacy of local control measures (ie, surgery and/or radiotherapy), prognostication studies and therapeutic and preventive trials. In the latter studies ipsilateral carcinoma in situ or new breast primary may be included
Regional recurrence free interval	Recurrence in the regional lymph nodes (ipsilateral axillary, infraclavicular, supraclavicular and internal mammary lymph nodes)	Recurrence in lymph nodes other than regional nodes. Recurrence in local and distant metastatic sites and deaths	Studies assessing efficacy of axillary control measures, prognostication studies and therapeutic trials

(*Continued*)

TABLE 1.—(*Continued*)

Outcome endpoints	Events included	Events not included	Suitability
Locoregional recurrence free interval	Recurrence in the ipsilateral breast, chest wall, mastectomy scar or regional lymph nodes	Recurrences in other sites and deaths	As above
Distant metastasis free interval	Recurrence at any site except those mentioned in the locoregional sites	New primary cancers and deaths	Most reliable recurrence-related event in prognostication studies and in clinical trials. It is a valid surrogate to patient survival
Breast cancer free interval	All breast cancer events including locoregional and distant recurrences, new primary breast cancer, in situ carcinomas, and contralateral breast cancer	Other non-breast primaries and deaths	Therapeutic and preventive trials. Less relevant in prognostication studies
Progression free interval	Time between diagnosis of the primary tumour or assignment into clinical trials and tumour progression (ie, increase in size; usually assessed clinically/radiologically)		Therapeutic trials. Prognostication studies in the setting of neoadjuvant therapy
Time-to-treatment failure	Time between commencing a treatment and tumour progression		Therapeutic trials

*Endpoints using interval instead of survival means that all events mentioned in the definition of these endpoints are included except death. Ipsilateral recurrence can be either local recurrence of the reference tumour or less frequently new primary invasive or in situ breast cancer. Contralateral breast cancer can be either metastasis from the reference tumour or new primary invasive or in situ breast cancer. Malignant tumours in the breast other than mammary carcinomas such as skin cancer, soft tissue sarcoma and metastasis should be considered as non-breast cancer in the outcome analysis.

Clinicopathological significance of CADM4 expression in invasive ductal carcinoma of the breast

Jang SM, Sim J, Han H, et al (Hanyang Univ, Seoul, South Korea)

J Clin Pathol 66:681-686, 2013

Aims.—Cell adhesion molecule 4 (CADM4) is a novel tumour suppressor involved in cell adhesion. Loss or decreased expression of CADM4 has been associated with the development and progression of some cancers. The purpose of this study was to investigate the clinicopathological significance of CADM4 expression in breast cancer.

Methods.—We constructed tissue microarrays to evaluate the immunohistochemical expression of CADM4 in 256 cases of invasive ductal carcinoma (IDC) and 45 cases of ductal carcinoma in situ (DCIS).

Results.—CADM4 was expressed in 37 (82.2%) DCIS cases, and in 173 (67.6%) IDC cases. CADM4 expression was higher in DCIS than in IDC ($P = 0.049$). Loss or decrease of CADM4 expression was significantly correlated with higher histological grade ($P = 0.020$), absence of oestrogen receptors ($P < 0.001$), absence of progesterone receptors ($P = 0.024$), and overexpression of c-erbB-2 ($P = 0.018$). In univariable and multivariable Cox regression analyses of all 256 IDC cases, CADM4 expression was not significantly associated with overall and disease-free survival. However, it showed a significant positive association with longer disease-free survival in 187 stages I and II IDC cases ($P = 0.039$, log-rank test).

Conclusions.—Loss or decrease of CADM4 expression seems to play an important role in breast cancer invasiveness, and it is associated with poorer biological parameters. CADM4 can be used as a novel marker predicting risk of recurrence and disease outcomes in stages I and II IDC.

▶ The authors' take-home message is that cell adhesion molecule 4 (CADM4) expression is significantly higher in ductal carcinoma in situ than in invasive ductal carcinoma, and loss or downregulation of CADM4 expression is correlated with higher histologic grade. In the future, CADM4 could be used as a marker to predict recurrence in stage I or II intraductal carcinoma. For additional reading, see the reference list.[1]

S. Raab, MD

Reference

1. Jang SM, Han H, Jun YJ, et al. Clinicopathological significance of CADM4 expression, and its correlation with expression of E-cadherin and Ki-67 in colorectal adenocarcinomas. *J Clin Pathol.* 2012;65:902-906.

Use of immunohistochemistry in the diagnosis of problematic breast lesions

Lee AHS (Nottingham Univ Hosps, UK)
J Clin Pathol 66:471-477, 2013

Most diagnoses in breast pathology can be made with H&E sections. Nevertheless immunohistochemistry plays a useful supplementary role. This article reviews the common uses of immunohistochemistry in diagnostic breast pathology. It is important to be aware of the limitations of individual antibodies. Such problems can often be overcome by using panels of antibodies. Quality control is also essential: internal and external controls should show appropriate staining. Immunohistochemistry must be interpreted in combination with the morphology seen on H&E sections. Myoepithelial markers, such as smooth muscle actin, smooth muscle myosin heavy chain and p63, are useful for distinguishing invasive carcinoma from sclerosing lesions and ductal carcinoma in situ (DCIS), and in the classification of papillary lesions. Basal cytokeratins can help distinguish epithelial hyperplasia of usual type (UEH) and clonal proliferations such as DCIS and lobular carcinoma in situ (LCIS). UEH usually shows patchy expression whereas DCIS and other clonal proliferations are typically negative. E-cadherin can usually separate DCIS and LCIS: DCIS typically shows membrane staining and most LCIS is negative. Cytokeratins can be used to detect small nodal metastases or subtle invasive carcinomas such as invasive lobular carcinomas. Immunohistochemistry plays a useful role in diagnosing spindle cell lesions such as a panel of cytokeratins to identify spindle cell carcinomas. Immunohistochemistry is helpful in recognising metastases to the breast. Different antibodies are useful for different tumours: WT1 for ovarian carcinoma; TTF1 for pulmonary adenocarcinoma; S100, melan-A and HMB45 for melanoma; and lymphoid markers for lymphoma.

► In this review article, Lee examines the use of immunohistochemistry in a variety of breast scenarios, such as distinction of epithelial hyperplasia of usual type from clonal lesions and distinction of ductal carcinoma in situ and lobular carcinoma in situ. Lee emphasizes the limitation of immunohistochemistry and the importance of quality control. For further reading, see reference list.[1,2]

S. Raab, MD

References

1. Hilson JB, Schnitt SJ, Collins LC. Phenotypic alterations in ductal carcinoma in situ-associated myoepithelial cells: biologic and diagnostic implications. *Am J Surg Pathol.* 2009;33:227-232.
2. Lee AHS. Recent developments in the histological diagnosis of spindle cell carcinoma, fibromatosis and phyllodes tumour of the breast. *Histopathology.* 2008; 52:45-57.

3 Gastrointestinal System

Filiform polyps and filiform polyp–like lesions are common in defunctioned or diverted colorectum resection specimens

Gill P, Chetty R (Oxford Univ Hosps and Univ of Oxford, UK)

Ann Diagn Pathol 17:341-344, 2013

We describe filiform polyps (FPs) in a series of defunctioned rectums with diversion colitis. A 6-year search of all defunctioned rectal resection specimens revealed 8 cases with 17 macroscopically observed FPs. They occurred in 4 females and 4 males aged between 12 and 64 years. Four had defunctioning colostomies for ulcerative colitis, 3 for Crohn disease and 1 for diverticular disease. Multiple lesions were seen in 6 of 8 cases: 1 case having 4 FPs, 1 patient with 3 lesions, and 4 cases with 2 lesions. The FP varied in length from 4 to 11 mm; mean length was 7.8 mm. No evidence of mucosal prolapse was seen in any of the polypoid lesions. In 65 cases without grossly observed polypoid lesions, prominent mucosal polypoid projections in keeping with FP were seen in 47 cases. These were observed in nonulcerated sections and were histologically identical to the 17 macroscopically observed FPs ranging from 3 to 8 mm, and 3 to 5 such polypoid lesions were seen in 20 cases. We suggest that FP and FP-like lesions are commonly encountered in defunctioned resection specimens (Fig).

► Gill and Chetty provide a nice review of the filiform polyp (FP), which is seen in a defunctioned rectum with diversion colitis. Good examples are shown in the Fig. Histologically, the FP mucosa and submucosa are indistinguishable from surrounding nonpolyp mucosa. There also is a lack of ulceration and the tubules display normal architecture. Gill and Chetty recommend that we do not confuse the FP with other types of polyps in the rectum. For additional reading, please see the reference list.[1,2]

S. Raab, MD

References

1. Lee CG, Lim YJ, Choi JS, et al. Filiform polyposis in the sigmoid colon: a case series. *World J Gastroenterol*. 2010;16:2443-2447.

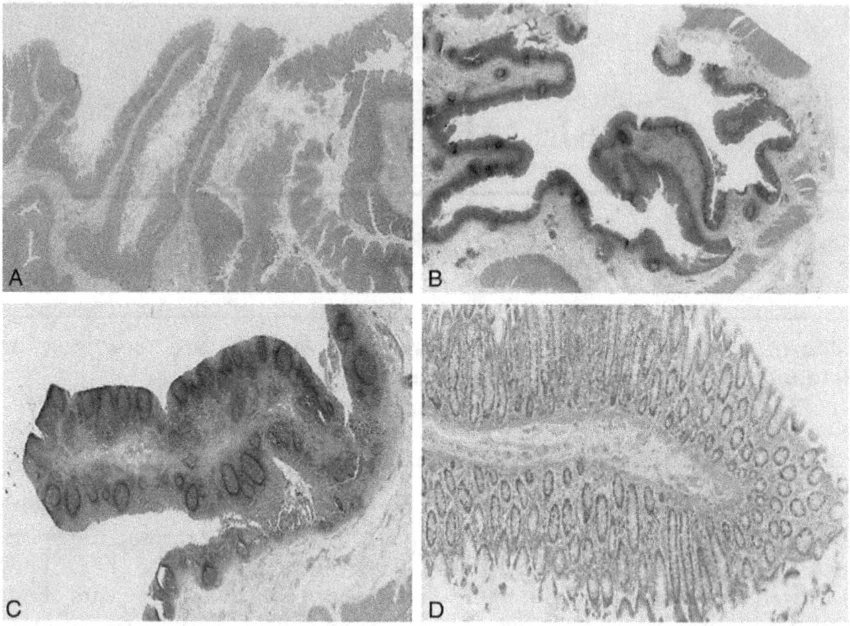

FIGURE.—A and B, Low-power images of cases 2 and 6. There are polypoid, finger-like projections into the lumen lined by normal mucosa and containing normal submucosa. These lesions most closely resemble FPs. Lymphoid aggregates are evident in B. C, Despite containing several reactive lymphoid aggregates within the mucosa and some in the submucosa, there is no distortion of mucosal architecture. The submucosa contains dilated vessels and a small amount of adipose tissue. D, An FP from case 8. The patient was defunctioned because of severe diverticular disease. Gland architecture is maintained, the lamina propria contains a normal complement of inflammatory cells, while the submucosa shows focal fibrosis and slightly dilated vessels aligned parallel to the long axis of the polyp. (Reprinted from Gill P, Chetty R. Filiform polyps and filiform polyp–like lesions are common in defunctioned or diverted colorectum resection specimens. *Ann Diagn Pathol.* 2013;17:341-344, with permission from Elsevier Inc.)

2. Appelman HD, Threatt BA, Ernst C, et al. Filiform polyposis of the colon: an unusual sequel of ulcerative colitis. *Am J Clin Pathol.* 1974;62:145-146.

Characterization of Perineural Invasion as a Component of Colorectal Cancer Staging

Ueno H, Study Group for Perineural Invasion projected by the Japanese Society for Cancer of the Colon and Rectum (JSCCR) (Natl Defense Med College, Tokorozawa, Japan; et al)

Am J Surg Pathol 37:1542-1549, 2013

Perineural invasion (PN) in colorectal cancer (CRC) is a site-specific prognostic marker, as mentioned by the AJCC Cancer Staging Manual, but it remains to be clearly defined. We aimed to identify an optimal characterization of PN as a component of cancer staging. On the basis of the anatomic features of the nervous system of the large bowel, site-specific

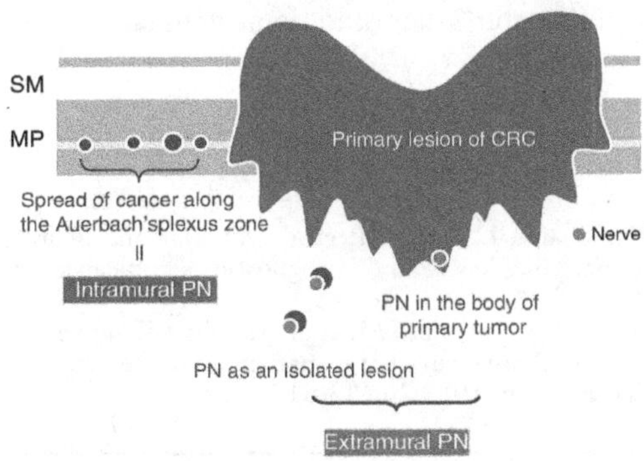

FIGURE 1.—A schema for the classification of PN in CRC. Horizontal spread of cancer along the Auerbach plexus zone was defined as intramural PN, and the histologic finding of tumor cells invading into or spreading along nerve fascicles external to the muscularis propria was defined as extramural PN. The latter is observed as an isolated lesion and is also observed in the body of the primary tumor. (Reprinted from Ueno H, Study Group for Perineural Invasion projected by the Japanese Society for Cancer of the Colon and Rectum (JSCCR). Characterization of perineural invasion as a component of colorectal cancer staging. *Am J Surg Pathol.* 2013;37:1542-1549, with permission from Lippincott Williams & Wilkins.)

pathologic criteria were assigned to PN according to the location of PN. Multi-institutional pathologic review based on these criteria was performed for 962 patients with stage I to III CRC at 2 institutions (1999 to 2004, cohort 1) and 1883 patients from 8 other institutions (2000 to 2004, cohort 2). In cohort 1, intramural and extramural PN were observed in 152 and 101 patients, respectively, which had a different impact on disease-free survival (hazard ratio, 2.6 [1.9 to 3.5] vs. 4.7 [3.4 to 6.5], respectively). A 3-tiered grading system (Pn0; Pn1a, intramural PN; Pn1b, extramural PN) distinguished 5-year disease-free survival as 88%, 70%, and 48%, respectively; and multivariate analysis identified PN grade as a significant prognostic marker independent of T or N stage. These results were similar in cohort 2. Interinstitutional difference of the prognostic impact of PN grade was acceptably small among all institutions. Interobserver study among 6 gastrointestinal pathologists showed superior judgment reproducibility for PN compared with vascular invasion. The results of our study indicate that PN is an important prognostic marker in CRC. The value of cancer staging could be enhanced by PN assessment using site-specific criteria and a simple grading system based on PN location within the bowel (Fig 1).

▶ Perineural invasion (PN) is a prognostic factor for colorectal cancer, but detailed study of this parameter is lacking. The literature indicates that up to 35% of colorectal carcinomas are associated with PN. Ueno et al wrote that there is a lack of standardized criteria for PN, there is no site-specific assessment rule for the large intestine (ie, intramurally or extramurally), and the prognostic value of PN in colorectal cancer has not been thoroughly evaluated. Ueno and colleagues carefully evaluate these 3 issues. Fig 1 shows a schema for the intramural and extramural classification PN in colorectal adenocarcinoma. The authors also show data that the 3-tier grading system is easy to use. For further reading, see the reference list.[1,2]

S. Raab, MD

References

1. Krasna MJ, Flancbaum L, Cody RP, et al. Vascular and neural invasion in colorectal carcinoma. Incidence and prognostic significance. *Cancer.* 1988;61: 1018-1023.
2. Knudsen JB, Nilsson T, Sprechler M, et al. Venous and nerve invasion as prognostic factors in postoperative survival of patients with resectable cancer of the rectum. *Dis Colon Rectum.* 1983;26:613-617.

Histologic Features and Cytologic Techniques That Aid Pathologic Stage Assessment of Colonic Adenocarcinoma

Panarelli NC, Schreiner AM, Brandt SM, et al (Weill Cornell Med College, NY; et al)

Am J Surg Pathol 37:1252-1258, 2013

Cancer involvement of the colonic serosa is designated pT4a by the *American Joint Committee on Cancer Staging Manual*, 7th edition. The manual defines criteria for pT4a as either tumor penetration of the serosa or comingling of cancer cells and mesothelial cells in histologic sections. Unfortunately, the pT4a grouping is inconsistently applied, because these guidelines are overly limited: fibroinflammatory changes near the serosa may be associated with peritoneal metastases even in the absence of overt peritoneal penetration. Thus, reliable ancillary techniques for detecting serosal penetration by the tumor and accurate criteria for stage assessment are needed. We evaluated the utility of cytologic preparations in determining tumor stage by comparing results of serosal scrape cytology with histologic stage assessment of 120 colon cancer resection specimens. We correlated our findings with the presence and type of inflammatory changes near the serosa to determine which, if any, are reliable indicators of peritoneal penetration. Cytologic smears from all pT1 and pT2 tumors were negative for carcinoma. However, 13 (19%) pT3 tumors showed cancer in cytologic smears, all of which were deeply invasive. In fact, 46% of pT3 cancers present ≤1 mm from a serosal tissue reaction were associated with cancer in cytologic preparations from the serosa, which was comparable to pT4a tumors (55%). We conclude that cytologic smears improve detection of peritoneal penetration among pT3 tumors compared with histology alone. Tumors close (≤1 mm) to a fibroinflammatory tissue reaction on the serosa are likely associated with peritoneal involvement by cancer. Peritumoral abscesses that communicate with the serosa and hemorrhage or fibrin on the serosa also predict cancer involvement of the peritoneum.

The presence of these findings among deeply invasive cancers should prompt their classification as pT4a lesions.

▶ Panarelli et al show the benefits of combining cytologic and histologic assessments in cases of identifying peritoneal involvement of a colonic tumor. The ability to grossly recognize the serosal regions to sample may be problematic and may take experience. The fact that scraping the area of concern produces a better sample (similar to the Pap test method, scraping the cervix and endocervix instead of first performing a biopsy increases sensitivity) seems intuitive. The potential pitfalls may be similar to those identified in peritoneal and pelvic washing specimens in which only a few groups of atypical cells are present. For further reading, see the reference list.[1,2]

S. Raab, MD

References

1. Leather AJ, Kocjan G, Savage F, et al. Detection of free malignant cells in the peritoneal cavity before and after resection of colorectal cancer. *Dis Colon Rectum.* 1994;37:814-819.
2. Ambrose NS, MacDonald F, Young J, et al. Monoclonal antibody and cytological detection of free malignant cells in the peritoneal cavity during resection of colorectal cancer—can monoclonal antibodies do better? *Eur J Surg Oncol.* 1989;15:99-102.

Microcystic/Reticular Schwannoma of the Proximal Sigmoid Colon: Case Report With Review of Literature

Trivedi A, Ligato S (Hartford Hosp, CT)

Arch Pathol Lab Med 137:284-288, 2013

We report a case of microcystic/reticular schwannoma of the proximal sigmoid colon in a 61-year-old man. A 12-mm polyp was detected while the patient was undergoing screening for colorectal neoplasm. This rare variant of schwannoma was initially described in 2008 and shows a predilection for the visceral organs, predominantly the gastrointestinal tract. We also review 11 other reported cases of microcystic/reticular schwannomas in the gastrointestinal tract. Unlike conventional gastrointestinal schwannomas, which are more common in the stomach, this variant appears to be more common in the large intestine. Histologic examination of this polyp showed predominant lipoblast-like vacuolated cells within a myxoid stroma with focal spindle cell areas. Features suggestive of malignancy, like nuclear pleomorphism, mitosis, or necrosis, were absent. Immunohistochemistry for S100 protein showed strong nuclear and cytoplasmic positivity, whereas cytokeratin and CD117 stains were negative. It is important to entertain microcystic/reticular schwannoma in the differential diagnosis of a signet ring cell adenocarcinoma or a myxoid gastrointestinal stromal tumor, particularly on small biopsy specimens.

▶ Trivedi and Ligato describe a colonic variant of a schwannoma that may mimic a myxoid variant of a gastrointestinal stromal tumor or a signet ring cell adenocarcinoma on biopsy specimen tissues. The keys to recognition are histologic (eg, vacuolated cells in myxoid stroma) and immunohistologic (reactivity for S100 and nonreactivity for cytokeratin and CD117). For additional reading, see reference list.[1,2]

S. Raab, MD

References

1. Liegl B, Bennett MW, Fletcher CD. Microcystic/reticular schwannoma: a distinct variant with predilection for visceral locations. *Am J Surg Pathol.* 2008;32: 1080-1087.
2. Hou YY, Tan YS, Xu JF, et al. Schwannoma of the gastrointestinal tract: a clinicopathological, immunohistochemical and ultrastructural study of 33 cases. *Histopathology.* 2006;48:536-545.

Reporting trends of right-sided hyperplastic and sessile serrated polyps in a large teaching hospital over a 4-year period (2009–2012)

Gill P, Wang LM, Bailey A, et al (Univ of Oxford, UK)

J Clin Pathol 66:655-658, 2013

Aim.—An audit of serrated polyps diagnosed over a 4-year period: 2009 to 2012 was undertaken to ascertain the reporting trends of sessile serrated polyps (SSP).

Methods.—All right sided hyperplastic polyps (HP) proximal to the splenic flexure and all polyps designated SSP were retrieved from the study period. Three pathologists blinded to the original diagnosis

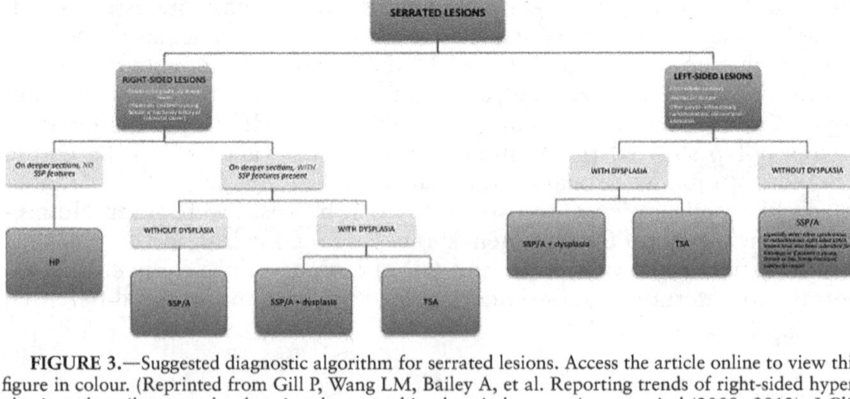

FIGURE 3.—Suggested diagnostic algorithm for serrated lesions. Access the article online to view this figure in colour. (Reprinted from Gill P, Wang LM, Bailey A, et al. Reporting trends of right-sided hyperplastic and sessile serrated polyps in a large teaching hospital over a 4-year period (2009–2012). *J Clin Pathol.* 2013;655-658.)

re-examined the slides. Recent American College of Gastroenterology guidelines for the diagnosis of SSP was utilised.

Results.—No cases of SSP were diagnosed in 2009. In 2010, 32 right-sided cases were encountered, 83 confirmed in 2011 and 134 confirmed in 2012. The vast majority of these were right-sided.

With regards to right-sided HP that were re-classified as SSP the data is as follows: 20 of 66 in 2009 (30%); 58 of 91 in 2010 (64%); 42 of 106 (40%) in 2011 and 69 of 206 in 2012 (33%).

Conclusions.—This study has demonstrated an almost exponential increase in the diagnosis of SSP over a 4-year period. In addition, 30 to 64% of right-sided HP were re-classified as SSP over the 4-year period suggesting that greater awareness of the diagnostic criteria for SSP is required.

SSP is an important precursor lesion in the serrated pathway of colorectal cancer. Its recognition is important for surveillance and therapeutic strategies (Fig 3).

▶ Sessile serrated polyps are thought to be precursor lesions to serrated adenocarcinomas, which compose up to 7.5% of colorectal adenocarcinomas. The American College of Gastroenterology described a sessile serrated polyp/adenoma to be a single unequivocal architecturally distorted, dilated, or horizontally branched crypt, particularly if it is associated with inverted maturation. Gill et al showed the frequency of reclassification of hyperplastic polyps to sessile serrated polyps/adenomas using the histologic criteria described by the World Health Organization (WHO). In Fig 3, Gill et al describe a diagnostic algorithm for right-sided and left-sided colorectal serrated lesions. The authors point out that right-sided hyerplastic lesions should be evaluated carefully to exclude a sessile serrated polyp and that because left-sided sessile serrated polyps are rare, mimics must be excluded. For further reading, please see reference list.[1,2]

S. Raab, MD

References

1. Rex DK, Ahnen DJ, Baron JA, et al. Serrated lesions of the colorectum: review and recommendations from an expert panel. *Am J Gastroenterol.* 2012;107:1315-1329.
2. Snover DC, Ahnen DJ, Burt RW, et al. Serrated polyps of the colon and rectum and serrated polyposis. In: Bosman FT, Carneiro F, Hruban RH, Theise N, eds. *WHO Classification of tumours. Pathology and genetics. Tumours of Digestive System.* 4th edition. Lyon, France: International Agency for Research on Cancer; 2010:160-165.

Clinicopathologic Features of Synchronous Colorectal Carcinoma: A Distinct Subset Arising From Multiple Sessile Serrated Adenomas and Associated With High Levels of Microsatellite Instability and Favorable Prognosis

Hu H, Chang DT, Nikiforova MN, et al (Univ of Pittsburgh Med Ctr, PA; Stanford Univ, CA)

Am J Surg Pathol 37:1660-1670, 2013

Analysis of synchronous colorectal carcinomas can provide a unique model to examine the underlying molecular alterations in colorectal

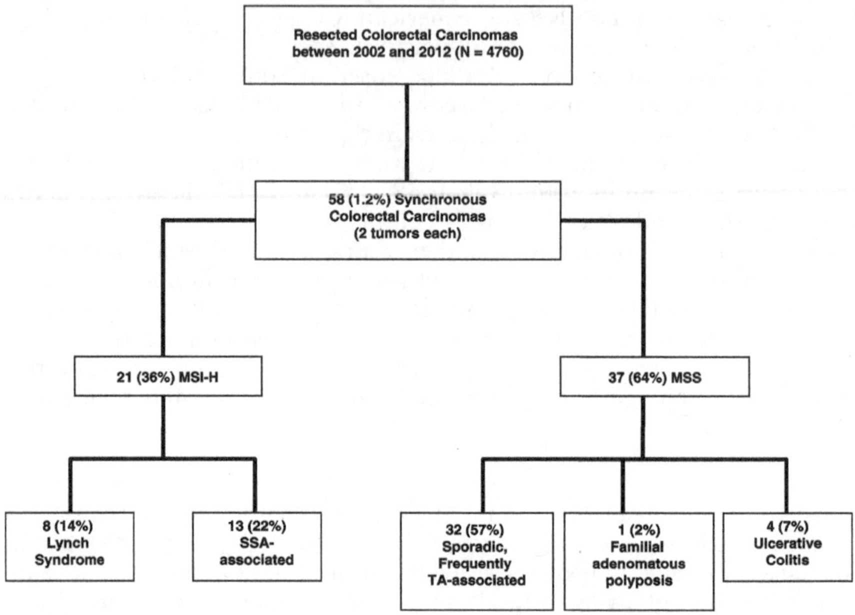

FIGURE 2.—Flowchart detailing the synchronous colorectal carcinoma study group further stratified into MSI-H and MSS groups and subgroups. (Reprinted from Hu H, Chang DT, Nikiforova MN, et al. Clinicopathologic features of synchronous colorectal carcinoma: a distinct subset arising from multiple sessile serrated adenomas and associated with high levels of Microsatellite instability and favorable prognosis. *Am J Surg Pathol.* 2013;37:1660-1670, with permission from Lippincott Williams &Wilkins.)

carcinoma, as synchronous tumors arise in a background of common genetic and environmental factors. We analyzed the clinicopathologic and molecular features of synchronous colorectal carcinomas compared with solitary carcinomas to correlate the histologic findings with molecular alterations and to identify the prognostic significance, if any, of synchronous colorectal carcinoma. Of the 4760 primary colorectal carcinomas resected for the years 2002 to 2012 at our institution, 58 patients (1.2%) harbored 2 invasive primary adenocarcinomas and comprise the synchronous colorectal carcinoma study group. A control group of consecutively resected solitary colorectal carcinomas from 109 patients was also analyzed. Compared with solitary colorectal carcinomas, synchronous colorectal carcinomas more frequently were identified in older patients (median age 70 vs. 60 y; $P = 0.001$), involved the right colon (42/58, 72% vs. 47/109, 43%; $P = 0.0003$), were more often microsatellite instability-high (MSI-H) (21/58, 36% vs. 13/109, 12%; $P = 0.0005$), and were more frequently associated with precursor sessile serrated adenomas (SSAs) (13/58, 22% vs. 2/109, 2%; $P = 0.0001$). A statistically significant difference in overall survival was identified between patients with synchronous and solitary colorectal carcinomas (5 y overall survival 92% vs. 56%, $P = 0.02$). A unique subgroup of 13 synchronous colorectal carcinomas demonstrated tumors arising from SSAs (SSA-associated). All SSA-associated synchronous colorectal carcinomas were seen in patients above 65 years of age, and 12/13 (92%) occurred in women. Most patients (12/13, 92%) with SSA-associated synchronous colorectal carcinomas demonstrated involvement of the right colon, and tumors were frequently stage I or II (9/13, 69%) and low grade (11/13, 85%). In 12/13 (92%) SSA-associated synchronous colorectal carcinomas, both tumors exhibited loss of MLH1 and PMS2 immunohistochemical expression with concurrent *BRAF* V600E mutation. Nine of 13 (69%) patients with SSA-associated colorectal carcinoma harbored additional SSAs. Three of 13 (15%) patients with SSA-associated synchronous colorectal carcinoma met the World Health Organization criteria for serrated polyposis. Notably, no patient with SSA-associated synchronous colorectal carcinoma developed disease recurrence or died of disease at last follow-up. In conclusion, synchronous colorectal carcinomas are enriched with MSI-H tumors, particularly those arising from SSAs, which contributes to the overall improved survival for patients with synchronous tumors compared with patients with solitary tumors. We demonstrate that SSA-associated synchronous colorectal carcinomas have a striking predilection for elderly women, are associated with a favorable prognosis, and are MSI-H and *BRAF* V600E positive (Fig 2).

▶ As molecular analysis begins to assess that categories of tumors may have different prognoses, depending on mutational differences, Hu et al provide an example in synchronous colorectal carcinomas. A take-home message comes from Fig 2, which shows the synchronous colorectal carcinoma study group further stratified into microsatellite instability-high and microsatellite stable groups. For additional reading, see the reference list.[1,2]

S. Raab, MD

References

1. Adloff M, Arnaud JP, Bergamaschi R, et al. Synchronous carcinoma of the colon and rectum: prognostic and therapeutic implications. *Am J Surg*. 1989;157:299-302.
2. Salaria SN, Streppel MM, Lee LA, et al. Sessile serrated adenomas: high-risk lesions? *Hum Pathol*. 2012;43:1808-1814.

Impact of Age on the Quality of Lymphadenectomy for Colorectal Cancer

Torre C, Paliogiannis P, Pulighe F, et al (Univ of Sassari, Italy)
Cancer Invest 31:39-42, 2013

The aim of this study was to evaluate the impact of patient age on the number of lymph nodes dissected during surgery for colorectal cancer. Clinical and histopathological data of 231 consecutive patients who underwent elective surgery for colorectal cancer were reviewed retrospectively. Patients were divided into those aged ≤70 years and >70 years. Our findings suggest that patient's age influences the number of lymph nodes

detected in surgical specimens; this number was lower in patients aged >70 years and decreased with further aging.

▶ Some investigators believe that at least 12 lymph nodes must be examined in a colorectal specimen for adequate staging. Torre et al report that colorectal specimens from patients older than 70 years have lower numbers of lymph nodes than those patients ≤70 years of age. Torre et al report that the reason for this lower number is unclear and could include patient-related factors and other factors not evaluated (eg, length of specimen). This issue has been a challenge to pathologists and gross room personnel who try to maximize the number of lymph nodes obtained. Most likely, the root causes are multifactorial and interrelated. Methods of maximizing the number of recovered lymph nodes are discussed elsewhere. For further reading, see the reference list.[1-3]

S. Raab, MD

References

1. Bilimoria KY, Stewart AK, Palis BE, et al. Adequacy and importance of lymph node evaluation for colon cancer in the elderly. *J Am Coll Surg*. 2008;206: 247-254.
2. Murphy J, Pocard M, Jass JR, et al. Number and size of lymph nodes recovered from Dukes B rectal cancers: correlation with prognosis and histologic antitumor immune response. *Dis Colon Rectum*. 2007;50:1526-1534.
3. Nelson H, Petrelli N, Carlin A, et al. National Cancer Institute Expert Panel. Guidelines 2000 for colon and rectal cancer surgery. *J Natl Cancer Inst*. 2001; 93:583-596.

4 Hepatobiliary System and Pancreas

Histologic Findings Predictive of a Diagnosis of De novo Autoimmune Hepatitis After Liver Transplantation in Adults

Sebagh M, Castillo-Rama M, Azoulay D, et al (AP-HP Hôpital Paul Brousse, Villejuif, France; Univ of Pittsburgh Med Ctr, PA; et al)

Transplantation 96:670-678, 2013

Background.—Autoimmune hepatitis (AIH) after liver transplantation has been defined histologically as a "hepatitic" pattern of injury, characterized by lymphoplasmacytic inflammation with necroinflammatory activity (NIA), comparable with findings seen in native livers. This definition, however, is difficult to apply in practice because specific histologic criteria are not clearly delineated. This study aimed to determine which histologic features correlated best with clinical and serologic features of dAIH.

Methods.—Index liver biopsies from patients with autoimmune-like hepatitis transplanted for non-AIH in two centers (n = 35 and 20) were reviewed. Histologic features were correlated with the clinical diagnosis of AIH based on a retrospective review of clinical and serologic data, including therapeutic response.

Results.—A clinical diagnosis of AIH was retrospectively assigned to 24 of 35 (68%) and 18 of 20 (90%) patients, respectively ($P = 0.10$). In multivariate analysis, centrilobular NIA and centrilobular plasma cell (PC) ratio of 30% to 50% were independently discriminating for a clinical diagnosis of AIH ($P = 0.04$ and 0.05, respectively). The best level of predictability (99.6%) was mathematically achieved when severe centrilobular NIA and centrilobular PC ratio of 30% to 50% were both present.

Conclusion.—A histologic pattern of centrilobular injury including increased NIA and increased PC infiltration correlates with measurements of autoimmunity in liver recipients. It could be used to segregate cases for further study and introduced into the AIH scoring systems when applied in the context of liver transplantation.

► Posttransplant plasma cell hepatitis (PCH) is a descriptive diagnosis for a wide spectrum of potential pathophysiologic entities, including late plasma cell—rich acute cellular rejection, de novo autoimmune hepatitis, recurrent autoimmune hepatitis, plasma cell—rich recurrent hepatotrophic viral infection, and an alloimmune-type phenomenon. Distinguishing the precise etiology usually requires fairly robust clinicopathologic and serologic correlation. This study sought to identify some histologic features that would be more specific for a diagnosis of posttransplant de novo autoimmune hepatitis. A benefit of this study was a clean population of post–liver transplant patients who underwent transplant for a history of liver disease other than autoimmune hepatitis. Therefore, recurrent autoimmune hepatitis could be reasonably excluded as a potential possibility. Surprisingly, in this cohort of PCH patients, a high percentage of patients had posttransplant de novo autoimmune hepatitis diagnosed (more than three-quarters from both of the centers combined). This number is higher than I would have predicted and underscores the importance of doing a complete clinical and serologic workup for patients presenting with posttransplant plasma cell hepatitis, including autoimmune serologies and immunoglobulin levels. It should be noted that this percentage may even be underestimated, as posttransplant patients are under immunosuppression and may show falsely negative or low serologic levels for auto-antibodies and immunoglobulins. One challenge to this report is the use of therapeutic response as inclusion criteria for patients with de novo autoimmune hepatitis. One could argue that any plasma cell–rich necroinflammatory lesion of the liver will likely respond to increased immunosuppression. Regardless, the histologic features of centrilobular necroinflammatory activity and centrilobular plasma cell–rich inflammation may suggest a unique etiologic entity that deserves further study at this point.

M. L. Smith, MD

The Hepatitis Aggressiveness Score (HAS): A Novel Classification System for Post–Liver Transplantation Recurrent Hepatitis C

Moreira RK, Salomao M, Verna EC, et al (Columbia Univ College of Physicians and Surgeons, NY)

Am J Surg Pathol 37:104-113, 2013

Several histopathologic features have been described in cases of fibrosing cholestatic hepatitis C (FCH-C). We investigated whether FCH-associated features can be utilized as the basis of a novel grading system for the entire population of post-liver transplantation (LT) recurrent hepatitis C virus (HCV) infection. Liver biopsies obtained at a median (interquartile range) of 12.3 (10.4-13.8) months post-LT from 170 patients with recurrent HCV were included. Biopsies were assessed for the following FCH features: (1) ductular reaction, (2) cholestasis, (3) hepatocyte ballooning, and (4) periportal sinusoidal fibrosis. A Hepatitis Aggressiveness Score (HAS) was assigned on the basis of the number of FCH features as follows: 0 features = HAS 1; 1 to 2 features = HAS 2; and 3 to 4 features = HAS 3. We analyzed the performance of this novel system in predicting clinicopathologic outcomes compared with conventional grading systems after a median (interquartile range) follow-up of 24 (13-45.5) months. The HAS classification was highly predictive of fibrosis progression ($P < 0.001$) and was the best predictor of graft loss in a multivariable analysis model, which included all conventional hepatitis grading systems (adjusted hazard ratio = 5.5, confidence interval 2.9-10.7, $P < 0.001$ for

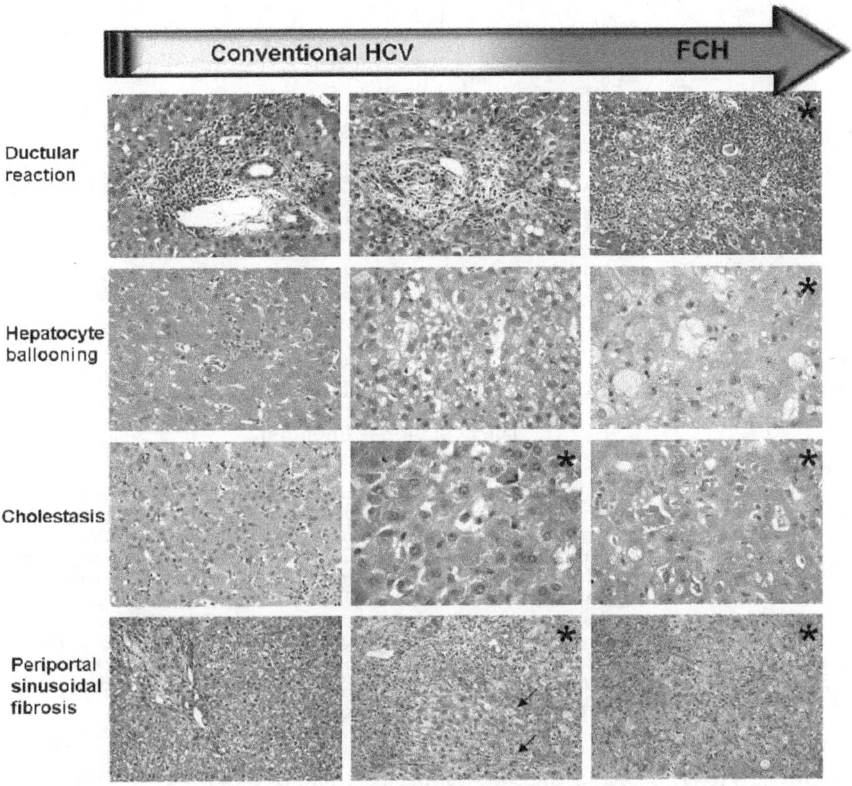

FIGURE 1.—Spectrum of FCH-C histopathologic changes in post-LT recurrent hepatitis C ranging from conventional histopathologic appearance (left column) to well-developed FCH-C (right column). Rows 1 through 4 illustrate increasing degrees of severity of ductular reaction, hepatocyte ballooning and lobular disarray, cholestasis, and periportal sinusoidal fibrosis (from left to right: none, moderate, and severe; rows 1 and 4, trichrome stain; rows 2 and 3 hematoxylin and eosin stain). Arrows indicate areas of periportal sinusoidal fibrosis (in contrast to areas of "usual" pattern of periportal fibrosis also shown in the image). *Degree of severity of each feature meeting the study criteria. (Reprinted from Moreira RK, Salomao M, Verna EC, et al. The Hepatitis Aggressiveness Score (HAS): a novel classification system for post—liver transplantation recurrent hepatitis C. *Am J Surg Pathol.* 2013;37:104-113, with permission from Lippincott Williams & Wilkins.)

HAS 3 vs. HAS 1 and 2, compared with adjusted hazard ratio = 1.0, confidence interval 0.5-1.9, $P = 0.94$ for the presence of moderate to severe necroinflammation by at least 1 conventional grading system). Presence of at least 3 of 4 FCH features (HAS 3 group) characterized a subset of patients with distinctly worse prognosis and severe cholestatic disease (ie, FCH-C). We propose a novel approach to the histologic grading of post-LT recurrent HCV based exclusively on FCH features. This system allows accurate identification of FCH-C cases and stratification of all recurrent HCV patients into distinct prognostic categories (Figs 1 and 6A).

▶ Fibrosing cholestatic hepatitis C virus infection is one of the most feared recurrent diseases in the post—liver transplant population because of its high rate of

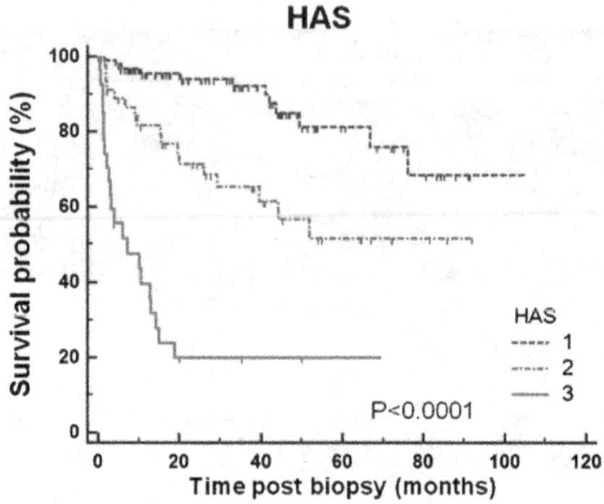

FIGURE 6A.—Comparison between the HAS classification (A) and other currently used hepatitis grading systems (B–E) in predicting graft loss in the setting of recurrent hepatitis C. Whereas all grading systems show prognostic utility, the HAS classification more accurately identifies the patient group at highest risk for graft loss (ie, HAS 3 or FCH-C). B–E, Blue dotted line, minimal activity (Batts-Ludwig grades 0 to 1, Scheuer grades 0 to 1, Ishak scores 0 to 4, and Metavir A0); green dotted line, mild activity (Batts-Ludwig grade 2, Scheuer grade 2, HAI scores 5 to 8, and Metavir A1); and red solid line, moderate to severe activity (Batts-Ludwig grades 3 to 4, Scheuer grades 3 to 4, HAI score >8, and Metavir A2 to 3). Kaplan-Meier survival analysis and log rank test. For Interpretation of the references to color in this figure legend, the reader is referred to web version of this article. (Reprinted from Moreira RK, Salomao M, Verna EC, et al. The Hepatitis Aggressiveness Score (HAS): a novel classification system for post-liver transplantation recurrent hepatitis C. *Am J Surg Pathol.* 2013;37:104-113, with permission from Lippincott Williams & Wilkins.)

progression to fibrosis and allograft failure. The pattern of recurrent viral hepatitis, classically described in patients with hepatitis B virus infection and immunosuppression, is characterized by widespread ballooning degeneration, a ductular reaction, cholestasis, and periportal subsinusoidal fibrosis. Interestingly, these histopathologic changes are not included in the most common hepatitis activity grading systems, including Batts-Ludwig, Metavir, and the modified hepatitis activity index. In this report, the authors propose a new scoring system that incorporates these histologic features. Fig 1 highlights the features, and the images with an asterisk in the corner should be noted as meeting study criteria for fibrosing cholestatic hepatitis, the degree of ductular reaction, hepatocyte ballooning, cholestasis, and periportal sinusoidal fibrosis is fairly significant. When the infections were stratified in this stringent morphology-based system and incorporated into the hepatitis aggressiveness score, the outcome is shown in Fig 6A and compared with some of the other common hepatitis activity grading systems. Obviously, this scoring system needs to be studied prospectively in multiple centers to confirm its validity; however, it certainly provides a nice framework for the evaluation of patients with potential fibrosing cholestatic hepatitis C virus infection. That being said, the recent US Food and Drug Administration approval of new anti–hepatitis C viral medications may drastically decrease the incidence of fibrosing cholestatic hepatitis C after liver transplantation.

M. L. Smith, MD

Acute Hepatitis With Periportal Confluent Necrosis Associated With Human Herpesvirus 6 Infection in Liver Transplant Patients

Buyse S, Roque-Afonso AM, Vaghefi P, et al (Centre Hépato-Biliaire, Villejuif, France; AP-HP, Hôpital Paul Brousse, Virology, Villejuif, France; et al)

Am J Clin Pathol 140:403-409, 2013

Objectives.—To correlate human herpesvirus 6 (HHV-6) viral load with pathologic features in graft acute hepatitis of unknown origin.

Methods.—Liver frozen samples from 26 patients with graft hepatitis of unknown origin were available for HHV-6 DNA quantification.

Results.—In 10 (38.5%) of 26 liver samples, HHV-6 DNA was detectable, with a median viral load of 3.84 $\log_{10}$ copies/10^6 cells. Confluent periportal necrosis was observed in 4 of 10 patients and associated with high viral load. These 4 patients responded to antiviral therapy. Mild unspecific hepatitis was observed in 4 patients with low intragraft viral load and in 2 patients with high viral load in a context of deep immunosuppression. Patients with HHV-6–negative graft hepatitis disclosed lobular necrotico-inflammatory activity without periportal necrosis.

Conclusions.—Our study provides data supporting the pathogenic role of HHV-6 for liver allografts. The presence of confluent periportal necrosis could be a clue for prompt diagnosis of HHV-6–induced graft hepatitis.

▶ This article describes for the first time histologic features of reactivation of human herpesvirus 6 (HHV-6) infection in liver allograft patients. Image 1 in the original article shows the severe periportal necrosis that was seen in 4 of 10 patients found to have HHV-6 DNA present within posttransplant biopsy specimens from 26 total patients with unexplained posttransplant hepatitis. This pattern of injury is rarely seen in the posttransplant setting or in the native liver biopsy setting. The primary differential diagnosis includes adverse drug reaction or other severe interface necroinflammatory activity from a viral infection. Most viral infections show fairly significant viral cytopathic changes. However, HHV-6 may not show any significant viral cytopathic change and may just show this fairly extensive periportal necrosis. This type of zone 1 confluent necrosis should be distinguished from zone 3 confluent necrosis, which is seen more commonly in adverse drug reaction and suboptimal hepatic blood flow. It is reasonable to consider HHV-6 as a potential etiology for an otherwise unexplained posttransplant hepatitis, particularly if there is significant zone 1 periportal necrosis.

For further investigation of the clinical implications of HHV-6 infection, I refer the reader to Abdel et al.[1]

M. L. Smith, MD

Reference

1. Abdel Massih RC, Razonable RR. Human herpesvirus 6 infections after liver transplantation. *World J Gastroenterol*. 2009;15:2561-2569.

Pathology report assessment of incidental gallbladder carcinoma diagnosed from cholecystectomy specimens: Results of a French multicentre survey

Chatelain D, Fuks D, Farges O, et al (Jules Verne Univ of Picardie, Amiens, France; Beaujon Hosp, Clichy, France; et al)

Dig Liver Dis 45:1056-1060, 2013

Aims.—To assess the accuracy of pathology reports on gallbladder specimens from patients operated on for incidental gallbladder carcinoma.

Methods.—Demographic data, details on pathological reports including gross and microscopic features section were recorded in 100 selected patients with incidental gallbladder carcinoma diagnosed from 2004 to 2007.

Results.—Pathology reports had a conventional format in 93% of cases, without any standardization. Turnaround time ranged from 1 to 35 days. Frozen sections were performed in 20% of cases. The reports failed to give information on prognostic histological factors: exact tumour site (missing in 55% of cases), depth of tumour infiltration within the gallbladder wall (missing in 10%), surgical margins (missing in 40% for the cystic duct margin), tumour differentiation (missing in 28%), vascular invasion (missing in 52%) and perineural invasion (missing in 51%). Lymph node status could be assessed in 44% of cases. Distances between the tumour and the cystic duct and circumferential margins were not specified in 68% and 84% of cases. Only 29% of the reports clearly stated the pTNM stage in the conclusion section. The pT stage with margin status and tumour site was only mentioned in 30% of the reports.

Conclusion.—Pathology reports on gallbladder carcinoma from participating centres frequently lacked important information on key prognostic histological factors.

▶ Although this type of study may not be of critical importance now, as pay per performance continues to encroach into the surgical pathology practice, studies such as this will be of increasing importance. Many surgical pathologists who review gallbladders do so with a mindset of "chronic cholecystitis and cholelithiasis" and do not approach them as typical carcinoma resection specimens. Because most of the gallbladders we review are resected for non-neoplastic disease, it is easy to get into the habit of signing these out in a minimalistic fashion. This article from multiple centers in France provides some data that support this impression. It was found that there was little standardization in reporting of incidentally identified carcinomas, and most cases were missing several critical elements for prognostication. These data highlight the importance of using a standard approach to the reporting of tumor specimens, even when the specimens are not usually associated with tumor, such as in gallbladder resections for assumed non-neoplastic disease. The use of standard reporting formats such as those provided by the College of American Pathologists can certainly help drive synoptic reporting and inclusion of all of the critical elements. The incorporation of these synoptic report checklists into pathology laboratory information systems is a critical next step for ease of use and efficiency.

M. L. Smith, MD

Hepatic Histological Findings in Suspected Drug-Induced Liver Injury: Systematic Evaluation and Clinical Associations

Kleiner DE, for the Drug-Induced Liver Injury Network (DILIN) (Natl Insts of Health, Bethesda, MD; et al)

Hepatology 59:661-670, 2014

Drug-induced liver injury (DILI) is considered to be a diagnosis of exclusion. Liver biopsy may contribute to diagnostic accuracy, but the histological features of DILI and their relationship to biochemical parameters and outcomes are not well defined. We have classified the pathological pattern of liver injury and systematically evaluated histological changes in liver biopsies obtained from 249 patients with suspected DILI enrolled in the prospective, observational study conducted by the Drug Induced Liver Injury Network. Histological features were analyzed for their frequency within different clinical phenotypes of liver injury and to identify associations between clinical and laboratory findings and histological features. The most common histological patterns were acute (21%) and chronic hepatitis (14%), acute (9%) and chronic cholestasis (10%), and cholestatic hepatitis (29%). Liver histology from 128 patients presenting with hepatocellular injury had more severe inflammation, necrosis, and apoptosis and more frequently demonstrated lobular disarray, rosette formation, and hemorrhage than those with cholestasis. Conversely, histology of the 73 patients with cholestatic injury more often demonstrated bile plugs and duct paucity. Severe or fatal hepatic injury in 46 patients was associated with higher degrees of necrosis, fibrosis stage, microvesicular steatosis, and ductular reaction among other findings, whereas eosinophils and granulomas were found more often in those with milder injury.

Conclusion.—We describe an approach for evaluating liver histology in DILI and demonstrate numerous associations between pathological findings and clinical presentations that may serve as a foundation for future studies correlating DILI pathology with its causality and outcome (Fig 1).

▶ This report represents a rare prospective histologic study in hepatic pathology. The main goal of the study was to correlate histologic features with clinical and biochemical features in patients with documented drug-induced liver injury. There are 2 primary findings in this study. The first is that there was only a minimal correlation between histologic features and biochemical findings. The extent of correlation is best shown in Fig 1, in which, despite the types of histologic patterns seen, there is a variety of hepatocellular, mixed, or cholestatic biochemical profiles. These findings suggest that biochemical profile of a patient does not necessarily predict the histologic features of drug-induced liver injury. The second main finding is really a confirmation of previous studies that found that the degree

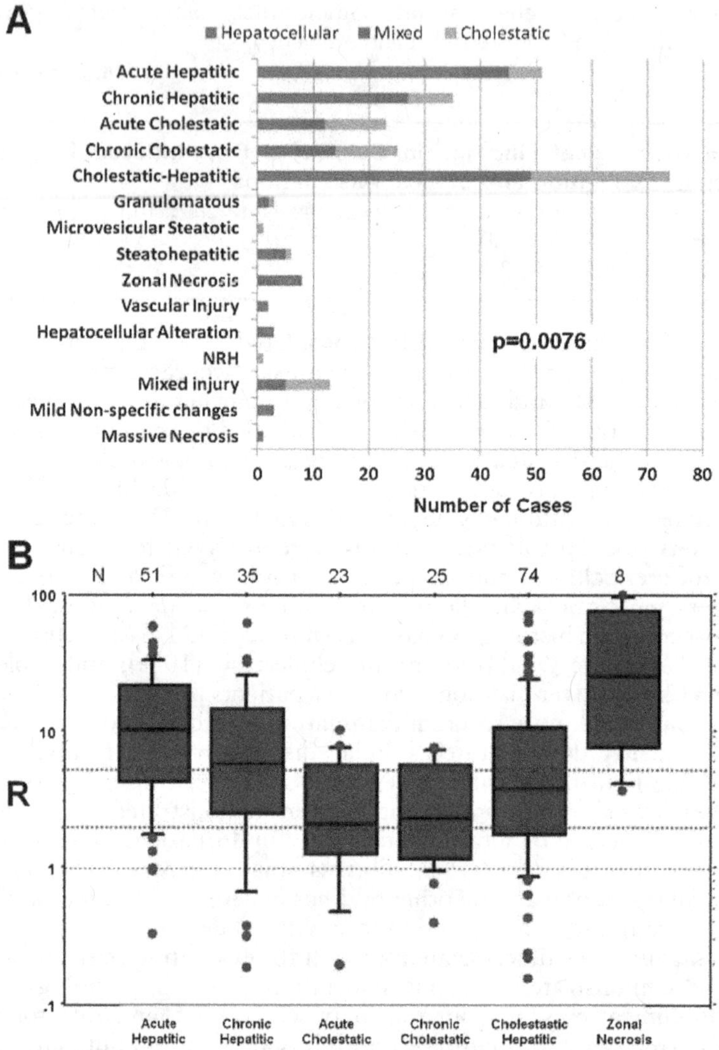

FIGURE 1.—Relationship between pathological injury patterns and biochemical presentation. (A) The association of particular patterns with biochemical presentation was significant by chi-square analysis. (B) box plot showing range of "R" for selected histological patterns of injury. "R" is defined as the normalized ratio of ALT to ALP. The number of cases of each pattern of injury is shown above each box plot. Red dotted lines indicate the dividing point between hepatocellular ($R > 5$), mixed ($R = 2\text{-}5$), and cholestatic ($R < 2$) reactions. For Interpretation of the references to color in this figure legend, the reader is referred to web version of this article. (Reprinted from Kleiner DE, for the Drug-Induced Liver Injury Network (DILIN). Hepatic histological findings in suspected drug-induced liver injury: systematic evaluation and clinical associations. *Hepatology.* 2014;59:661-670, with permission from Hepatology and John Wiley and Sons, www.interscience.wiley.com.)

of hepatocellular necrosis was associated with a bad outcome or poor prognosis, whereas the amount of eosinophils was associated with a more favorable outcome. However, I am not sure this finding will change the practice, as I am sure most pathologists already report these findings in their liver biopsy cases. If anything, I think the main findings of this study will encourage additional biopsies to document the histologic pattern of injury. One of the challenges associated with this study is that there was only one pathologist reviewer for all of the cases. Although this is good for internal standardization, the extrapolation of these histologic pattern designations to a population of general surgical pathologists is unknown. In addition, there was selection bias in this cohort, as only patients who had a clinical indication for liver biopsy underwent biopsy.

For additional investigation on this topic, I refer the reader to Ramachandran and Kakar.[1]

M. L. Smith, MD

Reference

1. Ramachandran R, Kakar S. Histologic patterns in drug-induced liver disease. *J Clin Pathol.* 2009;62:481-492.

Clinicopathologic Analysis of Combined Hepatocellular-Cholangiocarcinoma According to the Latest WHO Classification

Akiba J, Nakashima O, Hattori S, et al (Kurume Univ School of Medicine, Japan; Univ Hosp, Kurume, Japan; Kurume Univ, Japan)
Am J Surg Pathol 37:496-505, 2013

Combined hepatocellular-cholangiocarcinoma comprises <1% of all liver carcinomas. The histogenesis of combined hepatocellular-cholangiocarcinoma has remained unclear for many years. However, recent advances in hepatic progenitor cell (HPC) investigations have provided new insights. The concept that combined hepatocellular-cholangiocarcinoma originates from HPCs is adopted in the chapter "combined hepatocellular-cholangiocarcinoma" of the latest World Health Organization (WHO) classification. In this study, we conducted clinicopathologic analysis of combined hepatocellular-cholangiocarcinoma according to the latest WHO classification. Fifty-four cases were included in this study. Pathologic diagnosis was made according to the WHO classification. When a tumor contained plural histologic patterns, predominant histologic pattern (≥50%) was defined. Minor histologic patterns were also appended. Immunohistochemical staining with biliary markers (CK7, CK19, and EMA), hepatocyte paraffin (Hep-Par)-1, HPC markers (CD56, c-kit, CD133, and EpCAM), and vimentin was performed. Forty-five and 50 patients were analyzed for progression-free survival and overall survival, respectively. Ten, 1, 32, and 11 cases were diagnosed as: combined hepatocellular-cholangiocarcinoma, classical type; combined hepatocellular-cholangiocarcinoma, stem cell features, typical subtype; combined hepatocellular-cholangiocarcinoma, stem cell features,

TABLE 1.—Histologic Features of Combined Hepatocellular-Cholangiocarcinomas According to WHO Classification

Subtypes	Mucin Production	Stroma	Histologic Findings
CHC-classical			
HCC component	None	Scarce	Typical HCC, well to poorly differentiated type
ChC component	Observed	Intermediate-abundant	Typical adenocarcinoma, well to poorly differentiated type
CHC-SC-typical	None	Abundant	Nests of mature looking hepatocytes with peripheral clusters of small cells that have a high nucleus:cytoplasm ratio and hyperchromatic nuclei
CHC-SC-int	None	Intermediate-abundant	Tumor cells show features intermediate between hepatocytes and cholangiocytes. These tumor cells show strands, solid nests and/or trabeculae of small, uniform cells with scant cytoplasm and hyperchromatc nuclei
CHC-SC-CLC	None	Abundant	Tumor is composed of admixtures of small monotonous glands, antler-like anastomosing patterns. Each tumor cell is cuboidal, smaller in size than normal hepatocytes, with high nucleus:cytoplasm ratio, and distinct nucleoli

CHC indicates combined hepatocellular-cholangiocarcinoma; CHC-SC-typical, combined hepatocellular-cholangiocarcinoma, stem cell features, typical subtype; CHC-SC-int, combined hepatocellular-cholangiocarcinoma, stem cell features, intermediate cell subtype; CHC-SC-CLC, combined hepatocellular-cholangiocarcinoma, stem cell features, cholangiolocellular subtype.

intermediate cell subtype; and combined hepatocellular-cholangiocarcinoma, stem cell features, cholangiolocellular type, respectively. Combined hepatocellular-cholangiocarcinomas usually have high expression of biliary markers. CD56, c-kit, and EpCAM were expressed to various degrees in all combined hepatocellular-cholangiocarcinomas apart from the hepatocellular carcinoma component of combined hepatocellular-cholangiocarcinoma, classical type. The expression of CD133 and vimentin was observed only in combined hepatocellular-cholangiocarcinoma, stem cell features of intermediate cell subtype and cholangiolocellular subtype. The expression of CD133, EpCAM, and vimentin was significantly high in combined hepatocellular-cholangiocarcinoma, subtypes with stem cell features, especially cholangiolocellular subtype. Minor histologic patterns were significantly frequent in combined hepatocellular-cholangiocarcinoma, subtypes with stem cell features, compared with combined hepatocellular-cholangiocarcinoma, classical type. There was no significant difference in clinical outcome between each subtype. Combined hepatocellular-cholangiocarcinoma has wide histologic diversity and shows immunophenotypic expression of not only biliary markers but also HPC markers to various degrees, suggesting that the histogenesis of combined hepatocellular-cholangiocarcinoma could be strongly associated with HPCs. Our results pathologically validate the latest WHO classification of combined hepatocellular-cholangiocarcinoma. However, the complex mixture of histologic subtypes has presented a challenge to the classification of combined hepatocellular-cholangiocarcinoma. Further study should be conducted using a large cohort to support this classification (Table 1).

▶ The latest World Health Organization (WHO) classification schema involved a revision to the combined hepatocellular-cholangiocarcinoma diagnostic definitions and categories. The definition from the WHO of combined hepatocellular-cholangiocarcinoma is "a tumor containing unequivocal, intimately mixed elements of both hepatocellular carcinoma (HCC) and cholangiocarcinoma (CHC)."[1] Although additional subtypes to combined hepatocellular-cholangiocarcinoma were included in the classification scheme by the WHO (classical type and with stem cell features), there are insufficient data at this time to suggest that these distinctions carry any clinical or prognostic significance. Table 1 highlights the new WHO classification schema. Although the authors nicely show the immunohistochemical features of these subtypes of combined hepatocellular-cholangiocarcinoma, one of the major limitations of this study is the low overall number of patients. Because of the insufficient power, no prognostic significance was able to be determined. At this time, the subtype classification remains mainly an academic exercise.

For additional investigation, I refer the reader to Kim et al[2] and Zhang et al.[3]

M. L. Smith, MD

References

1. Theise ND, Nakashima O, Park YN, et al. *Combined Hepatocellular-Cholangiocarcinoma. WHO Classification of Tumors of the Digestive System.* Lyon: IARC Press; 2010. 225–227.
2. Kim H, Park C, Han KH, et al. Primary liver carcinoma of intermediate (hepatocyte-cholangiocyte) phenotype. *J Hepatology.* 2004;40:298-304.
3. Zhang F, Chen XP, Zhang W, et al. Combined hepatocellular cholangiocarcinoma originating from hepatic progenetor cells: immunohistochemical and double fluorescence immunostaining evidence. *Histopathology.* 2008;52:224-232.

Immunohistochemical characteristics of hepatocellular carcinoma in non-cirrhotic livers

Witjes CDM, ten Kate FJW, Verhoef C, et al (Erasmus Univ Med Centre, Rotterdam, The Netherlands)

J Clin Pathol 66:687-691, 2013

Hepatocellular carcinoma (HCC) typically develops in cirrhotic livers. In the absence of risk factors, for example, cirrhosis or hepatitis B or C virus infection, HCC diagnosis might be difficult. We aimed to explore the value of immunohistochemical characteristics to diagnostics and prognosis, and whether these immunohistochemical characteristics differ from those of HCC in a cirrhotic liver, possibly indicating an aberrant pathogenetic pathway. Paraffin-embedded, formalin-fixed tissue slides from liver

TABLE 2.—Staining Pattern of Immunohistochemical Markers in HCC in a Non-Cirrhotic Liver and in HCC in a Cirrhotic Liver According to Our Hospital and the Literature

	Staining	HCC in a Non-Cirrhotic Liver (Rotterdam) (%)	HCC in a Cirrhotic Liver (Rotterdam) (%)	HCC in a Cirrhotic Liver (Literature) (%)
AFP	Positive	30	35	25–40[15]
β-Cat	Positive	32	25	20–35[20,21]
CD34	Positive	88	95	88[22]
GPC-3	Positive	40	85	76–83[11,13,23]
GS	Positive		52	60[24]
	Positive diffuse	42		
	Positive focally	20		
CK7	Positive	44	59	22–40[25,26]
CK19	Positive	12	6	10–17[25,26]
MIB	1%–10% positive	22	17	51[27]
	≥10% positive	78	83	33[27]
	>10%–30% positive	28	26	
	≥30%–50% positive	28	34	
	≥50% positive	22	23	

β-Cat, β-catenin; AFP, α-fetoprotein; CK7, cytokeratin 7; CK19, cytokeratin 19; GPC-3, glypican-3;Ki67; GS, glutamine synthetase; HCC, hepatocellular carcinoma; MIB-1 = antigen.

Editor's Note: Please refer to original journal article for full references.

resection specimens of the patients with HCC in a non-cirrhotic liver were analysed. From January 2000 through April 2011, 799 patients with HCC were admitted to our hospital; in total, 47 patients with 50 HCCs in a non-cirrhotic liver were operated. These tumours were stained positive for α-fetoprotein (AFP) in 30%, CD34 in 88%, cytokeratine 7 (CK7) in 44%, CK19 in 12%, glypican-3 (GPC-3) in 40%, glutamine synthetase in 62% and β-catenin in 32%. There was similarity in immunohistochemical expression of several markers comparing HCC in a noncirrhotic liver with HCC in a cirrhotic liver. Moderate or poorly differentiated HCC more often expressed β-catenin and GPC-3 and showed a higher percentage of MIB-1-positive hepatocytes. A positive AFP immunohistochemical staining was significantly related with a high preoperative AFP serum level ($p=0.001$). None of the immunohistochemical stainings were associated with a worse overall survival. Of the patients treated with a surgical resection, 17 had recurrence of HCC and these patients more often had a positive CK19 staining ($p=0.048$). In conclusion, immunohistochemical expression of several markers in HCC in a non-cirrhotic and cirrhotic liver was comparable. Immunohistochemical markers have limited additional value to characterise HCC in non-cirrhoitc livers (Table 2).

▶ For general surgical pathologists who evaluate needle core biopsies of hepatic mass lesions, this article adds some important immunohistochemical staining data to the literature. In the past few years, there has been a robust proliferation of literature on additional immunohistochemical markers that can assist in the diagnosis of hepatocellular carcinoma, mainly glypican-3, glutamine synthetase, and β catenin. Most of these studies, understandably because of the incidence, have evaluated these markers in hepatocellular carcinomas arising in a setting of cirrhosis. This article attempts to compare the immunohistochemical staining profile of hepatocellular carcinoma arising in cirrhotic and noncirrhotic livers. The findings suggest that previous analyses of these immunohistochemical markers remain valid for hepatocellular carcinomas arising in noncirrhotic livers. Table 2 shows the percentage of reactivity in cirrhotic vs noncirrhotic hepatocellular carcinomas as well as a literature review of the reactivity rates. This study was not particularly well designed to evaluate the usefulness of these immunohistochemical studies in the diagnosis of hepatocellular carcinoma arising in noncirrhotic liver parenchyma. At our institution, when faced with a well-differentiated hepatocellular neoplasm, whether from a cirrhotic liver or a noncirrhotic liver, we typically use a panel of immunohistochemical stains, including β catenin, glutamine synthetase, glypican-3, HSP70, reticulin, and CD34 to assist in the analysis.

For additional investigation, I refer the reader to Wang et al,[1] Long et al,[2] and Tremosini.[3]

M. L. Smith, MD

References

1. Wang HL, Anatelli F, Zhai QJ, et al. Glypican-3 as a useful diagnostic marker that distinguishes hepatocellular carcinoma from benign hepatocellular mass lesions. *Arch Pathol Lab Med.* 2008;132:1723-1728.
2. Long J, Wang H, Lang ZW, et al. Expression level of glutamine synthetase is increased in hepatocellular carcinoma and liver tissue with cirrhosis and chronic hepatitis B. *Hepatol Int.* 2011;5:698-706.
3. Tremosini S, Forner A, Boix L, et al. Prospective validation of an immunohistochemical panel (glypican 3, heat shock protein 70, and glutamine synthetase) in liver biopsies for diagnosis of very early hepatocellular carcinoma. *Gut.* 2012; 61:1481-1487.

Histopathologic Distinction Between Fibrosing Cholestatic Hepatitis C and Biliary Obstruction

Salomao M, Verna EC, Lefkowitch JH, et al (Columbia Univ College of Physicians and Surgeons, NY; et al)
Am J Surg Pathol 37:1837-1844, 2013

The histopathologic distinction between posttransplantation fibrosing cholestatic hepatitis C (FCH-C) and biliary obstruction (BO) is challenging. We sought to identify histopathologic features that could be useful in the differential diagnosis between these 2 entities. A total of 38 cases of hepatitis C virus (HCV)-negative, cholangiography-proven BO (including 16 posttransplant and 22 nontransplant patients) and 13 patients with posttransplantation FCH-C were included. FCH-C patients were characterized by cholestatic disease, high HCV viral load, no evidence of biliary tract obstruction on imaging, and typical histopathologic findings (≥3 of the following: 1, prominent ductular reaction; 2, hepatocyte swelling with lobular disarray; 3, periportal sinusoidal fibrosis, and 4, cholestasis). Biopsies were evaluated with hematoxylin and eosin, Masson trichrome, Victoria blue, and rhodanine stains. Cytokeratin 7 (CK7) immunohistochemistry was

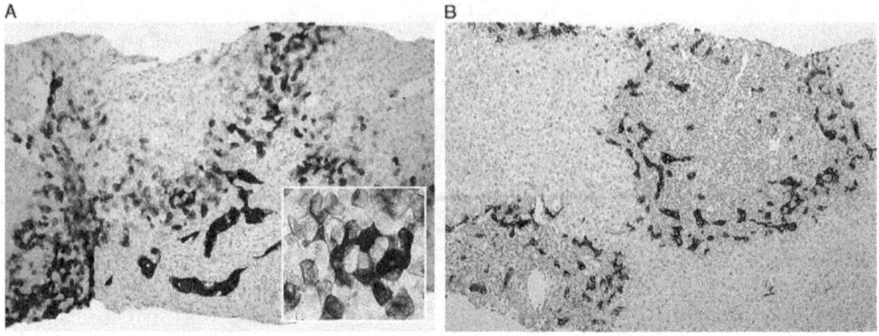

FIGURE 4.—CK7 immunohistochemistry. A, Bile ducts and ductules stain strongly positive for CK7. In addition, a significant number of CK7+ cells showing weak to moderate cytoplasmic staining (intermediate hepatobiliary cells) are seen in BO (inset). B, In FCH-C, few or no CK7+ intermediate cells are seen. (Reprinted from Salomao M, Verna EC, Lefkowitch JH, et al. Histopathologic distinction between fibrosing cholestatic hepatitis c and biliary obstruction. *Am J Surg Pathol.* 2013;37:1837-1844, with permission from Lippincott Williams & Wilkins.)

TABLE 4.—Distinguishing Features Between FCH-C and BO

Favors BO	Favors FCH-C
H&E and trichrome stains	
Bile duct dilatation	Hepatocyte swelling with lobular disarray
Portal edema	
Acute cholangitis	Periportal sinusoidal fibrosis
Bile infarcts	
Periductal fibrosis	
Copper/copper-binding protein stains	
Present, especially if abundant	Absent (despite pronounced ductular reaction)
CK7 immunohistochemistry	
Abundant CK7⁺ periportal intermediate hepatobiliary cells	No or few CK7⁺ intermediate cells in spite of pronounced ductular reaction

H&E indicates hematoxylin and eosin.

used to assess for the presence of CK7+ intermediate hepatobiliary cells. We found that portal edema (63.1% vs. 7.6%; $P < 0.0001$), bile duct dilatation (26.3% vs. 0%; $P = 0.0003$), acute cholangitis (15.7% vs. 0%; $P = 0.008$), bile infarcts (10.5% vs. 0%; $P = 0.03$), periductal fibrosis (23.6% vs. 0%; $P = 0.0007$), and periportal copper deposition (60.5% vs. 15.3%; $P = 0.0006$) are significantly more common in BO, whereas hepatocellular swelling with lobular disarray (84.6% vs. 5.2%; $P < 0.0001$) and periportal sinusoidal fibrosis (34.2% vs. 100%; $P < 0.0001$) are seen more frequently in FCH-C. Furthermore, marked ductular reaction with rare or absent CK7+ intermediate cells is highly suggestive of FCH-C in this context (73.6% vs. 7.6%; $P < 0.0001$). In summary, this study offers a comprehensive characterization of the histologic features discriminating FCH-C from BO (Fig 4, Table 4).

▶ This is a typical descriptive pathologic study comparing bile duct obstruction with fibrosing cholestatic hepatitis C (FCH-C), a differential diagnosis that any pathologist with experience in liver allograft pathology knows is fairly difficult. The authors use a relatively clean subset of patients for histopathologic analysis. The most important findings of this study suggest that although there is extensive overlap, there are some histopathologic features that may assist in distinguishing these 2 entities from each other. The study also looked at periportal copper deposition and CK7 immunohistochemistry as potential aids in the diagnosis. Although accumulation of copper within the periportal hepatocytes was more frequent in cases of bile duct obstruction than cases of FCH-C virus infection, there were still some cases of FCH that showed a moderate degree of periportal copper deposition. Fig 4 is perhaps the best take-home message from this article. In Fig 4 the demonstration of intermediate hepatobiliary cells in zone 1 is clearly shown in cases of bile duct obstruction, whereas cases of FCH-C show either no or very few periportal intermediate hepatobiliary cells. This distinction in the pattern of CK7 staining can also be used to assist in the differential diagnosis. Table 4 summarizes the features that favor bile duct obstruction or FCH and should be used when faced with this challenging differential diagnosis. Although these features may assist in your histologic interpretation, correlation with clinical studies, including ultrasound scan of the biliary tree and hepatitis C virus RNA levels, is critical for a definitive diagnosis.

M. L. Smith, MD

Hepatic steatosis estimated microscopically versus digital image analysis

Hall AR, Dhillon AP, Green AC, et al (Royal Free London NHS Foundation Trust, UK; UCL Med School, Royal Free Campus, London, UK; et al)

Liver Int 33:926-935, 2013

Background & Aims.—Evaluate in liver biopsies: (i) interobserver agreement of estimates of fat proportionate area (eFPA) and steatosis grading, (ii) the relationship between steatosis grades and measured fat proportionate area (mFPA, digital image analysis), (iii) the accuracy of eFPA, (iv) to present images to aid standardization and accuracy of eFPA.

Methods.—Twenty-one liver biopsies were selected from the Royal Free Hospital (RFH) histopathology archive to represent the full range of histopathological steatosis severity. As many non-overlapping fields of parenchyma as possible were photographed at ×20 objective magnification from the biopsies ($n = 651$). A total of 15 sample images were selected to represent the range of steatosis seen. Twelve hepatopathologists from 11 sites worldwide independently evaluated the sample images for steatosis grade [normal (none)/mild/ moderate/severe], and eFPA (% area of liver parenchyma occupied by fat).

Results.—The hepatopathologists had good linear correlation between eFPA and mFPA for sample images ($r = 0.924$, $P < .001$) and excellent concordance ($kappa = 0.91$, $P < 0.001$). Interobserver concordance of steatosis grade showed 'substantial agreement' ($kappa = 0.64$). There was significant difference between eFPA and mFPA in the sample images for

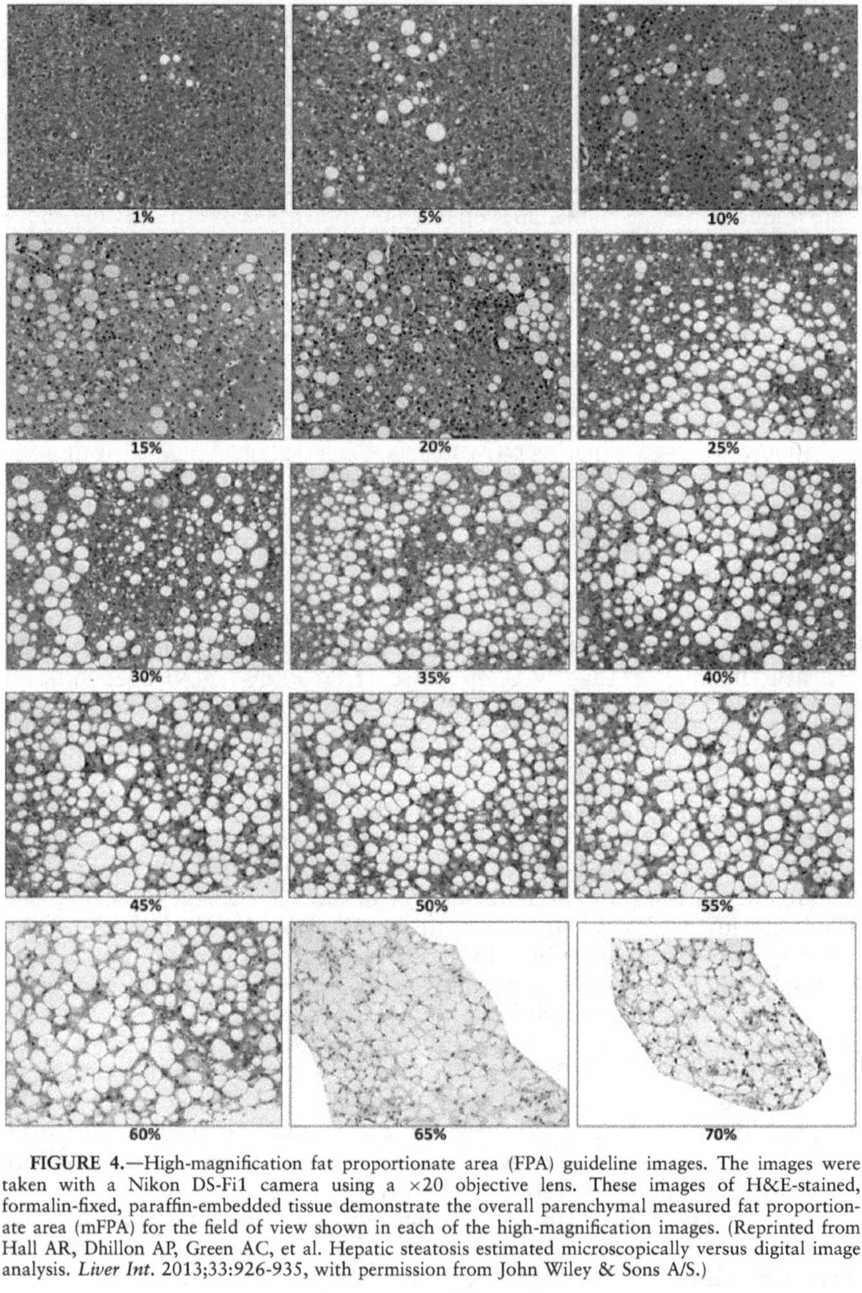

FIGURE 4.—High-magnification fat proportionate area (FPA) guideline images. The images were taken with a Nikon DS-Fi1 camera using a ×20 objective lens. These images of H&E-stained, formalin-fixed, paraffin-embedded tissue demonstrate the overall parenchymal measured fat proportionate area (mFPA) for the field of view shown in each of the high-magnification images. (Reprinted from Hall AR, Dhillon AP, Green AC, et al. Hepatic steatosis estimated microscopically versus digital image analysis. *Liver Int.* 2013;33:926-935, with permission from John Wiley & Sons A/S.)

mild, moderate and severe steatosis ($P = 0.024$, $P < 0.001$, $P < 0.001$ respectively): the observers consistently over-estimated the eFPA.

Conclusion.—Hepatopathologists showed 'excellent' interobserver agreement in eFPA and 'substantial' agreement in assigning steatosis grade (precision was high). However, compared with mFPA, eFPA was inaccurate. eFPA systematically exceeds mFPA; generally the overestimation increases with severity of steatosis. Considering that non-invasive technologies for estimating liver fat utilize histopathology as reference, such assessments would benefit from quantitative validation of visually estimated microscopic liver fat percentages (Fig 4).

▶ This excellent article addresses several issues with regard to grading the degree of steatosis in liver biopsies with fatty liver disease. First, it clarifies an important distinction in how pathologists characterize the amount of fat within liver biopsies. There are conflicting reports within the literature as to whether it is the surface area of involved fat that is graded or whether it is the percentage of involved hepatocytes that is graded. Although the scores may be similar, these are 2 very distinct approaches to the grading of steatosis. The authors make it clear that the current gold standard involves assessment for steatosis based on the percentage of the surface area of a histologic section involved. The other major contribution that this report makes to the field is seen in Fig 4, which provides a guideline for practicing pathologists in estimating the fat proportionate area in various biopsy samples. Although it is encouraging that they confirm prior reports that the grading of steatosis is relatively reproducible among pathologists, they also confirm the vast and systematic overestimation of the degree of steatosis. Fig 4 should assist pathologists in the appropriate percentage designation of the degree of steatosis. Furthermore, this figure can be used in prospective studies and at the time of assessment of organs for transplantation to create a more standardized practice.

M. L. Smith, MD

Diagnostic utility and limitations of glutamine synthetase and serum amyloid-associated protein immunohistochemistry in the distinction of focal nodular hyperplasia and inflammatory hepatocellular adenoma

Joseph NM, Ferrell LD, Jain D, et al (Univ of California, San Francisco; Yale Univ, New Haven, CT; et al)

Mod Pathol 27:62-72, 2014

Inflammatory hepatocellular adenoma can show overlapping histological features with focal nodular hyperplasia, including inflammation, fibrous stroma, and ductular reaction. Expression of serum amyloid-associated protein in inflammatory hepatocellular adenoma and map-like pattern of glutamine synthetase in focal nodular hyperplasia can be helpful in this distinction, but the pitfalls and limitations of these markers have not been established. Morphology and immunohistochemistry were analyzed in 54 inflammatory hepatocellular adenomas, 40 focal nodular hyperplasia, and 3 indeterminate lesions. Morphological analysis demonstrated that nodularity, fibrous stroma, dystrophic blood vessels, and ductular reaction were more common in focal nodular hyperplasia, while telangiectasia, hemorrhage, and steatosis were more common in inflammatory hepatocellular adenoma, but there was frequent overlap of morphological features. The majority of inflammatory hepatocellular adenomas demonstrated perivascular and/or patchy glutamine synthetase staining (73.6%), while the remaining cases had diffuse (7.5%), negative (3.8%), or patchy pattern of staining (15%) that showed subtle differences from the classic map-like staining pattern and was designated as pseudo map-like staining. Positive staining for serum amyloid-associated protein was seen in the majority of inflammatory hepatocellular adenomas (92.6%) and in the minority of focal nodular hyperplasia (17.5%). The glutamine synthetase staining pattern was map-like in 90% of focal nodular hyperplasia cases, with the remaining 10% of cases showing pseudo map-like staining. Three cases were labeled as indeterminate and showed focal nodular hyperplasia-like morphology but lacked map-like glutamine synthetase staining pattern; these cases demonstrated a patchy pseudo map-like glutamine synthetase pattern along with the expression of serum amyloid-associated protein. Our results highlight the diagnostic errors that can be caused by variant patterns of staining with glutamine synthetase and serum amyloid-associated protein in inflammatory hepatocellular adenoma and focal nodular hyperplasia (Tables 2 and 5).

▶ Numerous articles over the last few years have highlighted the importance of glutamine synthetase and serum amyloid-associated (SAA) protein or C-reactive protein in the distinction between focal nodular hyperplasia (FNH) and inflammatory hepatocellular adenoma. As with all new immunohistochemical studies, with increased use, exceptions to the typical results begin to appear over time. This is an important article that highlights the pitfalls associated with these 2 markers in this challenging differential diagnosis, particularly with respect to needle core biopsy specimens. The importance in the distinction between FNH and inflammatory hepatocellular adenoma is that although FNH can be followed, unless it is causing symptoms or its location is adversely affecting the liver, inflammatory hepatocellular adenomas are neoplastic and have a potential for intra-abdominal hemorrhage and transformation to hepatocellular carcinoma. Therefore, adenomas are more likely to be resected surgically. The authors nicely show in Table 2 the overlap in the histologic features of FNH and inflammatory hepatocellular adenoma. Although most of the features show a fairly significant statistical difference, none of them is perfect. Table 5 nicely highlights various pitfalls associated with SAA and glutamine synthetase staining, the potential pitfalls, and the approach that may be taken to avoid these pitfalls. Although not the specific goal of this study, the authors note that C-reactive protein had a higher sensitivity than SAA protein for the diagnosis of inflammatory hepatocellular adenoma. Any laboratory that receives needle core biopsies of mass lesions on a routine basis should probably have these immunohistochemical studies available, but a cautious approach to the interpretation is suggested.

TABLE 2.—Histological Features of Focal Nodular Hyperplasia (FNH) and Inflammatory Hepatocellular Adenoma (IHA)

	FNH (n = 40)	*IHA* (n = 54)	P-*value**	*Indeterminate* (n = 3)
Nodular architecture	34/40 (85)	4/54 (7.4)	<0.001	1/3 (33)
Fibrous bands	36/40 (90)	14/54 (26)	<0.001	1/3 (33)
Naked arterioles	8/36 (22)	30/50 (60)	0.001	1/3 (33)
Ductular reaction	33/40 (83)	23/54 (43)	<0.001	1/3 (33)
Pseudo-portal tracts	8/36 (22)	36/50 (72)	<0.001	0
Lymphocytic inflammation	19/40 (48)	32/53 (60)	0.08	1/3 (33)
Sinusoidal dilatation	7/39 (18)	44/53 (83)	<0.001	1/3 (33)
Hemorrhage	2/39 (5)	35/50 (70)	<0.001	0
Steatosis	8/39 (21)	31/54 (57)	<0.001	0

**P*-values reflect comparison between focal nodular hyperplasia (FNH) and inflammatory hepatocellular adenoma (IHA); numbers in parentheses reflect percentages.

TABLE 5.—Immunohistochemical Pitfalls and Suggested Approach in the Use of Glutamine Synthetase (GS) and Serum Amyloid-Associated (SAA) Protein in the Diagnosis of Focal Nodular Hyperplasia (FNH) and Inflammatory Hepatocellular Adenoma (IHA)

Feature	*Pitfall*	*Approach*
SAA staining in peritumoral liver in needle biopsy that missed the lesion	Misinterpreted as evidence of IHA, especially when other peritumoral features like inflammation and ductular reaction are also present	Positive SAA is not specific for IHA. Presence of interlobular bile ducts and absence of diffuse CD34 staining can help in confirming that the biopsy comprises non-neoplastic liver
SAA negative in a lesion that shows typical features of IHA	Misinterpreted as absolute evidence against IHA	SAA can be negative in 5–10% of IHA. Imaging and absence of map-like GS staining is needed to confirm IHA in these cases
SAA positive in a lesion that shows typical features of FNH	Misinterpreted as IHA	SAA can be seen in up to 17% of FNH. Map-like GS confirms FNH irrespective of SAA staining
Perivenous and patchy GS in a lesion that shows typical features of IHA	Misinterpreted as map-like pattern of FNH	This staining pattern is common in IHA. It is distinguished from map-like pattern by (i) lack of anastamosing pattern of staining and (ii) staining is heterogeneous and weak compared with homogeneous strong staining in map-like pattern
Diffuse GS staining	Misinterpreted as map-like pattern of FNH	Diffuse GS staining is seen in β-catenin-activated tumors and does not have areas of periseptal sparing typical of map-like pattern. Most of these cases also show nuclear β-catenin
Pseudo map-like GS pattern	Misinterpreted as map-like pattern of FNH	This pattern is seen at the periphery of IHA and 10% of FNH cases. When seen in biopsies, it is more likely to be FNH. Correlation with imaging and SAA staining is helpful. Diagnosis on needle biopsy may remain indeterminate in some cases

For additional investigation into this topic, I direct the reader to Bioulac-Sage et al.[1,2]

M. L. Smith, MD

References

1. Bioulac-Sage P, Balabaud C, Bedossa P, et al. Pathological diagnosis of liver cell adenoma and focal nodular hyperplasia: Bordeaux update. *J Hepatol.* 2007;46: 521-527.
2. Bioulac-Sage P, Laumonier H, Rullier A, et al. Over-expression of glutamine synthetase in focal nodular hyperplasia: a novel easy diagnostic tool in surgical pathology. *Liver Int.* 2009;29:459-465.

"Plasma Cell Hepatitis" in Liver Allografts: Identification and Characterization of an IgG4-Rich Cohort

Castillo-Rama M, Sebagh M, Sasatomi E, et al (Univ of Pittsburgh, Med Ctr, PA; AP-HP Hôpital Paul Brousse, Villejuif, France; et al)
Am J Transplant 13:2966-2977, 2013

Plasma cell hepatitis (PCH), also known as "*de novo autoimmune*" hepatitis, is an increasingly recognized, but suboptimally named and poorly understood, category of late allograft dysfunction strongly resembling autoimmune hepatitis (AIH): They share plasma-cell-rich necro-inflammatory activity on biopsy, autoantibodies and steroid responsiveness, but overlap with rejection is problematic. A retrospective study of clinical, serological, histopathological and IgG4 immunohistological features of PCH (n = 20) in liver allograft recipients, native liver AIH (n = 19) and plasma-cell-rich renal allograft rejection (n = 20) showed: (1) high frequency (44%) of HLA-DR15; (2) less female predominance ($p = 0.03$) and (3) n = 9/20 PCH recipients showed >25 IgG4+ plasma cells/high-power field (IgG4+ PCH) versus AIH (n = 1/19, $p = 0.008$) or plasma-cell-rich kidney rejection (n = 2/20, $p = 0.03$). The IgG4+ PCH (n = 9) subgroup showed lower alanine transaminase (ALT) ($p < 0.01$) and aspartate transaminase (AST) ($p < 0.05$) at index biopsy but (a) higher plasma cell number/percentage, (b) more aggressive-appearing portal/periportal and perivenular necro-inflammatory activity and (c) more severe portal/periportal fibrosis than IgG4– PCH (n = 11). Significant demographic, histopathologic and plasma cell phenotype differences between PCH and AIH suggest distinct pathogenic mechanisms for at least the IgG4+ PCH subgroup likely representing an overlap between allo- and auto-immunity. IgG4+ PCH was associated with fibrosis, but also highly responsive to increased immunosuppression (Fig 1).

► Although this study suffers from a small sample size, it is helpful in shedding some light on the pathogenesis of so-called plasma cell hepatitis. Fig 1 highlights the main finding of the study in which cases of plasma cell hepatitis generally showed a much higher percentage of immunoglobulin G4 (IgG4)-positive plasma cells than cases of native autoimmune hepatitis and kidney rejection–related plasma cell–rich inflammation. The group of plasma cell hepatitis cases with a high number of IgG4-positive plasma cells showed specific histologic features and epidemiologic features that suggest this represents a subgroup of

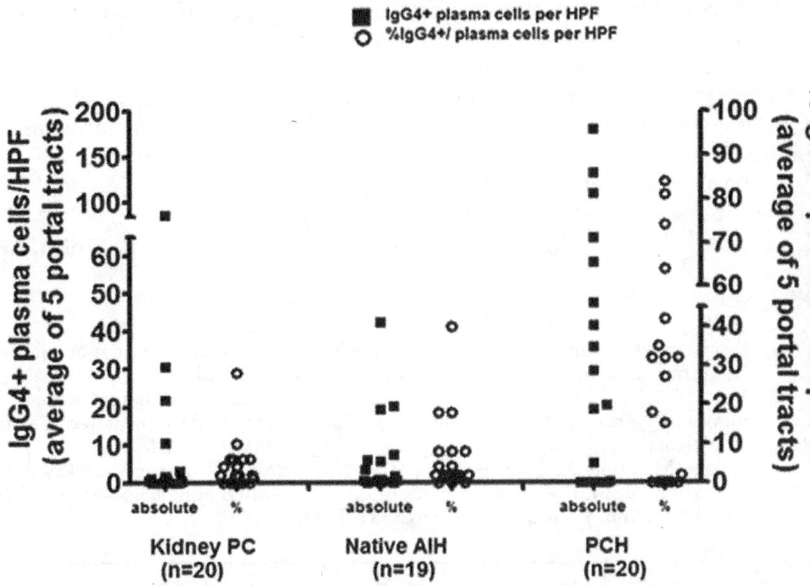

	Kidney (n=20)	Native liver AIH (n=19)	PCH livers (n=20)
Mean absolute number of IgG4+ cells (± SD)	7.9 (± 20.2)	5.8 (± 10.7)	37.14 (± 50.6)
Median absolute number of IgG4+ cells	0.4	0.8	19.8
Mean percent IgG4+/plasma cells (±SD)	4 (± 6.3)	6.7 (± 9.7)	27.1 (± 29)
Median percent IgG4+ cells	2	2	23

All mean values are an average of 5 portal tracts (livers) or 5 renal cortical interstitial areas (kidneys).
Exact Chi square test:
Absolute number of IgG4 cells: Kidney vs PCH: p= 0.03 ; Native liver AIH vs PCH: p= 0.008
Percent IgG4+/plasma cells: Kidney vs PCH: p=0.003 ; Native liver AIH vs PCH: p=0.003

FIGURE 1.—Absolute number of IgG4+ plasma cells per highpower field (filled squares; left Y-axis) and estimated percentage of IgG4+ plasma cells/total plasma cells (open circles; right Y-axis) comparing plasma-cell-rich kidney allograft rejection (left grouping), native liver autoimmune hepatitis (middle grouping) and plasma cell hepatitis in liver allografts (right grouping). Despite an overall similarity in the severity of portal inflammation, as scored by the mHAI portal inflammation component score (data not shown), about half of the PCH patients (n = 9) showed >25 IgG4+ plasma cells per portal tract high-power field or IgG4+ plasma cells comprised >25% of the total plasma cells present (n = 10). Other histopathological differences, based on a "blinded" review of the slides, are shown in Table 3. (Reprinted from Castillo-Rama M, Sebagh M, Sasatomi E, et al. "Plasma cell hepatitis" in liver allografts: identification and characterization of an IgG4-rich cohort. *Am J Transplant.* 2013;13:2966-2977, with permission from American Journal of Transplantation and John Wiley and Sons, www.interscience.wiley.com.)

traditional plasma cell hepatitis cases. It may be in the future that IgG4 testing be recommended in cases of plasma cell hepatitis, as at least this initial investigation showed a high responsiveness to increased immunosuppression. This subgroup also suggests the possibility of an allo-autoimmunity etiologic disease in this post–liver transplant population. It should be emphasized that the small sample number in this investigation limits the extrapolation to the general population. However, the initial results are intriguing, and further study in this IgG4-positive subgroup is necessary. Finally, it should also be noted that there was a relative paucity of serologic studies available within this patient population. This highlights the general lack of workup in the posttransplant plasma cell hepatitis population from a clinical perspective. Pathologists, when confronted with this histology, have an opportunity to encourage their clinical colleagues to perform a complete serologic workup as done in cases of native autoimmune hepatitis.

For further investigation, I refer the reader to Demetris and Sebagh,[1] Fiel et al,[2] and Sebagh et al.[3]

M. L. Smith, MD

References

1. Demetris AJ, Sebagh M. Plasma cell hepatitis in liver allografts: variant of rejection or autoimmune hepatitis? *Liver Transpl.* 2008;14:750-755.
2. Fiel MI, Agarwal K, Stanca C, et al. Post-transplant plasma cell hepatitis (de novo autoimmune hepatitis) is a variant of rejection and may lead to a negative outcome in patients with hepatitis C virus. *Liver Transpl.* 2008;14:861-871.
3. Sebagh M, Coilly A, Castillo-Rama M, et al. Centrilobular changes are key histological findings for segregating cases of de novo autoimmune hepatitis after liver transplantation. *J Hepatol.* 2012;56:S381-S382.

Revisiting the Topic of Histochemically Detectable Copper in Various Liver Diseases with Special Focus on Venous Outflow Impairment

Mounajjed T, Oxentenko AS, Qureshi H, et al (Division of Anatomic Pathology, Rochester, MN)

Am J Clin Pathol 139:79-86, 2013

We surveyed histochemically detectable copper in various liver diseases with emphasis on chronic biliary disease (CBD) and venous outflow impairment. Using rhodanine, we graded copper accumulation in 298 liver specimens: venous outflow impairment (n = 64), CBD (n = 123), Wilson disease (WD) (n = 12), chronic hepatitis C (n = 32), steatohepatitis (n = 28), sarcoidosis (n = 15), cholestatic hepatitis (n = 12), and acute large bile duct obstruction (n = 12). Copper was detected in 39% of specimens; all had chronic liver disease. Copper increased with increasing fibrosis. CBD accumulated copper more frequently than other chronic diseases (except WD), both in early (61% vs 3%) and late (94% vs 59%) stages and in larger amounts. Rhodanine was positive in 73% of livers with CBD, 20% with sarcoidosis, 9% with chronic hepatitis C, and 7% with steatohepatitis. Copper was detected in 14% of chronic venous outflow impairment specimens; with 1 exception, stainable copper was absent in early stages but detected in 38% of cirrhotic livers. In conclusion, rhodanine helps differentiate CBD from other conditions, including venous outflow impairment; in the absence of advanced fibrosis, rhodanine positivity strongly favors CBD.

In contrast, rhodanine positivity is nonspecific in cirrhosis, but the absence of copper in that setting excludes CBD.

► Common teaching in medical school and residency is that chronic biliary diseases are associated with copper accumulation within hepatocytes. What is not covered early in our training is that this finding is not specific, and there is a differential diagnosis. Perhaps the most important finding for practicing pathologists in this article is the high rate of copper accumulation present within cirrhotic livers (almost 40%). Therefore, it may not be reasonable to obtain copper staining in liver biopsies that show stage III or IV fibrosis with architectural distortion or regenerative nodules, because the specificity for a chronic biliary disease is markedly decreased. Although the sinusoidal changes of congestion, dilation, hemorrhage, and hepatocyte atrophy associated with venous outflow obstruction are usually present to assist in the diagnosis, there are some subtle portal-based changes such as inflammation and a ductular reaction that may contribute to confusion with chronic biliary diseases. Copper may be useful in the setting, as only 14% of biopsies with venous outflow impairment showed copper accumulation compared with 73% of livers with chronic biliary disease.

For additional investigation, I refer the reader to Kakar et al.[1]

M. L. Smith, MD

Reference

1. Kakar S, Batts KP, Poterucha JJ, et al. Histologic changes mimicking biliary disease in liver biopsies with venous outflow impairment. *Mod Pathol.* 2004;17: 874-878.

5 Lung and Mediastinum

Smoking-related interstitial fibrosis (SRIF): pathologic findings and distinction from other chronic fibrosing lung diseases

Katzenstein A-LA (SUNY Upstate Med Univ, Syracuse, NY)

J Clin Pathol 66:882-887, 2013

Smoking-related interstitial fibrosis (SRIF) is a common, histologically striking finding in smokers that must be distinguished from the idiopathic interstitial pneumonias and other chronic interstitial fibrosing lesions. It is characterised by marked thickening of alveolar septa by fibrosis composed of thick collagen bundles that have a distinctive hyalinised quality and often are admixed with variable numbers of hyperplastic smooth muscle fibres. There is minimal accompanying inflammation. This fibrosis is usually most prominent in subpleural and centrilobular parenchyma, but can be present elsewhere as well. It is accompanied by emphysema and respiratory bronchiolitis. Most patients are asymptomatic or only mildly symptomatic, and the clinical course is stable in most. This paper reviews the pathologic features of SRIF in detail, its differentiation from more ominous interstitial fibrosing processes, and the clinical implications of its diagnosis.

► This is an important review for any general surgical pathologist that encounters lung biopsies for interstitial lung disease. Dr Katzenstein clearly describes how to distinguish smoking-related interstitial fibrosis from some of the other more progressive interstitial lung diseases with worse prognosis. The first pearl is the nearly universal association of smoking-related interstitial fibrosis with respiratory bronchiolitis (pigmented macrophages primarily in a centrilobular distribution) and emphysematous change. The distinction from usual interstitial pneumonia (UIP) is typically less challenging, as UIP does not show this delicate dense interstitial fibrosis pattern, usually contains many more fibroblast foci, and contains areas of microscopic honeycomb remodeling, a feature not seen in smoking-related interstitial fibrosis. Probably the most difficult distinction is fibrotic nonspecific interstitial pneumonia. This distinction relies primarily on the identification of the densely eosinophilic and hyalinized collagen seen in smoking-related fibrosis, as opposed to the loose and often inflamed interstitial fibrosis of fibrosing nonspecific interstitial pneumonia. In addition, if the wedge biopsy is large enough, smoking-related interstitial fibrosis will have more of a subpleural and centrilobular distribution compared with a diffuse distribution of fibrosing nonspecific interstitial pneumonia. This may be a more common type of fibrosis seen in the non-neoplastic sections from patients with lung cancer.

For further investigation, I refer the reader to Katzenstein et al.[1]

M. L. Smith, MD

Reference

1. Katzenstein AL, Mukhopadhyay S, Zanardi C, et al. Clinically occult interstitial fibrosis in smokers: classification and significance of a surprisingly common finding in lobectomy specimens. *Hum Pathol.* 2010;41:316-325.

Fibrosing interstitial pneumonia predicts survival in patients with rheumatoid arthritis-associated interstitial lung disease (RA-ILD)

Solomon JJ, Ryu JH, Tazelaar HD, et al (Natl Jewish Health, Denver, CO; Mayo Clinic, Rochester, MN; Mayo Clinic, Scottsdale, AZ; et al)

Respir Med 107:1247-1252, 2013

Background.—Rheumatoid arthritis (RA) is a systemic autoimmune disorder with a variety of extra-articular manifestations. The lung is a common target and diffuse parenchymal lung disease can appear as any of the patterns found with idiopathic interstitial pneumonia. Controversy exists as to the prognostic significance of these patterns among patients with RA-ILD.

Methods.—We retrospectively identified 48 patients with a diagnosis of RA-ILD confirmed by surgical lung biopsy. The pathology was reviewed by four expert pulmonary pathologists. We examined survival after stratifying on the presence or absence of fibrotic ILD, and contrasted it with a matched idiopathic pulmonary fibrosis (IPF) population. The Cox proportional hazards model was used to identify independent predictors of survival.

Results.—The majority of subjects were male smokers with physiologic restriction. A usual interstitial pneumonia (UIP) pattern was identified in 31% of subjects. Median survival time for the entire cohort was 1360 days. Subjects with fibrotic ILD had worse survival than subjects with non-fibrotic ILD (log rank $p = 0.02$). There was no difference in survival between UIP-pattern RA-ILD subjects and IPF controls (log rank $p = 0.94$). Multivariable analysis revealed that age (hazard ratio [HR] = 1.04, $p = 0.01$) and fibrosis (HR = 2.1, $p = 0.02$) were independent predictors of mortality.

Conclusions.—Both cellular and fibrosing ILD patterns are common among RA-ILD patients who undergo surgical lung biopsy. These patients have a shortened survival when compared to the general population and all-comers with RA. Age and the presence of a fibrosing interstitial pneumonia predict shortened survival in these patients. Survival in UIP is similar to matched IPF patients (Fig 2).

▶ Autoimmune/connective tissue disease and particularly rheumatoid arthritis (RA) can be added to the differential diagnosis of essentially any pattern of lung injury, whether it be fibrotic or nonfibrotic. This study sought to identify

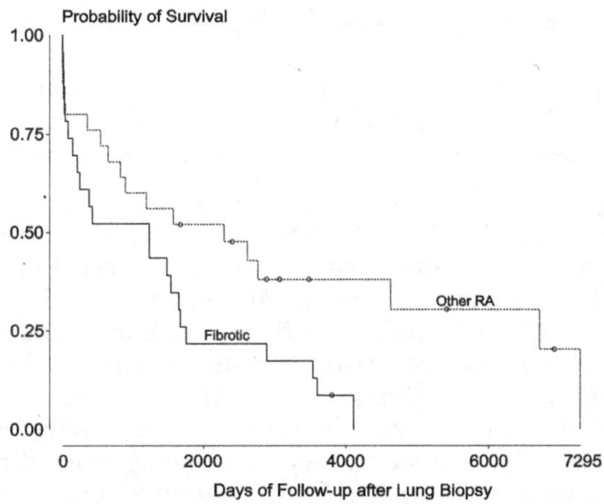

FIGURE 2.—Kaplan Meier curves comparing RA patients with and without fibrotic ILD (log rank $p = 0.02$). (Reprinted from Solomon JJ, Ryu JH, Tazelaar HD, et al. Fibrosing interstitial pneumonia predicts survival in patients with rheumatoid arthritis-associated interstitial lung disease (RA-ILD). *Respir Med.* 2013;107:1247-1252, Copyright 2013, with permission from Elsevier.)

independent prognostic factors in patients with RA-associated interstitial lung disease. One of the findings is shown in Fig 2 in which RA patients with fibrotic disease on lung biopsy show a worse prognosis compared with those with other types of disease on lung biopsy. In this study, the pathologies were reviewed blinded by 4 different expert pulmonary pathologists and were classified into different categories. Fibrosing categories including fibrotic nonspecific interstitial pneumonia, unclassifiable fibrosing interstitial lung disease, and usual interstitial pneumonia were combined. From a pathologic perspective, we spend a lot of time trying to distinguish between these various patterns of fibrosing interstitial pneumonia, with particular interest in the distinction of the usual interstitial pneumonia pattern of injury from the fibrotic nonspecific interstitial pneumonia pattern of injury. However, it seems from this report that regardless of the pattern of fibrosis, the presence of fibrosis in patients with rheumatoid arthritis is an independent negative predictor for survival, with a hazards ratio of 2:1. Perhaps in patients with clinical and serologic evidence of rheumatoid arthritis, instead of struggling over the pattern of fibrosis, pathologists need only to mention the presence or absence of fibrosis. This study does suffer from selection bias in that it is from two referral tertiary care centers and also has only evaluated patients with severe or atypical interstitial lung disease, which lead to biopsy.

For further investigation, I refer the reader to Olson et al[1] and Song et al.[2]

M. L. Smith, MD

References

1. Olson AL, Swigris JJ, Sprunger DB, et al. Rheumatoid arthritis-interstitial lung disease-associated mortality. *Am J Respir Crit Care Med.* 2011;183:372-378.
2. Song JW, Do KH, Kim MY, et al. Pathologic and radiologic differences between idiopathic and collagen vascular disease-related usual interstitial pneumonia. *Chest.* 2009;136:23-30.

End-stage Sarcoid Lung Disease Is Distinct From Usual Interstitial Pneumonia

Xu L, Kligerman S, Burke A (Univ of Maryland Med Ctr, Baltimore)
Am J Surg Pathol 37:593-600, 2013

Sarcoid lung disease may result in progressive lung failure, necessitating transplant. There is a debate on whether the scarring is similar to or distinct from that seen in other fibrotic lung disease such as usual interstitial pneumonia (UIP). We prospectively evaluated histologic sections from 9 lung explants with end-stage sarcoid lung disease diagnosed clinically and by chest computed tomographic scans. The study included 7 women and 2 men. Four lungs showed active granulomatous disease, with nonfibrotic nodular granulomas in the interstitium; the other 5 were predominantly fibrotic, of which 3 had areas of honeycombing (cysts lined by respiratory epithelium with surrounding scar). Chest computed tomographs of 8 cases were all read as either probable or definite sarcoid. Patients in the fibrotic phase were significantly older ($P = 0.016$). All cases showed dense acellular collagen, which was more extensive in the fibrotic phase. Granulomas were present in a lymphatic distribution (along bronchi, the lobular septa, and the pleura) and were predominantly small clusters of macrophages or giant cells embedded in scar in the fibrotic phase. Granulomas were not identified in 2 lungs in the fibrotic phase. In contrast to the honeycombing of UIP, the honeycombing was predominantly central, with prominent bronchiectasis. These end-stage sarcoid lungs were characterized by a fibrotic and active granulomatous pattern, both of which are very distinct from that seen in UIP.

► Usual interstitial pneumonia (UIP) is the most well-known of the fibrosing interstitial lung diseases to the general practicing pathologist. The classic description of UIP involves both temporal and geographic heterogeneity. What this means is that there are some areas of disease and fibrosis alternating with other areas that are relatively uninvolved (geographic heterogeneity). There are also some areas of relatively dense and mature scarring alternating with other areas of more active scarring and injury, such as the fibroblast focus (temporal heterogeneity). Unfortunately, using this general definition, there are actually a variety of fibrosing interstitial lung diseases that could potentially meet criteria for this entity. Therefore, because of its vague definition and easy name recognition, UIP often is overdiagnosed by the general practicing pathologist population. Any end-stage fibrosing interstitial lung disease may be confused with usual interstitial pneumonia, and sarcoidosis is no different. This article nicely highlights some of the distinctive features of fibrosing or end-stage sarcoidosis and its comparison with the usual interstitial pneumonia pattern of injury. In our experience, the distribution of fibrosis in UIP, being subpleural and paraseptal, the mature and dense fibrosis with smooth muscle proliferation, the relatively increased number of fibroblast foci, and the absence of giant cells or granulomas help confirm a diagnosis of UIP. Some of the limitations associated with this study include the use of explant lungs as opposed to surgical wedge biopsies and the relatively low number of patients. Nevertheless, the take-home message is clear: When central honeycomb changes are recognized and there is prominent associated airway damage, one should consider the possibility of an alternative fibrosing process to usual interstitial pneumonia, and, particularly if there are granulomas, sarcoidosis should be included in the differential diagnosis.

For further investigation of this topic, please refer to Nagai et al.[1]

M. L. Smith, MD

Reference

1. Nagai S, Nagao T, Hoshino Y, et al. Heterogeneity of pulmonary fibrosis: interstitial pneumonias and sarcoidosis. *Curr Opin Pulm Med.* 2001;7:262-271.

Bronchoscopic Cryobiopsy for the Diagnosis of Diffuse Parenchymal Lung Disease

Kropski JA, Pritchett JM, Mason WR, et al (Vanderbilt Univ School of Medicine, Nashville, TN)

PLoS One 8:e78674, 2013

Background.—Although in some cases clinical and radiographic features may be sufficient to establish a diagnosis of diffuse parenchymal lung disease (DPLD), surgical lung biopsy is frequently required. Recently a new technique for bronchoscopic lung biopsy has been developed using flexible cryo-probes. In this study we describe our clinical experience using bronchoscopic cryobiopsy for diagnosis of diffuse lung disease.

Methods.—A retrospective study of subjects who had undergone bronchoscopic cryobiopsy for evaluation of DPLD at an academic tertiary care center from January 1, 2012 through January 15, 2013 was performed. The procedure was performed using a flexible bronchoscope to acquire biopsies of lung parenchyma. H&E stained biopsies were reviewed by an expert lung pathologist.

Results.—Twenty-five eligible subjects were identified. With a mean area of 64.2 mm^2, cryobiopsies were larger than that typically encountered with traditional transbronchial forceps biopsy. In 19 of the 25 subjects, a specific diagnosis was obtained. In one additional subject, biopsies demonstrating normal parenchyma were felt sufficient to exclude diffuse lung disease as a cause of dyspnea. The overall diagnostic yield of bronchoscopic cryobiopsy was 80% (20/25). The most frequent diagnosis was usual interstitial pneumonia (UIP) ($n = 7$). Three of the 25 subjects ultimately required surgical lung biopsy. There were no significant complications.

Conclusion.—In patients with suspected diffuse parenchymal lung disease, bronchoscopic cryobiopsy is a promising and minimally invasive approach to obtain lung tissue with high diagnostic yield.

▶ As if the interpretation of surgical lung biopsies could be any more challenging, a new technique, recently described in 2009, involves a minimally invasive procedure in which bronchoscopic cryo biopsy is performed for the evaluation of interstitial lung disease. Anyone who routinely interprets transbronchial biopsies for interstitial lung disease knows that one of the most common diagnoses is nonspecific. This study sought to investigate the diagnostic potential of cryo biopsies for interstitial lung disease. The cryo biopsy results in a markedly increased surface area (64.2 mm^2) compared with the typical surface area of traditional transbronchial biopsies of 5 to 15 mm^2. It should be noted that in this study, a biopsy was considered diagnostic if a uniform diagnosis could be reached after the review of clinical information, radiology, and pathology by both the pathologist and the treating clinician. Therefore, the diagnosis often was not dependent on the pathologic features alone. One of the more feared complications of more extensive transbronchial biopsying such as cryo biopsy is intrabronchiolar bleeding. The safety outcomes were generally favorable in this study. The results suggest that cryo biopsy, in conjunction with extensive clinicopathologic correlation, may be sufficient for a diagnosis in interstitial lung disease and prevent the significant morbidity associated with open thoracotomy surgical lung biopsies. There is potential for cryo biopsies to offer the health care system a significant potential cost savings. Further investigation is required.

For additional investigation into this topic, I refer the reader to Babiac et al.[1]

M. L. Smith, MD

Reference

1. Babiac A, Hetzel J, Krishna G, et al. Transbronchial cryobiopsy: a new tool for lung biopsies. *Respiration.* 2009;78:203-208.

Nodular Pulmonary Amyloidosis Is Characterized by Localized Immunoglobulin Deposition and Is Frequently Associated With an Indolent B-cell Lymphoproliferative Disorder

Grogg KL, Aubry MC, Vrana JA, et al (Mayo Clinic, Rochester, MN)
Am J Surg Pathol 37:406-412, 2013

Nodular pulmonary amyloidosis, a rare localized form of amyloidosis, has been associated with immunoglobulin light chains (AL type) and variably with low-grade lymphoma. The clinicopathologic features of 18 cases were investigated; 5 of 14 had autoimmune disease. In 14 cases monotypic plasma cells could be demonstrated by immunohistochemistry. By mass spectrometry analysis of the amyloid deposits, all 18 cases showed a peptide profile with an abundance of immunoglobulin light chains (12 κ, 4 λ, and 2 mixed κ and λ), with 13 also showing significant codeposition of heavy chains (10 γ, 2 α, 1 δ). Of 14 patients with follow-up, 3 developed recurrent pulmonary amyloidoma, 2 had pulmonary recurrence plus cutaneous extranodal marginal zone lymphoma of mucosa-associated lymphoid tissue (MALT) type with and without amyloid, and 1 had a history of parotid gland MALT lymphoma. This study highlights the unique features of this localized form of amyloidosis. AL κ type is more frequent than AL λ type, with a ratio of 3:1, in contrast to the AL λ predominance that characterizes systemic AL amyloidosis. In addition, the majority of nodular pulmonary amyloid is of mixed AL/AH type, a rare finding in systemic amyloidosis. The association of nodular pulmonary amyloidoma with autoimmune disease and lymphoma indicate the majority of these lesions relate to an underlying lymphoplasmacytic neoplasm in the spectrum of MALT lymphoma.

▶ Nodular pulmonary amyloidosis is a relatively common, often incidental finding on lung biopsy. One of the benefits of this article is the detailed amyloid typing performed by mass spectroscopy as well as the association with clinical follow-up, indicating an association with underlying autoimmune disease and lymphoproliferative disease. Like other forms of amyloidosis, including systemic amyloidosis, nodular pulmonary amyloidosis is typically Congo red, and the diagnosis is rarely difficult. However, pulmonary light chain deposition disease may also be light chain restricted and show very similar morphology by hematoxylin and eosin staining. The only difference is the absence of congophilic on Congo red staining.[1] Despite the differences in Congo red staining, the distinction is unlikely to be of clinical significance, as both disease processes are associated with underlying lymphoproliferative disease and autoimmune disease.

M. L. Smith, MD

Reference

1. Bhargava P, Rushin JM, Rusnock EJ, et al. Pulmonary light chain deposition disease: report of five cases and review of the literature. *Am J Surg Pathol.* 2007;31: 267-276.

Molecular testing guideline for selection of lung cancer patients for EGFR and ALK tyrosine kinase inhibitors: guideline from the College of American Pathologists, International Association for the Study of Lung Cancer, and Association for Molecular Pathology

Lindeman NI, Cagle PT, Beasley MB, et al (Brigham & Women's Hosp, Boston, MA)

J Mol Diagn 15:415-453, 2013

Objective.—To establish evidence-based recommendations for the molecular analysis of lung cancers that are required to guide EGFR- and ALK-directed therapies, addressing which patients and samples should be tested, and when and how testing should be performed.

Participants.—Three cochairs without conflicts of interest were selected, one from each of the 3 sponsoring professional societies: College of American Pathologists, International Association for the Study of Lung Cancer, and Association for Molecular Pathology. Writing and advisory panels were constituted from additional experts from these societies.

Evidence.—Three unbiased literature searches of electronic databases were performed to capture published articles from January 2004 through February 2012, yielding 1533 articles whose abstracts were screened to identify 521 pertinent articles that were then reviewed in detail for their relevance to the recommendations. Evidence was formally graded for each recommendation.

Consensus Process.—Initial recommendations were formulated by the cochairs and panel members at a public meeting. Each guideline section was assigned to at least 2 panelists. Drafts were circulated to the writing panel (version 1), advisory panel (version 2), and the public (version 3) before submission (version 4).

Conclusions.—The 37 guideline items address 14 subjects, including 15 recommendations (evidence grade A/B). The major recommendations are to use testing for EGFR mutations and ALK fusions to guide patient selection for therapy with an epidermal growth factor receptor (EGFR) or anaplastic lymphoma kinase (ALK) inhibitor, respectively, in all patients with advanced-stage adenocarcinoma, regardless of sex, race, smoking history, or other clinical risk factors, and to prioritize EGFR and ALK testing over other molecular predictive tests. As scientific discoveries and clinical practice outpace the completion of randomized clinical trials, evidence-based guidelines developed by expert practitioners are vital for communicating emerging clinical standards. Already, new treatments targeting genetic alterations in other, less common driver oncogenes are being evaluated in lung cancer, and testing for these may be addressed in future versions of these guidelines.

▶ This article addresses several of the questions regarding molecular testing in lung cancers after the more widespread testing seen in the last few years. It is very common in our pulmonary pathology consult practice to receive questions regarding the molecular testing of lung cancer, and this article addresses several of these issues. Although the primary finding is discussed in the conclusion of the abstract, several pertinent questions for the general surgical pathologist are answered throughout the article, which is basically the result of expert consensus opinion and recommendations. With resection specimens, regardless of whether it is a wedge of a completion lobectomy specimen, it is recommended that all cases of adenocarcinoma be tested for epidermal growth factor receptor (EGFR) or anaplastic lymphoma kinase (ALK). Even in cases in which an adenocarcinoma component is not the majority, as long as there is some adenocarcinoma component present, the testing should be performed. For biopsy specimens, similarly, although it is not a formal recommendation to test, pathologists are encouraged to perform testing if a component of adenocarcinoma is not able to be excluded on the biopsy specimen. It is recommended that testing be performed on all high-stage lung cancers (stage IV), and it is encouraged to test the lower-stage lung cancers (stage I-III). Testing for both EGFR and ALK does not have to be performed at the same time but can be done sequentially, provided that all of the testing is completed in the recommended turnaround time of 10 days. It is best to set up an institutional protocol in collaboration with the oncologists and surgeons before starting optimal testing within your institution.

M. L. Smith, MD

Mesothelioma with signet-ring cell features: report of 23 cases

Ordóñez NG (The Univ of Texas, Houston)

Mod Pathol 26:370-384, 2013

Signet-ring cell mesothelioma is uncommon and only two case reports have been published on this mesothelioma variant, both of which were initially misdiagnosed as signet-ring cell carcinoma. Herein are reported 23 signet-ring cell mesotheliomas that were investigated by immunohistochemistry, 12 of which were also studied by electron microscopy. Twenty-one of the cases originated in the pleura and two in the peritoneum. For comparison purposes and in order to determine the value of these techniques in the differential diagnosis of these tumors, seven cases of signet-ring cell lung adenocarcinoma were also studied. All signet-ring cell mesotheliomas were positive for calretinin, keratin 5/6, keratin 7, and mesothelin, 93% for podoplanin, and 91% for WT1; whereas, none reacted for MOC-31, CEA, TAG-72, CD15, TTF-1, napsin A, or CDX2. Among signet-ring cell lung adenocarcinomas, 100% were positive for keratin 7, CEA, and napsin A, 86% each for TTF-1 and TAG-72, 71% for CD15, and 14% for mesothelin, while all were negative for calretinin, keratin 5/6, WT1, podoplanin, and CDX2. After analyzing the results, it is concluded that the panels of markers used in the differential diagnosis of this mesothelioma variant should include those markers that are usually expressed in mesotheliomas (eg, calretinin, keratin 5/6, WT1, and podoplanin), broad-spectrum carcinoma markers that are frequently expressed in adenocarcinomas regardless of their site of origin (eg, MOC-31 and CEA), and organ-associated markers (eg, TTF-1 and napsin A for lung), which allow the site of origin of a metastatic adenocarcinoma to be established. Electron microscopy can be very useful as it permits the identification of characteristic ultrastructural mesothelioma and adenocarcinoma markers, and it also allows a better understanding of the morphologic features seen on routine light microscopy. Pathologists should be aware of this mesothelioma subtype as it can potentially be confused with other tumors that exhibit signet-ring features.

▶ This is an important article for any general surgical pathology practice that encounters pleural-based biopsies for the evaluation of mesothelioma on a regular basis. It is exceedingly easy to misdiagnose signet ring cell lesions as invasive/metastatic signet ring cell adenocarcinoma. However, this descriptive clinicopathologic and immunohistochemical study helps solidify signet ring cell mesothelioma as an entity critical in the differential diagnosis for these pleural lesions. One of the key findings in this study is that a standard panel that is used for the distinction between adenocarcinoma and mesothelioma seems to work sufficiently, even in cases of this type of signet ring cell morphology. Although the author described how electron microscopy can be useful in the diagnosis because of the rarity of tissue available for electron microscopy, it is unlikely this will be used in widespread clinical practice. Mucin staining may also prove to be of some use.

M. L. Smith, MD

Intrapulmonary Solitary Fibrous Tumors: Clinicopathologic and Immunohistochemical Study of 24 Cases

Rao N, Colby TV, Falconieri G, et al (Med College of Wisconsin, Milwaukee; Mayo Clinic, Scottsdale, AZ; The MD Anderson Cancer Ctr, Houston, TX; et al)
Am J Surg Pathol 37:155-166, 2013

Solitary fibrous tumor (SFT) is a ubiquitous neoplasm that arises most commonly from the pleura. SFT arising within lung parenchyma (intrapulmonary SFT) has been rarely reported and is therefore not well recognized. We present a clinicopathologic and immunohistochemical study of 24 cases of primary intrapulmonary SFT. Patients' ages ranged from 44 to 83 years (mean, 58 y). None of the patients had evidence or history of a similar tumor elsewhere. Tumor size ranged from 2.3 to 22 cm (mean, 8.5 cm). On the basis of the degree of cytologic atypia, cellularity, mitotic activity, and areas of necrosis, the lesions were divided into low-grade, intermediate-grade, and high-grade histology. Twenty-one tumors showed the conventional features of SFT of low-grade histology (<5 mitoses per 10 high-power fields), with alternating bands of rope-like collagen flanked by a bland-appearing spindle cell proliferation. Hemangiopericytic, angiofibromatous, and a neural-like plexiform growth pattern were also observed. Five of 21 cases showed an "adenofibromatous" appearance imparted by entrapped normal airspaces at the advancing edges of the lesion. One intermediate-grade tumor showed overall increased cellularity with plump, pleomorphic nuclei, 5 to 10 mitoses per 10 high-power fields, and focal areas of classic SFT. Two cases showed high-grade features at initial presentation, with areas resembling a pleomorphic high-grade sarcoma admixed with foci of conventional, low-grade SFT. Immunohistochemical staining analyses performed in 13 cases showed positivity of the tumor cells for CD34, bcl-2, and CD99 in the majority of cases tested. Clinical follow-up was available in 18 patients, with long-term follow-up (>5 y) in 6. Fourteen (14/18) patients were alive and well without evidence of disease 1 month to 14 years after initial diagnosis. Three patients died of their tumors after 4, 5, and 7 years; in 2 of them the initial tumor was of low-grade histology, but the recurrence/metastases showed a high-grade histology; the third fatal case showed a tumor with high-grade histology at initial diagnosis. One patient with intermediate-grade histology also had chest wall metastases at 5 years but was subsequently lost to follow-up. The results of our study indicate that although tumors with overtly malignant histologic features can be expected to behave as high-grade sarcomas, tumors with bland-appearing morphologic features at presentation may also follow an aggressive behavior. Adequate excision with close clinical follow-up, thus, appears to be the most prudent course of action for the management of primary intrapulmonary fibrous tumors.

▶ This study is a valuable addition to the literature, as it describes for the first time a large series of a relatively rare intrapulmonary neoplasm, solitary fibrous tumor. In addition to increasing awareness and describing the clinicopathologic and immunohistochemical features of this lesion, a large differential diagnosis is also discussed. A large number of lesions may show spindle cells on needle core biopsies of the lung, including benign neural lesions, smooth muscle lesions such as leiomyoma and leiomyosarcoma, adenofibroma, synovial sarcoma, spindle cell thymoma, spindle cell carcinoid tumors, nerve sheath tumors, fibrosarcomas, sarcomatoid mesothelioma, and sarcomatoid carcinoma. One of the challenges with intrapulmonary solitary fibrous tumors is that the histologic spectrum from benign to malignant is quite broad, thus requiring the inclusion of a large number of potential etiologies in the differential diagnosis. The panel of stains, including CD34, bcl-2, and CD99, should help in most cases to confirm the diagnosis. It is interesting to note that in follow-up, although the obviously malignant lesions did show an aggressive behavior, aggressive behavior was also seen in lesions with relatively bland histologic features. Therefore, regardless of the histology, close clinical follow-up is warranted, as the authors suggest. This study excluded any cases of pleural involvement in an attempt to exclude pleural fibrous tumors invading the pulmonary parenchyma.

M. L. Smith, MD

Localized Pleuropulmonary Crystal-storing Histiocytosis: 5 Cases of a Rare Histiocytic Disorder With Variable Clinicoradiologic Features

Rossi G, De Rosa N, Cavazza A, et al (Azienda Ospedaliera Arcispedale Santa Maria Nuova/Istituto di Ricerca e Cura a Carattere Scientifico, Reggio Emilia, Italy; AORN Monaldi-Cotugno-CTO, Napoli, Italy; et al)

Am J Surg Pathol 37:906-912, 2013

Crystal-storing histiocytosis (CSH) localized to the thoracic region is a rare occurrence, often secondary to lymphoproliferative or plasma cell diseases. About 10 case reports have been previously published, and 3 of these have no relationship with clonal hematologic disorders. We collected here the first series of 5 consecutive cases of CSH involving lungs (4 cases) and pleura (1 case). There were 3 women and 2 men with a mean age at diagnosis of 65 years. All cases had an underlying hematologic disorder (2 B-cell marginal-zone lymphomas, 2 monoclonal gammopathy of undetermined significance and 1 pulmonary plasmacytoma). Despite a common morphology characterized by a dense and irregular growth of large eosinophilic histiocytes with intracytoplasmic refractile crystals, 2 cases presented with cystic changes at gross and imaging examinations, calcified amyloid was found in 2 cases, and 1 case showed an interstitial lung disease with nonspecific interstitial pneumonia pattern. Histiocytes were immunoreactive for CD68 (clones PGM-1 and KP-1) but were not for CD1a and

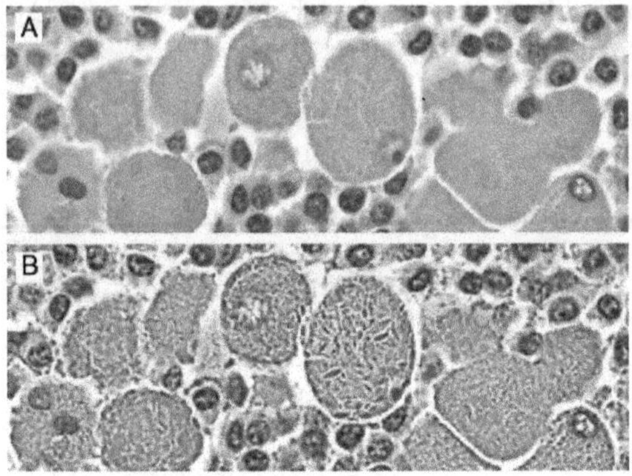

FIGURE 2.—High-magnification image of histiocytes (A) on removing the microscope condenser (B) highlights intracytoplasmic refractile crystals. (Reprinted from Rossi G, De Rosa N, Cavazza A, et al. Localized pleuropulmonary crystal-storing histiocytosis: 5 cases of a rare histiocytic disorder with variable clinicoradiologic features. *Am J Surg Pathol.* 2013;37:906-912, with permission from Lippincott Williams & Wilkins.)

S100; the associated lymphoplasmacellular disorder had a clonal profile on molecular analysis with κ light-chain restriction. Two cases were originally misdiagnosed as cystic fibrohistiocytic tumor and carcinoid tumor, thus confirming that CSH localized to this site may result in a diagnostic challenge with a broad spectrum of differential diagnoses. The presence of intracytoplasmic crystals and a plasma cell infiltrate around a histiocytic proliferation should alert the pathologist to consider CSH and to carefully investigate the presence of clonal hematologic disease (Fig 2).

► Pleuropulmonary crystal-storing histiocytosis (PCSH) is a rare disorder and is likely underdiagnosed. This article is the first to publish a series of consecutive cases of PCSH and highlights some important features for the practicing general surgical pathologist to keep in mind when evaluating macrophage-rich pulmonary lesions. One of the unique findings in this study was the identification of both nodular and cystic disease by radiographic imaging. Thus, it is reasonable to include PCSH in the differential diagnosis for cystic lung diseases along with Birt-Hogg Dube, pulmonary Langerhans' cell histiocytosis, cystic changes of advanced pulmonary fibrosis, and cysts of lymphoid interstitial pneumonia (Sjögren's syndrome). The article also highlights the challenge in diagnosing these lesions based on histologic analysis alone, recognizing that the differential diagnosis for macrophage-rich pulmonary lesions is broad and includes relatively common disorders, such as infections, and more rare disorders, such as inhaled crystalline materials, storage disease, Langerhans' cell histiocytosis, Rosai-Dorfman disease, and Erdheim-Chester disease. When present in the nodular form, PCSH may be mistaken for tumors with a histiocytoid appearance, in which case the consistent reactivity for CD68 becomes a helpful immunohistochemical feature. Finally, the authors note the use of dropping the microscope condenser to highlight the intracytoplasmic refractile crystals (Fig 2), which can be helpful in establishing the diagnosis. The importance in recognizing this disease, clearly, is its association with a clonal hematologic disease.

For additional investigation, I refer the reader to Ionescu et al.[1]

M. L. Smith, MD

Reference

1. Ionescu DN, Pierson DM, Qing G, et al. Pulmonary crystal-storing histiocytoma. *Arch Pathol Lab Med.* 2005;129:1159-1163.

Pathology of pulmonary antibody-mediated rejection: 2012 update from the Pathology Council of the ISHLT

Berry G, Burke M, Andersen C, et al (Stanford Univ, CA; Royal Brompton and Harefield NHS Foundation Trust, London, UK; Rigshospitalet, Copenhagen, Denmark; et al)

J Heart Lung Transplant 32:14-21, 2013

Background.—A significant complication after cardiac and renal transplantation is acute antibody-mediated rejection (AMR) of the allograft. AMR produces acute allograft dysfunction and predisposes patients to the rapid development of transplant vasculopathy and graft loss. The presence of AMR among patients having pulmonary transplants may be linked to persistent or recurrent acute cellular rejection of varying grades, lymphocytic bronchiolitis, and chronic rejection. A critical review and survey were undertaken to document the current morphologic and immunologic criteria for AMR, summarize current practices in the diagnosis and reporting of pulmonary AMR, and identify technical, interpretative, and reporting issues.

Diagnosis.—Pulmonary AMR is best diagnosed using a multidisciplinary approach. This includes identifying clinical allograft dysfunction, circulating donor-specific antibodies, and pathologic findings. This is termed the "triple test."

Histopathologic and Immunologic Findings.—The nonspecific patterns of injury found in AMR can occur in various disorders. However, such findings should prompt the use of subsequent, more specific immunopathologic studies. Capillary C4d immunoreactivity occurs both in the presence and in the absence of circulating donor-specific antibodies. Pathologists should be well-versed with C4d staining interpretation and able to recognize that serum and nonvascular septal staining can also occur. Positive capillary C4d staining is most accurately reported as "findings suggestive of AMR," while the final diagnosis is delayed until comprehensive clinical, serologic, and pathologic correlations are obtained.

Recommendations.—Centers that do not routinely obtain donor-specific antibody (DSA) studies should perform serologic studies close to the time of biopsy. Among the recommended protocols are those including frequent DSA and biopsy surveillance to develop experience in diagnosing AMR.

TABLE 1.—Comprehensive Review of Published Pathology Literature

First author/Year	# Pts	# TBBx/OLB	C4d IF/IP	% C4d+	DSA	AGD	High Grade ACR
Saint Martin GA/1996[28]	55	106/1	IF	ND	ND	NR	6/107
Badesch DB/1998[29]	5	3/3	IF	ND	ND	Yes	0/6
Magro CM/2002[30]	22	27/0	IF	100%	ND*	Yes	NR
Magro CM/2003[31]	25	52/0	IF	85%	Neg[†]	20/49	NWS
Miller GM/2004[33]	1	2/0	ND	ND	Pos	Yes	1/2
Girnita AL/2004[10]	54	423/0	ND	ND	Pos (10/54)	NR	28/83 TBBx
Astor TL/2005[37]	35	37/3	IF	ND	ND	Yes	12/40
Ionescu DN/2005[38]	32	192	IP	16%	Pos (16/32)	NR	28/171 (6/8 with C4d+)
Wallace WD/2005[36]	63	68/0	IP	25%	NR	NR	7/68
Magro CM/2006[34]	30	49/0	IF&IP	IF:36% IP:51%	ND	2/49	NR
Girnita AL/2006[18]	2	6/0	IP	50%	Pos	Yes	4/6 (2with C4d/HLA-ab+)
Westall GP/2008[35]	33	86/0	IP	73%	NR	NR	2/33 pts
Girnita AL/2008[39]	42	32/0	IP	28%	Pos (8/9 C4d +)	Yes	12/32 (all grades)
Astor TL/2009[19]	1	0/1	IF/IP	100%	Pos	Yes	0/1
Morrell MR/2009[41]	1	2/0	IP	100%	Pos	Yes	Absent
Neumann J/2010[42]	1	2/0	NR	1/1	Pos	Yes	2/2
Jacob EK/2011[20]	2*(only one LTr)	2/0	NWS	50%	Pos	No	Absent
Yousem SA/2012[40]	49	49/0	IP	74%	Pos	Yes	15/23 (11 with C4d/HLA-ab+)

LB	BOS	Mortality/ Graft Loss	Morphology Grading	IF/IP C4d Grading	Details
NR	NR	NR	ND	ND	
NR	NR	2 of 5	ND	ND	
NR	NR	NR	Yes (I-III)	Yes (Intensity: 1-3)	Bacteria/virus/fungus cultures in BAL in 22 specimens

NR	NWS	NR	Yes (I-III)	Yes (Intensity: 1-3; Distribution: 1:<30%; 2:30-50%; 3:>50%)	
NR	NR	0	ND	ND	
NR	NR	NR	ND	ND	
NR	NR	5 of 35	ND	ND	
20/32 (14 HLA-ab+)	15/32 (4 C4d/HLA-ab+)	NR	ND	ND	1/7/CMV+/2/11/DAD
NR	11/63	NR	ND	ND	
NR	16/30	NR	NR	IF: Distribution:1- < 30%; 2-30-50%; 3-> 50%IP: Low:<10 vessels/5HPF; Intermediate: 10-15; High >15	
NR	1/2	2/2	ND	ND	
NR	9/33	NR	ND	IP: Low:<10 vessels/5HPF; Intermediate: 10-15; High >15	15/33 bacterial infection
NR	NR	NR	ND	NR	1/9 CMV +
NR	Absent	0	ND	NR	
NR	NR	0	ND	NR	Pseudomonas A. at 2 nd TBBx
NR	NR	0	ND	NR	
NR	0	ND	NR	NR	Respiratory Infections at 1st biopsy (C4d+)
14/23 (10 with C4d/ HLA-ab +)	NR	NR	ND	Patchy: <50% capillaries + Diffuse: >50% capillaries +	6/26 C4d without HLA-Ab

ACR, acute cellular rejection; AGD, acute graft dysfunction; BOS, bronchiolitis obliterative syndrome; CMV, cytomegalovirus; DAD, diffuse alveolar damage; DSA, donor specific antibodies; IF, immunofluorescence; IP, immunoperoxidase; LB, lymphocytic bronchiolitis; LTr, lung transplant recipient; ND, not done; NR, not reported; NWS, not well specified; OLB, open lung biopsy; POS, positive; PTS, patients; TBBx, transbronchial biopsies.

*PRA only.

†ELISA and flow cytometry only.

TABLE 2.—Histopathologic Indications for Immunopathologic Evaluation

1. Neutrophilic capillaritis
2. Neutrophilic septal margination
3. High-grade acute cellular rejection (≥A3)
4. Persistent/recurrent acute cellular rejection (any A Grade)
5. Acute lung injury pattern/diffuse alveolar damage
6. High-grade lymphocytic bronchiolitis (Grade B2R)
7. Persistent low-grade lymphocytic bronchiolitis (Grade B1R)
8. Obliterative bronchiolitis (Grade C1)
9. Arteritis in the absence of infection or cellular rejection
10. Graft dysfunction without morphologic explanation
11. Any histologic findings in setting of de novo DSA positivity

DSA, donor-specific antibodies.

Conclusions.—AMR is a relatively infrequent finding based on the current definitions and the experience of most transplant pathologists. The current experience should be broadened by the use of digital pathology slide technology, so that many pathologists can assess cases and manipulate images in real time through virtual microscopy on desktop computers. Through this broader dissemination of cases, pathologists can identify morphologic patterns, intensity, and distribution profiles of C4d staining; characterize novel histopathologic manifestations; and evaluate unusual antibody or ancillary technique results (Tables 1 and 2).

▶ This is an important article for any general surgical pathologist who is involved in the interpretation of lung biopsies in the posttransplant setting. This editorial statement comes from the 2012 Pathology Council of ISHLT and formally recognizes pulmonary antibody-mediated rejection (AMR). The summary conclusions are shown in Box 1 of the original article, which are the consensus points for the pathologic diagnosis of pulmonary AMR. There is an emphasis throughout the article on the need for a multidisciplinary approach, including pathologic findings, the presence of clinical allograft dysfunction, and the presence of circulating donor-specific antibodies (DSA). Unfortunately, the histopathologic findings in AMR are entirely nonspecific, and the differential diagnosis for the acute lung injury seen is often very broad. Table 2 shows the variety of different histopathologic findings that should prompt testing for C4d within the biopsy as well as DSAs within the patient's serum. As with the other organ systems, the consensus opinion was that the interpretation of C4d would require multifocal or diffuse staining patterns (> 50% of the interstitial capillaries). It was suggested that an outright diagnosis of acute AMR within the lung allograft should not be made by the pathologist alone but should be done at the clinician level after clinicopathologic correlation. Future directions involved developing protocols within transplant centers to increase the amount of DSA screening being performed to increase the collective experience with DSA and AMR within lung allografts. The take-home summary is that the histopathology of pulmonary AMR is nonspecific, and the pathologist should have a low threshold to obtain

C4d immunohistochemistry/immunofluorescence and to suggest correlation with DSA testing.

For additional investigation into this topic, I refer the reader to Witt et al.[1]

M. L. Smith, MD

Reference

1. Witt CA, Gaut JP, Yusen RD, et al. Acute antibody-mediated rejection after lung transplantation. *J Heart Lung Transplant.* 2013;32:1034-1040.

Immunohistochemical Study of 36 Cases of Pulmonary Sarcomatoid Carcinoma—Sensitivity of TTF-1 is Superior to Napsin

Terra SBSP, Aubry MC, Yi ES, et al (Mayo Clinic, Rochester, MN)

Hum Pathol 2013 [Epub ahead of print]

Immunohistochemistry is often used to distinguish pulmonary sarcomatoid carcinoma from morphologic mimics. Napsin-A is a pulmonary adenocarcinoma marker, but literature on expression in sarcomatoid carcinoma is limited. Thirty-six cases of sarcomatoid carcinoma were stained for napsin, TTF-1, Oscar, CAM5.2, AE1/AE3, desmin, SMA, S-100, CK5/6, calretinin, D2-40, and WT1. Patients were 24 men and 12 women (mean, 70 years; range, 46-93). There were 27 pleomorphic carcinomas, 5 spindle cell carcinomas, 3 carcinosarcomas, and 1 giant cell carcinoma. Cases were positive for at least 1 keratin: AE1/3 was positive in all 36 cases; Oscar, in 34 cases (94%); and CAM5.2, in 32 cases (89%, weaker/ more focal). Napsin was positive in 14 cases (39%): 8 diffuse, 3 focal, and 3 rare cells. TTF-1 was positive in 22 cases (61%): 15 diffuse, 3 focal, and 4 rare cells. No cases were napsin positive and negative for TTF-1. Variable staining for mesothelial markers was observed, including positivity for calretinin (12 cases, 33%), WT1 (6 cases, 17%), D2-40 (5 cases, 14%), and CK5/6 (9 cases, 25%). Mesenchymal markers were also sometimes positive (usually focal), including S-100 (4 cases, 11%), desmin (4 cases, 11%), and SMA (7 cases, 19%, 1 diffuse). In conclusion, TTF-1 is more sensitive than napsin for detection of sarcomatoid carcinoma, and no cases were positive for napsin but negative for TTF-1. CAM5.2 is less sensitive than AE1/AE3 and Oscar. Use of a thoughtful immunohistochemical panel is important in the evaluation of sarcomatoid carcinoma because mesothelial and mesenchymal markers can be expressed.

▶ Sarcomatoid neoplasms of the thorax can be extremely challenging to diagnose and usually result in a high number of immunohistochemical stains, often with conflicting results. As the health care system moves to a capitated payment system, unique reports such as this will be required to develop immunohistochemical panels that not only are diagnostically efficient but also result in wise use of resources. The key finding from this study was that no cases of sarcomatoid carcinoma of the lung that were positive for napsin were negative for TTF-1; therefore, TTF-1 was far more sensitive than napsin for the distinction of pulmonary origin. This article also highlights the high percentage (33%, 17%, 14%, 25%) of markers traditionally thought of as mesothelioma markers in this population of highly selected sarcomatoid carcinomas of the lung. One could argue that this high rate of reactivity of these mesothelial markers suggests they may not be necessary and may actually cloud the diagnostic picture in many cases.

For further investigation of this topic, I refer the reader to Ye et al[1] and Travis.[2]

M. L. Smith, MD

References

1. Ye J, Findeis-Hosey JJ, Yang Q, et al. Combination of napsin-A and TTF-1 immunohistochemistry helps in differentiating primary lung adenocarcinoma from metastatic carcinoma in the lung. *Appl Immunohistochem Mol Morphol.* 2011; 19:313-317.
2. Travis WD. Sarcomatoid neoplasms of the lung and pleural. *Arch Pathol Lab Med.* 2010;134:1645-1658.

Diffuse Intrapulmonary Malignant Mesothelioma Masquerading as Interstitial Lung Disease: A Distinctive Variant of Mesothelioma

Larsen BT, Klein JRH, Hornychová H, et al (Mayo Clinic, Rochester, MN; Univ of Manitoba, Winnipeg, MB, Canada; Charles Univ in Prague, Hradec Kralove, Czech Republic; et al)

Am J Surg Pathol 37:1555-1564, 2013

Malignant mesothelioma typically encases lungs as a thick rind, while relatively sparing lung parenchyma. We describe an unusual presentation of mesothelioma characterized by diffuse intrapulmonary growth, with absent or inconspicuous pleural involvement, clinically simulating interstitial lung disease (ILD). We identified 5 patients (median age 56 y, all men) with diffuse intrapulmonary malignant mesothelioma in our pathology consultation practice from 2009 to 2012. Clinical history, imaging, and pathology materials were reviewed. Symptoms included chronic dyspnea (4 cases), cough (3), and acute dyspnea with bilateral pneumothorax (1). Chest imaging showed irregular opacities (5), reticulation (4), pleural effusions (2), and subpleural nodular densities (1), without radiologic evidence of pleural disease or masses. A clinicoradiologic diagnosis of ILD was made in all cases, and wedge biopsies were performed. Histologic evaluation revealed a neoplastic proliferation of bland epithelioid or spindled cells, showing various growth patterns simulating silicotic nodules, desquamative interstitial pneumonia, organizing pneumonia, and Langerhans cell histiocytosis. Some areas mimicked adenocarcinoma, with lepidic, acinar, micropapillary, and solid patterns. Initial diagnoses by referring pathologists included reactive changes (1), hypersensitivity pneumonitis versus drug reaction (1), desquamative interstitial pneumonia versus neoplasm (1), and mesothelioma (2). Microscopic pleural involvement was identified in 4 cases. Immunohistochemistry confirmed the characteristic immunophenotype of mesothelioma in all cases. Median survival of 3 patients treated with chemotherapy was

28 months. Two patients received no therapy and survived 3 and 4 weeks, respectively. "Diffuse intrapulmonary malignant mesothelioma" is a rare variant with a distinctive presentation that clinically mimics ILD. Recognition is essential to avoid misdiagnosis.

▶ Although diffuse intrapulmonary malignant mesothelioma is an exceedingly rare entity, the authors nicely summarize a series of 5 patients from their consult practice and also include 4 additional patients from case reports to collate the largest case series of diffuse intrapulmonary malignant mesothelioma to date. The importance of this entity is the clinical and radiographic mimicry of interstitial lung disease as well as the histologic pitfalls, highlighted by the referring pathologist's initial differential diagnosis of hypersensitivity pneumonitis, drug reaction, desquamative interstitial pneumonia, neoplasm, and mesothelioma. For those unfamiliar with the natural history of malignant mesothelioma, involvement of the lung parenchyma is rare and usually occurs only very late in the disease progression. Therefore, in the absence of pleural nodules or a pleural effusion, there are no clinical or radiographic clues to a diagnosis of neoplasm, much less malignant mesothelioma. The clinical presentation is relatively nonspecific, including cough and shortness of breath. Some of the histopathologic patterns of the cases presented in this study also were reminiscent of organizing pneumonia, Langerhans' cell histiocytosis, and pneumoconiosis.

For further investigation of this entity, I refer the reader to Oviedo et al[1] and Nind et al.[2]

M. L. Smith, MD

References

1. Oviedo SP, Cagle PT. Diffuse malignant mesothelioma. *Arch Pathol Lab Med.* 2012;136:882-888.
2. Nind NR, Attanoos RL, Gibbs AR. Unusual intraparenchymal growth patterns of malignant pleural mesothelioma. *Histopathology.* 2003;42:150-155.

6 Soft Tissue and Bone

Impact of Molecular Analysis on the Final Sarcoma Diagnosis: A Study on 763 Cases Collected During a European Epidemiological Study

Neuville A, Ranchère-Vince D, Dei Tos AP, et al (Univ of Bordeaux, Bordeaux Cédex, France; Univ of Lyon, France; Hosp of Treviso, Italy; et al)

Am J Surg Pathol 37:1259-1268, 2013

Sarcomas are rare, heterogenous, and often difficult to classify. A large proportion of sarcomas are associated with specific molecular genetic lesions such as translocations, mutations, and amplifications, which are helpful in the diagnosis of individual cases. However, the exact impact of molecular genetics on the final diagnosis of sarcomas is unknown. In this study, all soft tissue and visceral sarcomas arising in patients living in 3 European regions in 2 countries (representing 13 million inhabitants) were collected and reviewed during 2 consecutive years. A molecular analysis was performed for all suspicions of sarcomas with specific genetic lesions [mutations of *KIT/PDGFRA* in gastrointestinal stromal tumors (GISTs), reciprocal translocation, or amplification of *MDM2* in atypical lipomatous tumors, well-differentiated liposarcoma-dedifferentiated liposarcoma (ALT/WDLPS-DDLPS)]. To evaluate the impact of molecular tests, a premolecular analysis diagnosis was proposed with 3 categories of certainty: certain, probable, or possible. A molecular analysis was performed in 763/1484 tumors corresponding to 295 cases in which GIST was suspected, 248 sarcomas with a suspicion of translocation, and 220 cases in which ALT/WDLPS-DDLPS was suspected. Molecular analysis was found to be useful (confirms a probable diagnosis) in 11 (4%) GISTs, 62 (26%) suspicions of translocation, and 66 (31%) suspicions of ALT/WDLPS-DDLPS; and necessary (allows a possible diagnosis) in 2 (<1%) GISTs, 31 (12%) suspicions of translocation, and 19 (9%) suspicions of ALT/WDLPS-DDLPS. This study performed in an epidemiological setting demonstrates the significant impact of molecular analysis on the final sarcoma diagnosis and favors such an analysis on any tumor with a suspicion of a specific genomic abnormality and for which the diagnosis is uncertain (Table 2).

▶ Sarcomas often pose considerable challenges for many pathologists because of their relative rarity. Neuville and coauthors show the transformational nature of molecular testing for several sarcomas. Table 2 shows the molecular testing results stratified by the clinical certainty of a specific sarcoma type before obtaining molecular testing results. In 248 cases in which molecular testing was performed, 153 cases showed positive results and 83 showed negative results

TABLE 2.—Results of Molecular Analyses According to the Diagnostic Certainty in Sarcomas With a Suspicion of Translocation

Diagnostic Certainty	Certain	Probable	Possible	Total
Alveolar rhabdomyosarcoma	2	9	30	41
Molecular analysis done	2	9	25	36
Molecular analysis positive	0	7	3	10
Molecular analysis negative	1	2	22	25
Molecular analysis ni	1	0	0	1
DFSP	86	6	3	95
Molecular analysis done	55	6	3	64
Molecular analysis positive	47	4	1	52
Molecular analysis negative	2	1	2	5
Molecular analysis ni	6	1	0	7
Ewing/PNET	0	10	16	26
Molecular analysis done	—	10	16	26
Molecular analysis positive	—	10	8	18
Molecular analysis negative	—	0	8	8
Molecular analysis ni	—	0	0	0
Myxoid liposarcoma	18	14	2	34
Molecular analysis done	17	14	2	33
Molecular analysis positive	15	14	1	30
Molecular analysis negative	0	0	1	1
Molecular analysis ni	2	0	0	2
Synovial sarcoma	7	28	33	68
Molecular analysis done	7	28	33	68
Molecular analysis positive	7	22	2	31
Molecular analysis negative	0	6	29	35
Molecular analysis ni	0	0	2	2
DSRCT	3	1	3	7
Molecular analysis done	3	1	3	7
Molecular analysis positive	3	1	2	6
Molecular analysis negative	0	0	1	1
Molecular analysis ni	0	0	0	0
LGFMS	0	8	7	15
Molecular analysis done	—	7	7	14
Molecular analysis positive	—	4	2	6
Molecular analysis negative	—	3	5	8
Molecular analysis ni	—	0	0	0
Total	116	76	94	286
Molecular analysis done	84	75	89	248
Molecular analysis positive	72	62	19	153
Molecular analysis negative	3	12	68	83
Molecular analysis ni	9	1	2	12

ni indicates noninterpretable.

(12 were indeterminate). For some of the tumor types, the authors felt certain of the diagnosis, even if the molecular test results were negative. The critical scenarios may be when a pathologist thinks that a specific sarcoma diagnosis is possible or probable (and is not certain), and the molecular test result assists with more definitive confirmation. For further reading, please see reference list.[1,2]

S. Raab, MD

References

1. Antonescu CR. The role of genetic testing in soft tissue sarcoma. *Histopathology.* 2006;48:13-21.
2. Arbiser ZK, Folpe AL, Weiss SW. Consultative (expert) second opinions in soft tissue pathology. Analysis of problem-prone diagnostic situations. *Am J Clin Pathol.* 2001;116:473-476.

Fibrosarcoma-like Lipomatous Neoplasm: A Reappraisal of So-called Spindle Cell Liposarcoma Defining a Unique Lipomatous Tumor Unrelated to Other Liposarcomas

Deyrup AT, Chibon F, Guillou L, et al (Univ of South Carolina School of Medicine-Greenville; Dept of Pathology and INSERM U916 Institut Bergonié, Bordeaux, France; Univ Hosp, Lausanne, Switzerland; et al)
Am J Surg Pathol 37:1373-1378, 2013

The term "spindle cell liposarcoma" has been applied to liposarcomas (LPSs) composed predominantly or exclusively of spindled cells. These tumors have been considered variants of well-differentiated LPS (WDL), myxoid LPS, and spindle cell lipoma, suggesting that this is a heterogenous group of lesions. Using strict morphologic criteria and molecular and immunohistochemical analyses, we have identified a homogenous group of spindle cell lipomatous tumors, histologically and genetically distinct from other forms of LPS, which we have called "fibrosarcoma-like lipomatous neoplasm." Cases classified as "spindle cell LPS" or "low-grade LPS with spindle cell features" were reviewed. Final selection criteria included: (1) an exclusive low-grade spindle cell component resembling fibrosarcoma; (2) a mixture of bland fibroblastic cells resembling the preadipocyte and early-adipocyte stage of embryonic fat; and (3) molecular-genetic analysis that excluded other forms of lipomatous tumors. Of the initial 25 cases identified, comparative genomic hybridization (CGH) was uninformative in 2 cases; 5 were reclassified as WDL on the basis of molecular data (MDM2 amplification) and 6 as spindle cell lipoma (CGH profiles with a few gains and losses including a constant loss of chromosome 13 and frequent losses of chromosomes 16 and 6). The 12 remaining cases showed flat CGH profiles; of these cases, 11 were negative for *DDIT3* gene rearrangements, and 1 result was uninterpretable. Patients ranged in age from 15 to 82 years (mean 50 y); male patients were affected slightly more often (7:5). Tumors arose in the deep (6) and superficial (3) soft tissue of the groin (4), buttock (3), thigh (2), flank (1), shoulder (1), and paratesticular tissue (1) and ranged in size from 2 to 20 cm (mean 7.5 cm). Clinical follow-up in 11 patients (9 mo to 20 y; mean 68 mo) showed no recurrences or metastases. As defined above, "fibrosarcoma-like lipomatous neoplasm" is a unique lipomatous tumor that should be distinguished from WDL/(low-grade) dedifferentiated

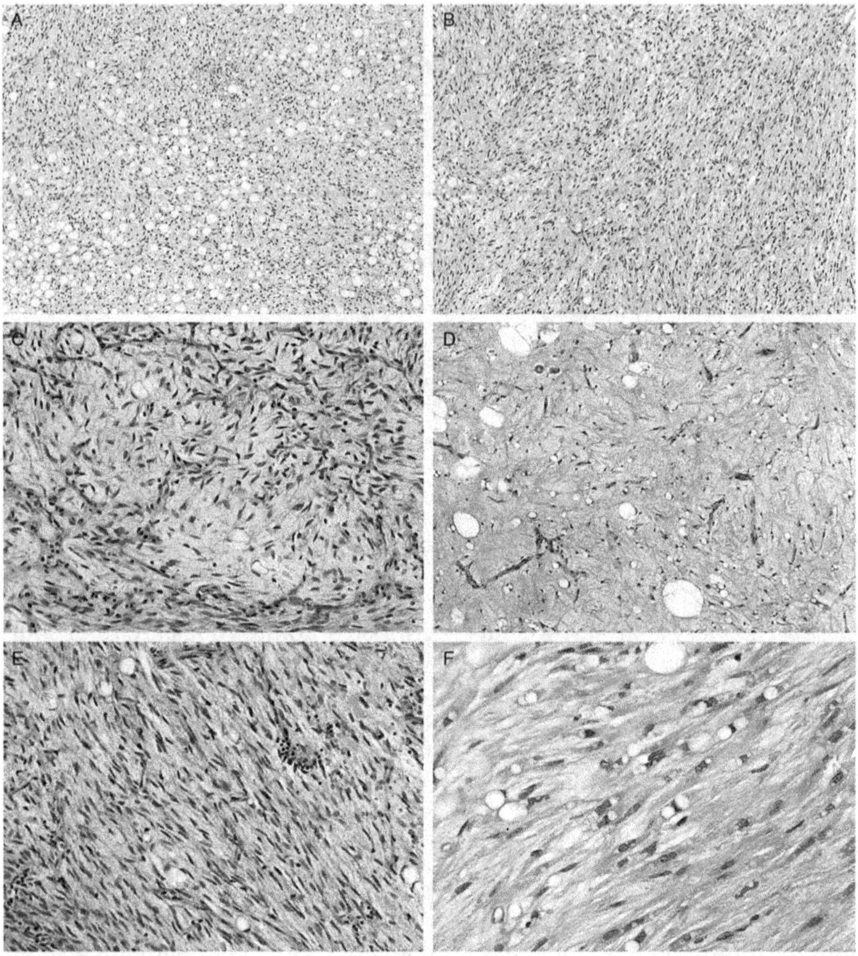

FIGURE 1.—Microscopic appearance of fibrosarcoma-like lipomatous tumor. Tumors were composed of slender bipolar spindled cells resembling fibroblasts and arranged parallel to one another with a spectrum of lipoblastic differentiation (A and B) and loosely separated by a variably myxoid stroma with arborizing capillaries (C). D, Rarely, myxoid change was prominent. E, The least differentiated cells resemble preadipocytes with a symmetrically tapered shape and an elongated nucleus with finely stippled chromatin and no atypia. F, The more-differentiated cells showed a dominant vacuole that indented the nucleus (ice cream cone lipoblast) or 2 vacuoles resembling an hourglass. (Reprinted from Deyrup AT, Chibon F, Guillou L, et al. Fibrosarcoma-like lipomatous neoplasm: a reappraisal of so-called spindle cell liposarcoma defining a unique lipomatous tumor unrelated to other liposarcomas. *Am J Surg Pathol.* 2013;37:1373-1378, with permission from Lippincott Williams & Wilkins.)

LPS and myxoid LPS on combined histologic/molecular features because of its better prognosis (Fig 1).

▶ Deyrup and colleagues claim that a category described as fibrosarcoma-like lipomatous tumor is unique in the spectrum of spindle cell liposarcomas based on histopathologic features and molecular analysis (ie, flat genomic hybridization profile and negative for *DDIT3* gene rearrangements). Fig 1 shows some histopathologic examples of fibrosarcoma-like lipomatous tumor. Deyrup et al indicate that these tumors have a better prognosis. For the practicing pathologist, the better recognition of this entity could result in obtaining molecular testing to assist in the confirmation. For additional reading, see the reference list.[1,2]

S. Raab, MD

References

1. Mentzel T, Palmedo G, Kuhnen C. Well-differentiated spindle cell liposarcoma ('atypical spindle cell lipomatous tumor') does not belong to the spectrum of atypical lipomatous tumor but has a close relationship to spindle cell lipoma: clinicopathologic, immunohistochemical, and molecular analysis of six cases. *Mod Pathol.* 2010;23:729-736.
2. Bartuma H, Nord KH, Macchia G, et al. Gene expression and single nucleotide polymorphism array analyses of spindle cell lipomas and conventional lipomas with 13q14 deletion. *Genes Chromosomes Cancer.* 2011;50:619-632.

7 Female Genital Tract

Interobserver Agreement for Assessing Invasion in Stage 1A Vulvar Squamous Cell Carcinoma

Abdel-Mesih A, Daya D, Onuma K, et al (Juravinski Hosp, Hamilton, Ontario, Canada)

Am J Surg Pathol 37:1336-1341, 2013

Invasive squamous cell carcinoma of the vulva with ≤1 mm stromal invasion is classified as stage 1A. Cancer staging systems state that the depth of invasion should be measured from the epithelial-stromal junction of the adjacent most superficial dermal papilla to the deepest point of the invasive tumor. Measurement of the depth of invasion guides patient management. Even though this measurement is critical, no studies have reported the reliability among pathologists for determining the cutoff point of ≤1 mm stromal invasion in vulvar cancer. We assessed agreement among pathologists for determining whether a vulvar tumor is invasive, for the depth of invasion, and for tumor thickness. Forty-five cases of vulvar squamous cell carcinoma with a depth of invasion of ≤5 mm were chosen. Eleven gynecologic pathologists independently reviewed the slides and, for a subset of cases, pictorially recorded measurements on photographs. The number of cases that were reported as invasive by the 11 pathologists ranged from 21 to 44. The number of cases that were reported as showing a depth of invasion of ≤1 mm ranged from 7 to 27. Eight pathologists provided measurements for all lesions reported as invasive, the remaining 3 pathologists stated that they were unable to measure 2, 7, and 16 lesions, respectively. Mean κ for diagnosing vulvar carcinoma as invasive was 0.24 and for measuring the depth of invasion and thickness was 0.51 and 0.49, respectively. There was only fair agreement in determining whether the lesion was invasive. In cases in which pathologists agreed upon the diagnosis of invasion, agreement on depth was moderate. When using the recommended cancer staging method, interpretation of the location of the most superficial dermal papilla varied among pathologists. Measuring thickness did not improve agreement. This is the first study that has assessed the reliability of the diagnosis of invasion in vulvar cancer among gynecologic pathologists, the interobserver agreement for reporting the critical 1 mm threshold of depth of stromal invasion, and the way in which the International Federation of Gynecology and Obstetrics method is used by pathologists (Figs 2 and 3).

▶ Determining the presence or absence of invasion as well as the depth of invasion in squamous cell carcinoma of the vulva critically impacts tumor staging and

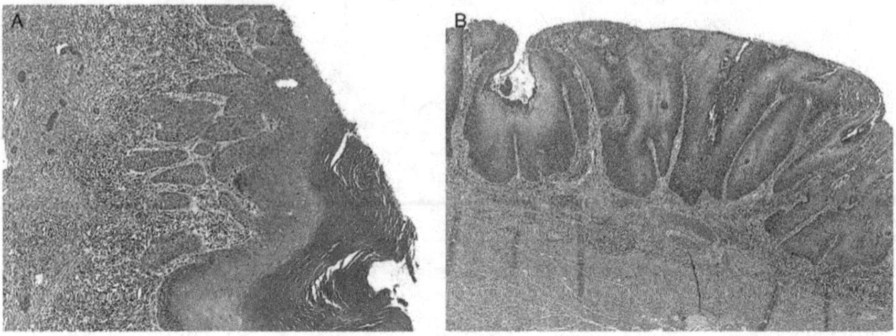

FIGURE 2.—Examples of 2 cases in which pathologists differed in their interpretation of whether stromal invasion was present. A, 7 pathologists diagnosed the case as invasive, 3 pathologists as noninvasive, and 1 pathologist as undecided (H&E stain). B, 4 pathologists diagnosed the case as invasive, 6 pathologists as noninvasive, and 1 pathologist as undecided (H&E stain). H&E indicates hematoxylin and eosin. (Reprinted from Abdel-Mesih A, Daya D, Onuma K, et al. Interobserver agreement for assessing invasion in stage 1A vulvar squamous cell carcinoma. *Am J Surg Pathol.* 2013;37:1336-1341, with permission from Lippincott Williams & Wilkins.)

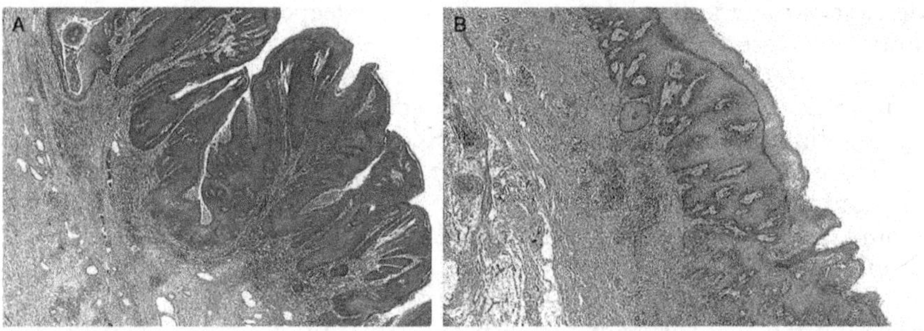

FIGURE 3.—Examples of 2 cases in which the depth of stromal invasion was reported as ≤1 mm and >1 mm by different pathologists (H&E stain). A, 4 pathologists diagnosed invasion as >1 mm, and 4 pathologists diagnosed invasion as ≤1 mm. B, 3 pathologists diagnosed invasion as >1 mm, and 6 pathologists diagnosed invasion as ≤1 mm. H&E indicates hematoxylin and eosin. (Reprinted from Abdel-Mesih A, Daya D, Onuma K, et al. Interobserver agreement for assessing invasion in stage 1A vulvar squamous cell carcinoma. *Am J Surg Pathol.* 2013;37:1336-1341, with permission from Lippincott Williams & Wilkins.)

thus clinical treatment. The American Joint Committee on Cancer defines a stage 1A vulvar squamous cell carcinoma as a lesion that is 1 cm or less in size and with stromal invasion of 1 mm or less. Squamous lesions that are 2 cm or less in size but have a depth of invasion greater than 1 mm are stage 1B. Based on AJCC and International Federation of Gynecology and Obstetrics (FIGO) criteria, depth of invasion is to be measured from the adjacent most superficial dermal papilla to the deepest point of invasion. Stage is a critical distinction because patients with stage 1B lesions have a higher rate of lymph node metastasis[1] and as such are treated with wide local excision plus lymph node dissection, whereas stage 1A lesions are treated with wide local excision only. In this article, the authors examined 45 cases of vulvar squamous cell carcinoma with a depth of invasion of ≤5 mm, a diagnosis that has previously been reported as having excellent interobserver agreement.[2] These cases were then reviewed independently by 11 gynecologic pathologists who assessed for presence or absence of invasion as well as depth of invasion. None of these measures turned out to be straightforward, as there was variability on a number of cases (Figs 2 and 3). The average interobserver agreement on the presence or absence of invasion for each lesion was only fair ($\kappa = 0.24$) and agreement on the depth of invasion as ≤ 1 mm was only moderate ($\kappa = 0.51$). When analyzing only the lesions that were agreed to be invasive, the agreement on depth of invasion improved to substantial ($\kappa = 0.67$). Additionally, the authors found that there was variability in the pathologists' determinations of what constituted the "adjacent most superficial dermal papilla" used for measuring the depth of invasion. These findings suggest that there is a need for improvement in the histologic criteria for the presence of invasion as well as a need for clarification of the FIGO method for measuring depth of invasion.

M. C. O'Keefe, MD

References

1. Oonk MH, Hollema H, de Hullu JA, et al. Prediction of lymph node metastases in vulvar cancer: a review. *Int J Gynecol Cancer.* 2006;16:963-971.
2. Yoder BJ, Rufforny I, Massoll NA, et al. Stage IA vulvar squamous cell carcinoma: an analysis of tumor invasive characteristics and risk. *Am J Surg Pathol.* 2008;32: 765-772.

A comparison of cervical histopathology variability using whole slide digitized images versus glass slides: experience with a statewide registry

Gage JC, Joste N, Ronnett BM, et al (Natl Insts of Health, Bethesda, MD; Univ of New Mexico Health Sciences Ctr, Albuquerque; The Johns Hopkins Univ School of Medicine, Baltimore, MD; et al)

Hum Pathol 44:2542-2548, 2013

Whole slide imaging is increasingly used for primary and consultative diagnoses, teaching, telepathology, slide sharing, and archiving. We compared pathologist evaluations of glass slides and corresponding digitized images within the context of a statewide surveillance effort. Cervical specimens collected by the New Mexico HPV Pap Registry research program targeted cases diagnosed between 2006 and 2010. Two samples of 250 slides each were digitized with the ScanScope XT (Aperio, Vista, CA) microscope and reviewed with Aperio ImageScope reader. (1) A "random set" had a distribution of community diagnoses: 70% from cases of cervical intraepithelial neoplasia grade 2 or higher, 20% from cases of cervical intraepithelial neoplasia grade 1 and 10% from negative cases. (2) A "discrepant set" was represented by difficult cases where 2 study pathologists initially disagreed. Within the regular workflow of the New Mexico HPV Pap Registry, 3 pathologists read the slides 2 to 3 times each without knowledge of clinical history, previous readings or sampling scheme. Pathologists also read each corresponding image twice. For within- and between-reader comparisons we calculated unweighted κ statistics and asymmetry χ^2 tests. Across all comparisons, slides and images yielded similar results. For the random set, almost all within-reader and between-reader Kappa values ranged between 0.7 and 0.8 and 0.6 and 0.7, respectively. For the discrepant set, most within- and between-reader κ values were 0.4 to 0.6. As cervical intraepithelial neoplasia diagnostic terminology changes, pathologists may need to re-read histopathology slides to compare disease trends over time, eg, before/after introduction of human papillomavirus vaccination. Diagnosis of cervical intraepithelial neoplasia differed little between slides and corresponding digitized images.

▶ This article attempted to determine whether whole-slide imaging (WSI) provides a viable alternative to glass slide review in the context of cervical histomorphology. The authors note that comparison studies of cervical biopsies over time will require extensive review of histology, as changing terminology and definitions somewhat alter the diagnoses that can be rendered. Because pulling glass slides from archives is time consuming and burdensome, they sought to explore the utility of the digital image review instead. The study should be considered a success in that in most instances there was substantial within-reader and moderate between-reader agreement with glass slides vs digital images. There was a slight tendency for lower calls on the digital images, particularly in difficult cases in which the readers had initially shown disagreement with one another or the initial interpretation.

This represents the largest study of its type thus far evaluating cervical histomorphology (500 cases), lending strength to the findings that overall there is good agreement between glass slide and image review. The authors note several limitations of digital review, however, including extensive up-front effort on the part of laboratories to develop a system of archiving and image viewing options, exceedingly long periods required for digitization of slides (described as many hours per 100 slides), requirements for reimaging in cases of inadequate capture on the first attempt (3%—5% for the registry utilized in this study), and a substantial learning period for pathologists who evaluate digital images. Despite these limitations, the field of pathology seems to be increasingly moving toward digitized images, particularly given their utility in evaluating cases remotely or from historical archives where retrieval of glass slides would take enormous effort. Having preliminary data suggesting that such a review shows consistency with the more traditional glass slide viewing supports additional efforts to make WSI a viable and perhaps ultimately more efficient alternative.

M. D. Post, MD

Cervical Squamocolumnar Junction–specific Markers Define Distinct, Clinically Relevant Subsets of Low-grade Squamous Intraepithelial Lesions

Herfs M, Parra-Herran C, Howitt BE, et al (Brigham and Women's Hosp, Boston, MA; et al)

Am J Surg Pathol 37:1311-1318, 2013

Low-grade cervical squamous abnormalities (low-grade squamous intraepithelial lesions [LSIL, CIN1]) can be confused with or followed by high-grade (HSIL, CIN2/3) lesions, expending considerable resources. Recently, a cell of origin for cervical neoplasia was proposed in the squamocolumnar junction (SCJ); HSILs are almost always SCJ^+, but LSILs include SCJ^+ and SCJ^- subsets. Abnormal cervical biopsies from 214 patients were classified by 2 experienced pathologists (panel) as LSIL or HSIL using published criteria. SILs were scored SCJ^+ and SCJ^- using SCJ-specific antibodies (keratin7, AGR2, MMP7, and GDA). Assessments of interobserver agreement, $p16^{ink4}$ staining pattern, proliferative index, and outcome were compared. The original diagnostician agreed with the panel diagnosis of HSIL and SCJ^- LSIL in all cases (100%). However, for SCJ^+ LSIL, panelists disagreed with each other by 15% and with the original diagnostician by 46.2%. Comparing SCJ^- and SCJ^+ LSILs, 60.2% and 94.9% were $p16^{ink4}$ positive, 23% and 74.4% showed strong (full-thickness) p16 staining, and 0/54 (0%) and 8/33 (24.2%) with follow-up had an HSIL outcome, respectively. Some SCJ^+ LSILs are more likely to both generate diagnostic disagreement and be associated with HSIL. Conversely, SCJ^- LSILs generate little observer disagreement and, when followed, have a very low risk of HSIL outcome. Thus, SCJ biomarkers in conjunction with histology may segregate LSILs with very low risk of HSIL outcome and conceivably could be used as a management tool to reduce excess allocation of resources to the follow-up of these lesions (Fig 1).

▶ The purpose of the study was to explore the clinical relevance of the recently proposed squamocolumnar junction (SCJ) cell as the origin of squamous intraepithelial lesions. These cells, located at the junction between the endocervical cells and the ectocervical/transition zone squamous cells, have a unique gene expression profile that can be detected using immunohistochemistry for keratin 7, AGR2, MMP7, and GDA. Based on previous studies, high-grade squamous intraepithelial lesions (HSILs) are nearly always positive for the SCJ markers, thereby implying SCJ origin, but low-grade squamous intraepithelial lesions (LSILs) may be either positive or negative (SCJ^+ or SCJ^-, respectively). After re-reviewing 214 cervical biopsies and staining them with the SCJ markers, the authors found nearly half (46.2%) of what they called LSIL had originally been classified as HSIL when these cases were found to be positive for SCJ markers; in contrast, no cases diagnosed by the expert panel as SCJ^- LSIL had originally been called HSIL. Between the 2 experts, there was originally a 15% disagreement for SCJ^- LSIL. In contrast, there was no disagreement between the reviewing pathologists for SCJ^+ LSILs. This shows the diagnostic heterogeneity for squamous intraepithelial lesions arising from the SCJ. That is, SCJ^+ (junctional) LSIL appears more closely linked to an HSIL than LSIL arising from the ectocervix/transition zone.

A minor weakness of this study is that whenever the reviewing pathologists disagreed, the disagreement was resolved by group review of the same 2 pathologists. A more rigorous approach would have included at least a third pathologist to lend a majority opinion. However, to counteract this potential bias, any follow-up biopsies of original LSIL cases were not considered high-grade unless the 2 pathologists agreed in their independent review. Additionally, disagreement

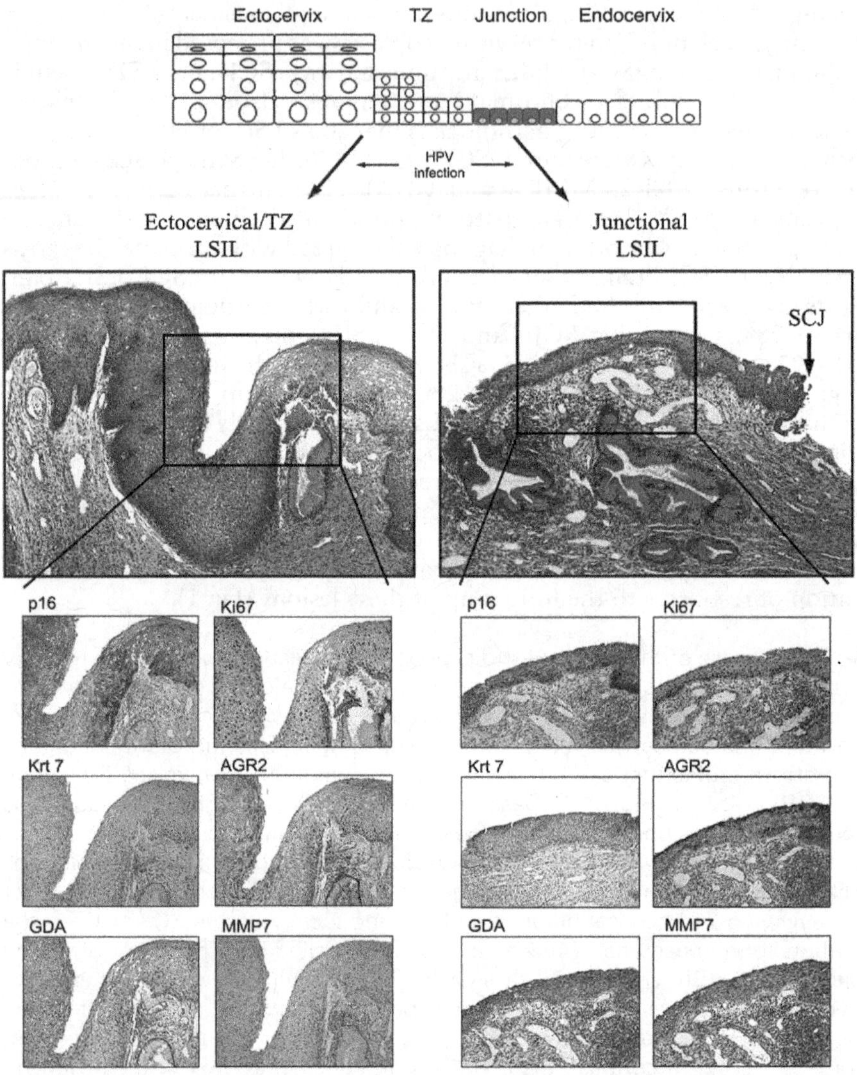

FIGURE 2.—LSILs (CIN1s) stained for p16^{ink4}, Ki67 and the SCJ-specific markers. A schematic showing proposed origin is at the top. Note the absence of staining of the ectocervical/TZ LSILs and uniform staining of junctional LSILs. (Reprinted from Herfs M, Parra-Herran C, Howitt BE, et al. Cervical squamocolumnar junction–specific markers define distinct, clinically relevant subsets of low-grade squamous intraepithelial lesions. *Am J Surg Pathol.* 2013;37:1311-1318, with permission from Lippincott Williams & Wilkins.)

between the 2 pathologists was quite rare; they agreed on an HSIL diagnosis in 96 of 97 cases and an LSIL diagnosis in 111 of 117 cases.

Immunohistochemistry for p16 and Ki67 as well as polymerase chain reaction (PCR) for HPV16 and 18 was performed to assess their concordance with histologic diagnoses. Only 1 of 39 (2.6%) cases of SCJ^{+} LSIL was found to have human papillomavirus (HPV)-8 (21 were HPV-16+), begging the question of whether different HPV types may have different tropism preferences within the cervical epithelium. There are, however, an insufficient number of HPV-18+ cases in this study to answer that question.

Review of follow-up specimens from patients with LSIL was performed to see which progressed to high-grade lesions. The authors found that 8 of 33 (24%) of SCJ^+ LSIL cases did show HSIL on a subsequent excisional procedure, whereas no SCJ^- low-grade squamous intraepithelial lesion cases did. A caveat is that nearly one-third of SCJ^- LSIL cases did not have follow-up information available.

Immunohistochemical markers for SCJ cells can reliably distinguish SCJ^+ SIL vs SCJ^- SIL (Fig 2). However, the authors make 2 critical points regarding the use of SCJ markers. One, positive SCJ markers along with positive p16 and positive HPV-16 PCR still cannot reliably differentiate between CIN1 and CIN2 and should not be used to decide whether to upgrade from a CIN1 (LSIL) to a CIN2 (HSIL) lesion. Second, the absence of SCJ markers in an LSIL lesion does not always confer a low-risk LSIL, as the rare SCJ^- LSIL will become high grade. This risk may be low enough, however, to justify reducing surveillance frequency for women who demonstrate SCJ^- LSIL, and additional studies are needed.

D. R. Olson, MD

Implementation of tumor testing for lynch syndrome in endometrial cancers at a large academic medical center

Moline J, Mahdi H, Yang B, et al (Cleveland Clinic, OH)

Gynecol Oncol 130:121-126, 2013

Objectives.—Lynch syndrome (LS) is a hereditary condition that increases the risk for endometrial and other cancers. Recognizing women at risk for LS based on personal/family history is burdensome and imprecise. Tumor testing using microsatellite instability (MSI) testing and immunohistochemistry (IHC) for mismatch repair protein expression can be an effective strategy for identifying potential LS in patients presenting with colorectal or endometrial cancer. Here we describe our experience implementing a screening program for endometrial cancers.

Methods.—Endometrial cancers diagnosed ≤50 years or those with suspicious personal history or histopathologic features were screened with MSI/IHC, June 2009–June 2011. Criteria were later (July 2011–July 2012) expanded to patients diagnosed <60 years, or at any age with suspicious features, and finally (after August 2012) universal screening was implemented. Screening techniques began with both MSI and IHC for every tumor, and later converted to IHC for two proteins, and *MLH1* promoter methylation analysis when indicated. A genetic counselor contacted patients directly to offer genetic counseling appointments.

Results.—Two hundred and forty-five endometrial cancers (average age, 57 years) were screened. Sixty-two patients (25%) had abnormal results, and 42 patients were referred for genetic counseling. Of the 42 patients,

34 underwent genetic counseling, 28 pursued genetic testing, and 11 were diagnosed with LS. When age and pathology criteria were used, 27 eligible cases were overlooked for screening and 3 cases of LS were found only because a clinician requested screening.

Conclusions.—Universal screening of endometrial cancers for LS is practical and successfully implemented with collaboration among genetic counselors, gynecologic oncologists, and pathologists (Table 3).

► The authors describe their experience implementing a screening program at the Cleveland Clinic for Lynch syndrome (LS) in women presenting with endometrial cancer. Although screening guidelines have been well established for screening patients with colorectal cancer for LS, they are lacking for endometrial cancers, despite the fact that approximately 50% of women with LS present with endometrial cancer as their first malignancy. Early studies suggested that screening should be reserved for women presenting at less than 50 years of age, but it has since been shown that most women with LS presenting with endometrial cancer are diagnosed after the age of 50. The authors used an evolving screening program that originally started with women diagnosed at ≤50 years of age or with suspicious medical history, but it became universal toward the end of the study period. This resulted in a total of 245 cases being screened, of which, 11 ultimately were proven or likely cases of LS (Table 3).

This changing screening protocol is both a strength and weakness of the study. It allowed the protocol to change in accordance with insights made by the genetic counselors, who noticed that 6 of 8 patients during the initial timeframe were older than 50 years when they were diagnosed with LS. Conversely, the universal screening protocol was only in effect for 5 months. As the authors point out, this short period is insufficient to develop a complete picture of the prevalence of LS in patients older than 60 years (which became the age cutoff during the first change of the screening protocol). Although LS testing originally included microsatellite instability (MSI) testing followed by immunohistochemistry (IHC) for all 4 mismatch repair proteins, the protocol changed to testing only for PMS2 and MSH6. If both are present, then all 4 proteins will be intact in at least 95% of cases. Although a high proportion, that still leaves up to 5% of false-negative cases. Testing for only 2 proteins does reduce testing costs but counteracts the utility of a screening program intended to detect all cases of the disease of interest. As a side note, from a genetic counseling perspective, IHC for proteins is preferable to MSI testing, as it pinpoints the missing protein immediately, as opposed to MSI, which simply indicates a protein may be missing.

For institutions looking to establish a similar universal screening program, the authors emphasize the necessity of a strong genetic counseling program (the study institution had same-day appointments and outreach clinics) as well as good communication of genetic counseling results or conferment with gynecologic oncologists.

The need for stronger LS screening guidelines in women presenting with endometrial cancer is clear, and this study makes progress toward establishing more helpful guidelines. Questions still remain about whether universal screening is truly needed or practical for smaller institutions or if an age cut-off beyond

TABLE 3.—Characteristics of Patients with Proven or Likely Lynch Syndrome

Patient No.	Age	Histology	FIGO Grade	Met Amsterdam Criteria	Met Revised Bethesda Criteria	Family History FDR	Personal History of Other Cancer	Met MSI/IHC Screening Criteria or Ordered	MSI	Absent MMR Protein	GC Visit	Genetic Testing Results
1	54	Endometrioid	1	No	Yes	Yes	Colon dx 42	Met criteria[b]	5/5	MSH2	Yes	MSH2 c.1012G > C p.G338R
2	55	Endometrioid	1	No	No	No	No	Ordered	5/5	MSH2	Yes	No mutation in MSH2, EPCAM, or MSH6
3	49	Endometrioid	3	No	No	No	TCC bladder dx 49	Met criteria	ND	MSH2/MSH6	Yes	No mutation in MSH2, EPCAM, or MSH6
4	55	Mixed serous/ endometrioid	High	No	No	Yes	No	Met criteria	4/5	MLH1(eq)/ PMS2	Yes	PMS2 c.2113G > A p.E705K
5	59	Endometrioid	3	No	No[c]	No	Colon dx 61	Met criteria	5/5	MLH1/PMS2	No[a]	MLH1 exon 16–19 del
6	55	Endometrioid	1	No	No	No	No	Met criteria	ND	MSH2/MSH6	Yes	No mutation in MSH2, EPCAM, or MSH6
7	56	Endometrioid	3	No	No	Yes	No	Ordered	0/5	MSH6	Yes	MSH6 c.1176_ 1178delTGCinsGGAA
8	50	Mixed endometrioid/ clear cell	High	Yes	No	Yes	No	Met criteria	ND	MLH1/PMS2	Yes	MLH1 c.1489delC
9	45	Endometrioid	2	No	No	No	No	Met criteria	ND	PMS2	Yes	PMS2 c.861_864delACAG
10	45	Endometrioid	1	No	No[c]	Yes	Rectal dx 46	Met criteria	ND	MSH2/MSH6	No[a]	MSH2 exon 8 del
11	60	Endometrioid	1	No	No	No	No	Met criteria	ND	MSH2(eq)/ MSH6	Yes	MSH6 c.1421_1422dupTG

GC = genetic counseling; ND = not done; TCC = transitional cell carcinoma; eq = equivocal results.
[a]GC pursued after colorectal cancer diagnosis.
[b]Met screening criteria but initially missed by pathology and later ordered by surgeon.
[c]Met revised Bethesda criteria after second cancer diagnosis.

60 years would be sufficient, and further large-scale studies are needed as practice evolves.

D. R. Olson, MD

Histologic and Immunohistochemical Analyses of Endometrial Carcinomas: Experiences From Endometrial Biopsies in 358 Consultation Cases

Wei J-J, Paintal A, Keh P (Northwestern Univ, Chicago, IL)

Arch Pathol Lab Med 137:1574-1583, 2013

Context.—Uterine serous carcinoma is biologically more aggressive than the endometrioid carcinoma. Because uterine serous carcinoma has a high propensity for lymphovascular invasion and intraperitoneal and extraabdominal spread, accurate diagnosis of this tumor type in endometrial biopsies/curettings is critical for appropriate clinical management.

Objective.—To share our experience in the evaluation of endometrial biopsy specimens in type I and type II endometrial adenocarcinoma.

Design.—We retrospectively reviewed 358 biopsies containing endometrial carcinoma during a recent 3-year period of our consultation records. In cases in which our interpretation differed from the submitting diagnosis, a panel of immunostains was performed. The performance characteristics of each antibody in our panel was calculated in this group of challenging cases.

Results.—Among the endometrial carcinomas we examined, a diagnosis of type I carcinoma accounted for 91% of cases (327 of 358) and type II carcinoma for 9% of cases (31 of 358); 41 cases (11.5%) were ambiguous or discordant (differing from submitted diagnoses and reviewed) based on histology alone. All 41 ambiguous and discordant cases were further evaluated with a battery of immunohistochemical markers. Of the 41 cases, 36 (88%) were ultimately classified (10 cases [24%] were endometrioid carcinoma; 18 cases [44%] were uterine serous carcinoma; 8 cases [20%] resulted in various other outcomes) and 5 cases (12%) remained indeterminate.

Conclusions.—Making the distinction between type I and II endometrial carcinoma remains a common problem in general practice. Although no one biomarker provides excellent statistical performance, a panel of immunohistochemical markers is often useful in difficult cases.

▶ Endometrial cancer is the most common gynecologic malignancy in the developed world, and it is increasing in incidence. Endometrial cancers are broadly divided into 2 histologic groupings: type 1, including endometrioid carcinoma (EMC) and variants, and type 2, including uterine serous carcinoma (ESC) and the more rare clear cell carcinoma and carcinosarcoma. Although EMC accounts for approximately 80% to 85% of uterine cancers compared with ESC (10%), ESC is more aggressive and more likely to present with extrauterine spread or lymphovascular invasion; it accounts for 50% of stage III or IV disease and 40% of all deaths from uterine cancer. This highlights how critical it is to accurately identify the histologic subtype on endometrial biopsy and curettage specimens so that clinical management can be appropriately targeted, as the management of ESC is more aggressive and often includes a combination of surgery, radiation, and chemotherapy, whereas EMC can often be managed surgically. Histologic features often make the distinction between these 2 cancers relatively straightforward; however, there is sometimes ambiguity in the diagnosis because of specimen size, histologic ambiguity, necrosis, or the tumor showing characteristics of both histologic variants. The authors show that in such cases, using a panel of immunohistochemical stains can help pathologists to render an accurate diagnosis. To assure reliability of the selected immunohistochemical markers, they reviewed the expression patterns in 56 well-characterized endometrial carcinomas (30 EMC, 26 ESC). They then reviewed 358 referral specimens of endometrial carcinomas. Of these, 41 (11%) showed discordance between their diagnosis and that of the submitting pathologist. For all 41 cases, immunohistochemical stains were performed for ER, PR, p16, p53, and vimentin, as well as certain others in select cases.

After staining, 36 (88%) were given a diagnosis (24% EMC, 44% ESC, 20% other), whereas the others (12%) remained uncharacterized. The authors found that none of the individual markers were sensitive or specific enough to be used alone in assessing these tumors. In particular, there is significant overlap in the staining patterns of International Federation of Gynecology and Obstetrics (FIGO) grade 3 endometrioid adenocarcinoma and ESC. However, they did find that this panel of markers in combination with careful histologic examination allowed them to classify 88% of the ambiguous results (Fig 3 in the original article). The authors note that in the future, molecular markers may be more valuable than immunohistochemical markers in distinguishing EMC from ESC. Different patterns of molecular alterations and mutations may be responsible for the different pathogenesis of these 2 cancers of the uterus. The most common genetic abnormalities in EMC are MSI as well as PTEN, β-catenin, PIK3CA, and K-ras mutations, whereas ESC typically shows p53 mutations and ERBB2 overexpression. Making an accurate distinction between EMC and ESC is essential for the patient's clinical management and outcome. For further reading, please see reference list.[1,2]

M. E. Quinn, MD

References

1. Ueda SM, Kapp DS, Cheung MK, et al. Trends in demographic and clinical characteristics in women diagnosed with corpus cancer and their potential impact on the increasing number of deaths. *Am J Obstet Gynecol.* 2008;198:218.e1-218.e6.
2. Lax SF. Molecular genetic pathways in various types of endometrial carcinoma: from a phenotypical to a molecular-based classification. *Virchows Arch.* 2004; 444:213-223.

Toward standard HER2 testing of endometrial serous carcinoma: 4-year experience at a large academic center and recommendations for clinical practice

Buza N, English DP, Santin AD, et al (Yale Univ School of Medicine, New Haven, CT)

Mod Pathol 26:1605-1612, 2013

HER2 overexpression and/or amplification have been reported in endometrial serous carcinoma, suggesting that HER2 may be a promising therapeutic target. However, there is considerable variation in the reported rates of HER2 overexpression and amplification, likely—at least in part—resulting from variability in the testing methods, interpretation, and scoring criteria used. Unlike in breast and gastric cancer, currently there are no established guidelines for HER2 testing in endometrial carcinoma. A total of 108 endometrial carcinoma cases—85 pure serous carcinomas and 23 mixed endometrial carcinomas with serous component—were identified over a 4-year period. All H&E and HER2 immunohistochemical slides were reviewed and HER2 FISH results (available on 52 cases) were retrieved from pathology reports. HER2 immunohistochemical scores were assigned according to the FDA criteria and the current breast ASCO/CAP scoring criteria. Clinical information was retrieved from the patients' medical records. Thirty-eight cases (35%) showed HER2 overexpression and/or gene amplification, 20 of which (53%) had significant heterogeneity of protein expression by immunohistochemistry. Lack of apical membrane staining resulting in a lateral/basolateral staining pattern was observed in the majority of HER2-positive tumors. Five of the HER2-positive cases (13%) demonstrated discrepant immunohistochemical scores when using the FDA *versus* ASCO/CAP scoring system. The overall concordance rate between HER2 immunohistochemistry and FISH was 75% (39/52) when using the FDA criteria, compared with 81% (42/52) by the ASCO/CAP scoring system. In conclusion, in this largest comprehensive study, 35% of endometrial serous carcinoma harbors HER2 protein overexpression and/or gene amplification, over half of which demonstrate significant heterogeneity of protein expression. The current breast ASCO/CAP scoring criteria provide the highest concordance between immunohistochemistry and FISH. Assessment of HER2 immunohistochemistry on multiple tumor sections or sections with large tumor areas is recommended, due to the significant heterogeneity of HER2 protein expression (Fig 2).

▶ Endometrial serous carcinoma represents an aggressive, chemoresistant malignancy. Identification of HER2 overexpression in these tumors may provide a therapeutic target, based on the success of HER2-directed therapies applied to other cancers. While well-defined HER2 testing guidelines have been developed for breast and gastric cancers, no such directives exist for endometrial serous carcinoma. The authors of this study aimed to characterize HER2 overexpression, identified by immunohistochemistry (IHC) and fluorescence in situ hybridization (FISH) to optimize guidelines for standard testing. Two gynecologic pathologists,

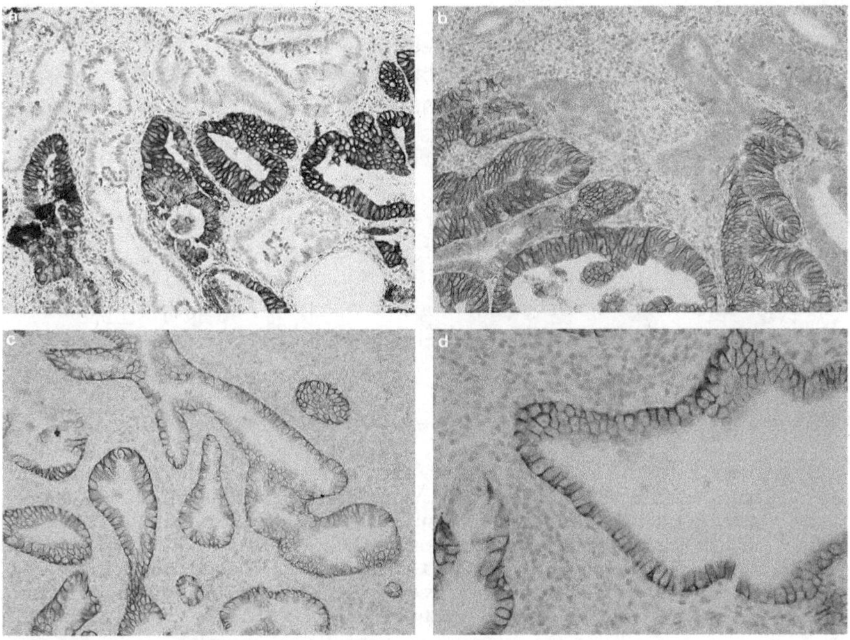

FIGURE 2.—Tumor heterogeneity and membrane staining pattern of HER2 immunohistochemistry in endometrial serous carcinoma. (**a, b**) Heterogeneous HER2 expression in serous carcinoma. (**c–d**) Lack of apical HER2 immunostaining results in a lateral or basolateral ('U-shaped') staining pattern. (Reprinted from Buza N, English DP, Santin AD, et al. Toward standard HER2 testing of endometrial serous carcinoma: 4-year experience at a large academic center and recommendations for clinical practice. *Mod Pathol.* 2013;1-8, Copyright 2013, by USCAP, Inc, http://www.nature.com/modpathol/.)

blinded to HER2 status, reviewed HER2 IHC slides from each case and assessed the percentage of tumor cells with complete and incomplete membrane staining, staining intensity, and staining heterogeneity. HER2 scores were then assigned according to 2 systems developed for breast cancer: the older US Food and Drug Administration (FDA) criteria and the 2007 The American Society of Clinical Oncology and the College of American Pathologists (ASCO/CAP) guidelines. A greater concordance rate between HER2 IHC scores and FISH was observed when using the ASCO/CAP criteria compared with the FDA criteria, but in contrast to most breast carcinomas, approximately half of HER2-positive cases showed heterogeneous HER2 protein expression by IHC. HER2-positive tumors with glandular or pseudoglandular architecture almost invariably lacked apical staining on IHC (at least focally), demonstrating so-called U-shaped or basolateral staining (Fig 2). Based on the above results, a number of conclusions can be drawn. First, although the ASCO/CAP guidelines provide better concordance between HER2 IHC and FISH, the rate is still below that which is reported for breast cancer, suggesting a need for criteria unique to cancers arising in the endometrium. Second, intratumoral heterogeneity of HER2 status is common in endometrial serous carcinoma, similar to gastric cancer but rare in breast cancer. Guidelines allowing for 3+ HER2 IHC score if any cell clusters show strong membranous staining, such as in the gastric cancer guidelines, may be appropriate for endometrial serous carcinoma. Also, tumor heterogeneity underscores the importance of adequate sampling when assessing HER2 status. Third, the FDA or ASCO/CAP guidelines do not address basolateral (U-shaped) staining pattern, which is a prominent feature in endometrial serous carcinoma with glandular architecture. The authors recommend a 3+ HER2 IHC score in tumors that stain strongly in this manner. This study shows the need for new HER2 scoring criteria specific for endometrial serous carcinoma. A system similar to that used in gastric cancer, which allows for tumor heterogeneity and incomplete membranous staining, may be more appropriate than the breast guidelines. There is not yet sufficient evidence that universal HER2 IHC should be performed on all endometrial serous carcinomas; however, additional research may offer further support for this approach. For further reading, see reference list.[1,2]

A. M. Richmond, MD

References

1. Singh P, Smith CL, Cheetham G, Dodd TJ, Davy ML. Serous carcinoma of the uterus-determination of HER-2/neu status using immunohistochemistry, chromogenic in situ hybridization, and quantitative polymerase chain reaction techniques: its significance and clinical correlation. *Int J Gynecol Cancer.* 2008;18:1344-1351.
2. Togami S, Sasajima Y, Oi T, et al. Clinicopathological and prognostic impact of human epidermal growth factor receptor type 2 (HER2) and hormone receptor expression in uterine papillary serous carcinoma. *Cancer Sci.* 2012;103:926-932.

The Pattern of Myometrial Invasion as a Predictor of Lymph Node Metastasis or Extrauterine Disease in Low-grade Endometrial Carcinoma

Euscher E, Fox P, Bassett R, et al (The Univ of Texas MD Anderson Cancer Ctr, Houston; et al)

Am J Surg Pathol 37:1728-1736, 2013

The purpose of this study was to examine predictors of lymph node (LN) metastases or extrauterine disease (ED) in low-grade (FIGO grade 1 or 2) endometrioid carcinoma (LGEC) in a multi-institutional setting. For LGEC with and without LN metastasis or ED, each of the 9 participating institutions evaluated patients' age, tumor size, myometrial invasion (MI), FIGO grade, % solid component, the presence or absence of papillary architecture, microcystic, elongated, and fragmented glands (MELF), single-cell/cell-cluster invasion (SCI), lymphovascular invasion (LVI), lower uterine segment (LUS) and cervical stromal (CX) involvement, and numbers of pelvic and para-aortic LNs sampled. A total of 304 cases were reviewed: LN^+ or ED^+, 96; LN^-/ED^-, 208. Patients' ages ranged from 23 to 91 years (median 61 y). Table 1 summarizes the histopathologic variables that were noted for the LN^+ or ED^+ group: tumor size ≥2 cm, 93/96 (97%); MI>50%, 54/96 (56%); MELF, 67/96 (70%); SCI, 33/96 (34%); LVI, 79/96 (82%); >20% solid, 65/96 (68%); papillary architecture present, 68/96 (72%); LUS involved, 64/96 (67%); and CX involved, 41/96 (43%). For the LN^-/ED^- group, the results were as follows: tumor size ≥2 cm, 152/208 (73%); MI>50%, 56/208 (27%); MELF, 79/208 (38%); SCI, 19/208 (9%); LVI,

TABLE 1.—Summary of Histologic Variables in Cases With and Without LNMs or ED

Variables	LN⁺ or ED⁺ (n = 96)	LN⁻ or ED⁻ (n = 208)
Tumor ≥2.0 cm	93 (97)	152 (73)
LUS involvement	64 (67)	77 (37)
CX stromal invasion	41 (43)	24 (12)
>20% solid	65 (68)	160 (77)
Papillary architecture present	68 (72)	122 (59)
>50% MI	54 (56)	57 (27)
MELF pattern invasion present	67 (70)	79 (38)
SCI present	33 (34)	19 (9)
LVI present	79 (82)	56 (27)

TABLE 3.—Multivariate Logistic Regression Results Modeling LNMs or ED

Variable	Odds Ratio (95% CI)	*P*
Tumor (per cm)	1.10 (0.97-1.24)	0.1505
LUS involvement	1.92 (0.96-3.87)	0.067
CX stromal invasion	3.15 (1.12-8.35)	0.0211
% solid component (continuous, per 1%)	0.99 (0.97-1.02)	0.6704
%MI (per 10%)	1.15 (1.02-1.30)	0.0280
MELF pattern invasion present	1.34 (0.64-2.82)	0.4422
SCI present	3.46 (1.56-7.67)	0.0022
LVI	4.92 (2.37-10.19)	<0.0001

CI indicates confidence interval.

56/208 (27%); >20% solid, 160/208 (77%); papillary architecture present, 122/208 (59%); LUS involved, 77/208 (37%); CX involved, 24/208 (12%). There was no evidence of a difference in the number of pelvic or para-aortic LNs sampled between groups ($P = 0.9$ and 0.1, respectively). After multivariate analysis, the depth of MI, CX involvement, LVI, and SCI emerged as significant predictors of advanced-stage disease. Although univariate analysis pointed to LUS involvement, MELF pattern of invasion, and papillary architecture as possible predictors of advanced-stage disease, these were not shown to be significant by multivariate analysis. This study validates MI, CX involvement, and LVI as significant predictors of LN⁺ or ED⁺. The association of SCI pattern with advanced-stage LGEC is a novel finding (Tables 1 and 3).

▶ This study sought to validate existing and identify new predictors of advanced-stage disease in low-grade (International Federation of Gynecology and Obstetrics [FIGO] grade 1 or 2) endometrioid endometrial carcinoma. The low incidence of lymph node metastases and extrauterine disease in clinical stage I, low-grade, endometrioid adenocarcinoma may obviate the need for lymph node dissection in all but a subset of these patients. This report helps identify the subset of patients who would benefit from surgical staging. The investigators reviewed cases of FIGO grade 1 or 2 endometrioid endometrial adenocarcinoma from 9 institutions over a 10-year period and classified the following histopathologic variables: tumor size, percent myometrial invasion, FIGO grade, percentage solid component, papillary architecture, pattern of myometrial invasion, lymphovascular invasion, lower uterine segment involvement, and cervical stromal involvement (Table 1). Although univariate analysis found multiple features to be significantly associated with lymph node metastasis or extrauterine disease, multivariate analysis showed only deep myometrial invasion, lymphovascular invasion, cervical stromal involvement, and single-cell/cell-cluster invasion (SCI) to be statistically significant independent predictors of advanced-stage disease (Table 3). A strength of this study is the breadth of material covered both in geographic variability and number of characteristics evaluated. A potential weakness is the inclusion into multivariate analysis of only those factors found to be statistically significant in univariate analysis, as such variables may become significant in a multivariate analysis. A number of conclusions can be drawn. First, the traditional risk factors of myometrial invasion, lymphovascular invasion, and cervical stromal involvement are valid, significant predictors of lymph node metastases and extrauterine disease. Of these, myometrial invasion is readily evaluated intraoperatively and may guide the decision to surgically stage a patient. Second, SCI is a novel predictor of advanced-stage disease and should alert the pathologist to take extra care when evaluating lymph nodes, as metastases associated with this pattern of invasion may be composed of only single cells. Third, it is noteworthy that the authors found no difference in the risk for lymph node metastases or extrauterine disease between FIGO grade 1 and 2 tumors, and continued to find no difference when FIGO grade 2 tumors were subdivided based on a 20% solid architecture threshold. These findings may favor a revision from a 3-tier to a 2-tier grading system for endometrioid endometrial adenocarcinoma. For further reading, refer to Akbayir et al[1] and Quick et al.[2]

A. M. Richmond, MD

References

1. Akbayir O, Corbacioglu A, Goksedef B, et al. The novel criteria for predicting pelvic lymph node metastasis in endometrioid adenocarcinoma of endometrium. *Gynecol Oncol.* 2012;125:400-403.
2. Quick CM, May T, Horowitz NS, Nucci MR. Low-grade, low-stage endometrioid endometrial adenocarcinoma: a clinicopathologic analysis of 324 cases focusing on frequency and pattern of myoinvasion. *Int J Gynecol Pathol.* 2012;31:337-343.

Prediction of lymph node and distant metastasis in patients with endometrial carcinoma: A new model based on demographics, biochemical factors, and tumor histology

Luomaranta A, Leminen A, Loukovaara M (Helsinki Univ Central Hosp, Finland)
Gynecol Oncol 129:28-32, 2013

Objective.—To develop a model that might predict the probability of lymph node and distant metastasis (stages IIIC–IV) in endometrial carcinoma.

TABLE 4.—The Capability of Various Risk Factors and Their Combined Score to Predict Lymph Node and Distant Metastasis in Endometrial Carcinoma

	AUC	*P* (Two-Tailed) vs. Total Score
Leukocytosis[1]	0.603	<0.0001
Thrombocytosis[2]	0.580	<0.0001
Elevated CA125[3]	0.721	0.026
High-risk histology[4]	0.636	<0.0001
Total score[5]	0.823	

[1]Leukocytes >8.2×10⁹/L.
[2]Thrombocytes >360×109/L.
[3]CA125 >35 U/mL.
[4]BMI <25 kg/m²; grade 3 endometrioid, clear cell, serous, undifferentiated, neuroendocrine.
[5](2×leukocytosis)+(3×thrombocytosis)+(7×elevated CA125)+(4×high-risk histology).

Methods.—We studied 774 patients with endometrial carcinoma treated in a single institution. Demographic factors, biochemical factors and preoperative tumor characteristics, identified as potential risk factors for advanced carcinoma in unadjusted analyses, were used to create a logistic regression model with lymph node and distant metastasis as the dependent variable. Statistically significant odds ratios in the regression model were rounded to the nearest whole number. These rounded values were the estimated weights for each factor that were summed to generate a score that might predict the probability of stage IIIC—IV carcinoma.

Results.—Biochemical factors and preoperative tumor characteristics predicted lymph node and distant metastasis in the regression model, whereas demographic factors were without effect. The score combining weighted risk factors was: (2×leukocytosis)+(3×thrombocytosis)+(7×elevated CA125)+(4×high-risk histology). The area under curve (AUC) for this total score was 0.823, with 71.6% sensitivity, 75.2% specificity, 25.9% positive predictive value, and 95.7% negative predictive value, using 6 as cutpoint. After excluding stage IV carcinomas from the dataset, the AUC was 0.813 for the total score in predicting nodal involvement ($P = 0.82$ vs. total score in predicting stage IIIC—IV carcinomas in the complete dataset).

Conclusions.—Based on the high negative predictive value, this prediction model could be applied for identifying patients who may not benefit from lymphadenectomy for endometrial carcinoma staging (Table 4).

▶ Endometrial cancer is the most common gynecologic malignancy in the developed world, and it is increasing in incidence. Currently, surgery is the mainstay of treatment, and traditional staging for endometrial cancers includes total hysterectomy, bilateral salpingo-oophorectomy, retroperitoneal lymph node dissection, and peritoneal washings. The necessity of lymph node dissection in patients with low risk of disease extension beyond the uterus is currently a topic of debate, given the risk of metastases weighed against the associated complications and morbidity of full node dissection. General practice is to perform a combined retroperitoneal and para-aortic lymph node dissection on women with intermediate and high-risk cancers, including grade 1 to 2 endometrial cancers in which lymphovascular invasion is identified, superficial grade 3 endometrioid and non-endometrioid carcinomas, and those with deep myometrial invasion. Current methods to assess myometrial involvement are transvaginal ultrasound scan and positron emission tomography/computed tomography (PET/CT), all of which have limitations and can be costly. Ideally, clinicians would be able to utilize a low-cost, predictive model to identify women who would (or would not) be good candidates for lymph node dissection to aid in the planning of surgical staging.

The authors evaluated demographic factors (age, body mass index, and endometrial thickness), biochemical markers (CA125, Hb, WBC, Plt), and pathologic features (separated as high risk and low risk) to create a model to predict the probability of lymph node or distant metastases (stage IIIC–IV). Their cohort included 774 women treated at Helsinki University Central Hospital. The high-risk pathology subset included those with grade 3 endometrioid, clear cell, serous, undifferentiated, and neuroendocrine tumors. Biochemical markers were based on the reference ranges for Finnish adult women. Only leukocytosis, thrombocytosis, elevated serum CA125 concentration, and high-risk pathology were significant independent factors influencing lymph node and distant metastasis. The predictive power of each variable was low, except for CA125, with an odds ratio of 6.5 (95% confidence interval, 3.7–11). However, by combining the features in a weighted fashion and performing regression analysis, the authors found a 95.7% negative predictive value for lymph node/distant metastasis (Table 4). This model could be helpful to determine preoperatively whether lymphadenectomy is appropriate or necessary. Given that the negative predictive value of other methods (magnetic resonance imaging, PET/CT) is no better, this is a cost-effective method with little interpretive variability that would be useful to gynecologic-oncology teams in planning the surgical staging of tumors in women who may not be good candidates for aggressive surgery.

M. E. Quinn, MD

Comparison of Current Staging Systems and a Novel Staging System for Uterine Leiomyosarcoma

Giuntoli RL II, Lessard-Anderson CR, Gerardi MA, et al (The Johns Hopkins Medicine, Baltimore, MD; Mayo Clinic and Foundation, Rochester, MN; et al)
Int J Gynecol Cancer 23:869-876, 2013

Objectives.—Uterine leiomyosarcoma (LMS) was traditionally staged by modified 1988 International Federation of Gynecology and Obstetrics (FIGO) staging criteria for endometrial adenocarcinoma. Contemporary methods of staging include the 2009 FIGO system for uterine LMS and the 2010 American Joint Committee on Cancer (AJCC) soft tissue sarcoma system. The aim of this study was to compare the accuracy of these 3 staging systems and a novel system in predicting disease-specific survival for patients with uterine LMS.

Methods.—Patients, evaluated at our institution with uterine LMS from 1976 to 2009, were identified. Stage was assigned retrospectively based on

TABLE 1.—Three Staging Systems for Uterine LMS

Stage	Modified 1988 FIGO Endometrial	2009 FIGO Uterine LMS	2010 AJCC Soft Tissue
I	Confined to uterine corpus	Limited to uterus and/or cervix	
IA		<5 cm	T1a or b, N0, M0, G1
IB		>5 cm	T2a or b, N0, M0, G1
II	Involves uterine cervix	Extends to pelvis	
IIA		Adnexal involvement	T1a or b, N0, M0, G2,3
IIB		Extrauterine pelvic tissue	T2a or b, N0, M0, G2
III	Positive cytology, serosa or pelvis involved		T2a or b, N0, M0, G3
	Retroperitoneal lymph nodes		Any T, N1, M0, Any G
IIIA		Invades abd (not just protruding) 1 site	
IIIB		Invades abd (not just protruding) >1 site	
IIIC		Involvement of pelvic and/or PA nodes	
IV	Involves bladder or rectal mucosa		Any T, Any N, M1, Any G
	Distant metastasis		
IVA		Involves bladder or rectum	
IVB		Distant metastasis	

Modified 1988 FIGO staging system for endometrial adenocarcinoma,[4] 2009 FIGO staging system for uterine LMS,[7] and 2010 AJCC staging system for soft tissue sarcoma.[9]

2010 AJCC staging system TMN classification for soft tissue sarcoma.[9] G, is grade: T, primary tumor: T1a, superficial tumor 5 cm or smaller; T1b, deep tumor 5 cm or smaller; T2a, superficial tumor larger than 5 cm; T2b, deep tumor larger than 5 cm. All pelvic sarcomas are classified as deep tumors. N is lymph nodes: N0, negative; N1, positive. M is metastases: M0, absent; M1, present.

Abd, Abdomen; PA, para-aortic.

Editor's Note: Please refer to original journal article for full references.

operative and pathology reports. Staging systems performance was compared using confidence indices.

Results.—We identified 244 patients with uterine LMS with sufficient information to be staged by all 3 systems. For each staging method, lower stage was associated with significantly improved disease-specific survival, $P < 0.001$. Patients with 2010 AJCC stage IA disease (low-grade, ≤5 cm) experienced no disease-specific deaths. We created a novel staging system, which used size and grade to stratify patients with disease confined to the uterus and/or cervix and combined the remaining patients with extrauterine disease as stage IV. Based on confidence index, the 2010 AJCC system and our novel system provided more accurate prognostic information than either of the 2 FIGO systems.

Conclusions.—Uterine LMS remains a clinically aggressive malignancy. Size and grade provided accurate prognostic information for patients with disease confined to the uterus and/or cervix. Patients with small, low-grade uterine LMS do not benefit from adjuvant therapy (Table 1).

▶ Uterine leiomyosarcoma (LMS) is a rare but highly aggressive sarcoma with survival rates of 20% to 60%. Given this wide variability and the question often raised about whether a particular patient will benefit from adjuvant therapy (as LMS responds poorly to most conventional chemotherapeutic regimens), providing a prognostically significant staging system is crucial. There are currently 3 separate systems in use (Table 1): International Federation of Gynecology and Obstetrics (FIGO) endometrial adenocarcinoma (1988), FIGO uterine LMS (2009), and American Joint Committee on Cancer (AJCC) LMS (2010). The predictive value of the 2 newer systems had not been directly compared, which this study attempted to do using disease-specific survival from diagnosis as the endpoint.

A total of 244 patients had sufficient data recorded for the authors to retrospectively assign stages in all 3 systems. Forty-one patients had a low-grade LMS, whereas the remaining 203 tumors were classified as high grade. Median greatest tumor dimension was 8 cm. A total of 157 (64%) patients had disease confined to the uterus or cervix. Ninety-three patients (38%, including 41 with localized disease) received postoperative therapy, including chemotherapy (49), radiation (41), or both (3). The authors constructed Kaplan-Meier curves to evaluate the influence of specific variables. The overall median disease-specific survival was 4.5 years, but a variety of factors were associated with longer survival, including lower grade, younger age, ovarian preservation, and smaller tumor size. Neither form of adjuvant therapy improved survival for those patients with disease confined to the uterus or cervix. The greatest differences in survival noted between the 3 staging systems was that stage I disease based on the 2010 AJCC system had significantly improved disease-specific survival, indicating that applying these criteria may allow for identification of patients who will do better. Across systems, both tumor size and grade were important prognostic variables, and these 2 elements should be considered mandatory for any reporting of LMS.

Based on their findings, the authors developed a novel staging system in which stages I to III apply to disease confined to the uterus or cervix, and stage IV encompasses all cases with extrauterine spread, as these cases are noted to have nearly uniformly poor outcomes. Lower stage correlated with better survival. Although the findings in this study may seem intuitively obvious and may make the creation of yet another staging system onerous, several important points are made. The authors point out the need for a simple system that incorporates prognostically significant elements. Each of the 2 most recent systems fails in this regard, as the 2009 FIGO system divides those patients with extrauterine disease into multiple categories (no prognostic significance) and the 2010 AJCC system has complex criteria, including division of high-grade tumors into grades 2 and 3. There is limited evidence that adjuvant therapy for primary disease is more effective than that given for recurrence, and the 100% survival rate for patients with low-grade tumors less than 5 cm indicates that they in particular likely do not benefit from postsurgical treatment. Adoption of any single staging system worldwide is a daunting challenge, but one that would allow for greater ease in effectively comparing patients with this rare disease, with the ultimate hope to offer patients the most effective and evidence-based therapy and prognosis for their particular disease. For additional reading, refer to Zivanovic et al[1] and Hensley et al.[2]

M. D. Post, MD

References

1. Zivanovic O, Leitao MM, Iasonos A, et al. Stage-specific outcomes of patients with uterine leiomyosarcoma: a comparison of the international federation of gynecology and obstetrics and american joint committee on cancer staging systems. *J Clin Oncol.* 2009;27:2066-2072.
2. Hensley ML, Ishill N, Soslow R, et al. Adjuvant gemcitabine plus docetaxel for completely resected stages I-IV high grade uterine leiomyosarcoma: results of a prospective study. *Gynecol Oncol.* 2009;112:563-567.

Endometrial Stromal Sarcomas With Sex Cord Differentiation Are Associated With *PHF1* Rearrangement

D'Angelo E, Ali RH, Espinosa I, et al (Univ of Barcelona, Spain; Univ of British Columbia, Vancouver, Canada; et al)
Am J Surg Pathol 37:514-521, 2013

Endometrial stromal tumors may pose diagnostic challenges particularly when they exhibit variant histologic appearances, involve extrauterine sites, or present as metastatic disease. In such cases, use of immunohistochemical markers and identification of specific nonrandom chromosomal rearrangements may be helpful. Over the last decade, fluorescence in situ hybridization (FISH) has been progressively incorporated as a diagnostic tool for the evaluation of endometrial stromal tumors. The purpose of this study was to review a series of these tumors and compare the results of FISH analysis with the clinicopathologic characteristics. Three endometrial stromal nodules (ESNs), 13 endometrial stromal sarcomas (ESSs), and 7 undifferentiated endometrial sarcomas (UESs) were reviewed. Three metastases from 1 of the ESS cases were also analyzed. Nine of these tumors (1 ESN, 8 ESSs, and 1 UES) exhibited unusual histologic features, including smooth muscle (3), sex cord (7), epithelioid (1), fibromyxoid (1), and skeletal muscle (2) differentiation. A tissue microarray was prepared, and FISH analysis was performed using break-apart and fusion probes for *JAZF1, SUZ12, EPC1*, and *PHF1* genes. FISH was successful in 22 cases, and rearrangements involving *JAZF1, SUZ12, EPC1*, and *PHF1* genes were detected in 10 of the 22 (45%) uterine tumors, including 2 of the 3 ESNs and 8 of 12 ESSs. Genetic rearrangements were found neither in the 3 metastases of the ESS nor in any of the UESs. It is noteworthy that a correlation between sex cord differentiation and *PHF1* rearrangement was encountered in ESSs ($P = 0.008$). In our series, all ESSs showing sex cords had *PHF1* genetic rearrangement, suggesting that such rearrangements may induce sex cord differentiation (Fig 1).

► Endometrial stromal tumors (ESTs) may present with several histologic variants, creating diagnostic challenges. The last decade has seen a development in the identification of specific chromosomal alterations characteristic of these stromal tumors; however, our understanding of the link between genotype and phenotype is still evolving. The authors of this study investigated the frequency of 4 gene rearrangements (*JAZF1, SUZ12, EPC1*, and *PHF1*) in 26 ESTs with

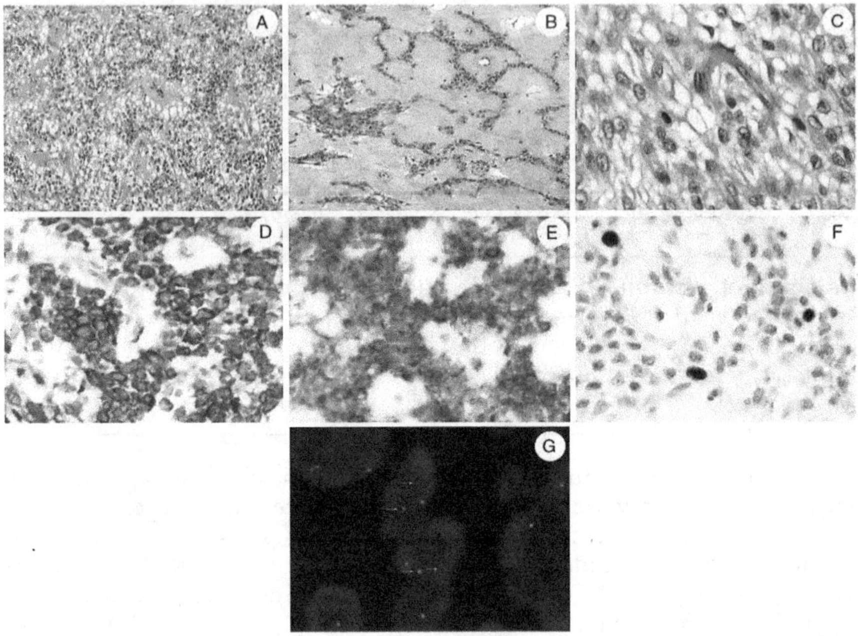

FIGURE 1.—ESS with sex cord–like and fibromyxoid differentiation. A, The medium-sized tumor cells are distributed in anastomosing cords and show round to oval nuclei with eosinophilic cytoplasms. The cords are intersected by fibromyxoid stroma. B, Elongated cords of tumor cells separated by hyalinized fibrous stroma. C, The tumor cells exhibit only mild nuclear atypia. An MF is seen. D, Strong caldesmon immunoreaction. E, Strong CD10 immunoreaction. F, Low Ki67 index. G, PHF1 rearrangement by break-apart FISH assay (green centromeric and red telomeric PHF1 probes). The presence of separate green and red signals indicates rearrangement in this region (arrows). For Interpretation of the references to color in this figure legend, the reader is referred to web version of this article. (Reprinted from D'Angelo E, Ali RH, Espinosa I, et al. Endometrial stromal sarcomas with sex cord differentiation are associated with PHF1 rearrangement. *Am J Surg Pathol.* 2013;37:514-521, with permission from Lippincott Williams & Wilkins.)

several histologic variations from those phenotypes most commonly seen. Fluorescence in situ hybridization (FISH) analysis found rearrangements in 33% of endometrial stromal nodules (ESNs) and 54% of endometrial stromal sarcomas (ESSs). Notably, the authors found a significant correlation between sex cord differentiation and *PHF1* gene rearrangement. In fact, all ESTs in the study with sex cord–like histology harbored a *PHF1* genetic rearrangement, suggesting its role in the induction of sex cord differentiation in ESTs (Fig 1). This finding supports the utility of FISH in the diagnosis of these tumors. To highlight this point, the authors provided 2 examples of ESSs with sex cord differentiation that were originally diagnosed as a leiomyosarcoma and uterine tumor resembling ovarian sex cord tumor. In both cases, immunohistochemistry results were misleading or limited, and it was not until FISH found a *PHF1* rearrangement that the tumors were reclassified. This report provides compelling evidence supporting the role of FISH in the diagnosis of ESTs. However, the study is limited by a small sample size. Further research is warranted before this application of FISH is used in day-to-day practice. In addition to serving as an ancillary tool for diagnosis, molecular markers may also shed light on prognosis. The authors mention a recently described genetic fusion, YWHAE-FAM22A/B, present in ESSs that behave more aggressively than the *JAZF1*-rearranged ESSs. These aggressive ESSs have a higher histologic grade, but do not have features of undifferentiated endometrial sarcomas. The authors postulated that they likely represent the old "high-grade ESS," a classification that will be reintroduced in the new World Health Organization classification of tumor being published in 2014. As the molecular characteristics of ESTs are better defined, classification and diagnoses will become more accurate. For further reading, please see reference list.[1,2]

A. M. Richmond, MD

References

1. Micci F, Panagopoulos I, Bjerkehagen B, Heim S. Consistent rearrangement of chromosomal band 6p21 with generation of fusion genes JAZF1/PHF1 and EPC1/PHF1 in endometrial stromal sarcoma. *Cancer Res.* 2006;66:107-112.
2. Huang HY, Ladanyi M, Soslow RA. Molecular detection of JAZF1-JJAZ1 gene fusion in endometrial stromal neoplasms with classic and variant histology: evidence for genetic heterogeneity. *Am J Surg Pathol.* 2004;28:224-232.

An Immunohistochemical Panel to Distinguish Ovarian From Uterine Serous Papillary Carcinomas

Zhang Y, Garcia-Buitrago MT, Koru-Sengul T, et al (Univ of Miami-Jackson Memorial Hosp, FL)

Int J Gynecol Pathol 32:476-481, 2013

Serous papillary carcinomas (SPCs) share a similar morphology regardless of whether they originate from the ovary or the uterus. Identification of the site of origin of the tumor can be a challenging and a diagnostic dilemma, particularly, in the setting of a pelvic mass or peritoneal carcinomatosis. Recognition of the site of origin influences the staging, management, and prognosis of these malignancies. The purpose of this study is to identify a panel of markers to distinguish the ovarian serous papillary carcinomas (OSPC) from the uterine serous papillary carcinomas (USPC). Formalin-fixed, paraffin-embedded archival tissue from 46 cases of SPCs (33 uterine and 13 ovarian) were stained using antibodies for estrogen receptor (ER), WT1, insulin-like growth factor-II mRNA-binding protein 3 (IMP3), p53, and p16. The OSPC expressed ER (92%), WT1 (100%), IMP3 (92%), p53 (92%), and p16 (92%). The USPCs expressed ER (30%), WT1 (64%), IMP3 (85%), p53 (64%), and p16 (76%). Only ER expression was significantly higher in OSPC compared with USPCs ($P < 0.001$). The combined ER^+WT1^+ phenotype was present in 92% of the OSPC, whereas only 18% of the USPCs had the same phenotype ($P < 0.001$). Furthermore, 71% of the OSPCs expressed ER^+, $p53^+$, $WT1^+$, $IMP3^+$, and $p16^+$ immunophenotype, whereas in USPCs, the tumor cells showed immunophenotypic diversity, with only 6% of the USPCs expressing reactivity to all the 5 markers ($P < 0.001$). This study

TABLE 1.—ER, WT1, IMP, p53, and p16 Expression in Ovarian and Uterine SPCs

	Case	ER (%)*	WT1 (%)	IMP3 (%)	p53 (%)	p16 (%)	ER+WT+ (%)*
Ovarian SPCs	13	92	100	92	92	92	92
Uterine SPCs	33	30	64	85	64	76	18

ER indicates estrogen receptor; IMP3, insulin-like growth factor-II mRNA-binding protein 3; SPC, serous papillary carcinoma.
*$P<0.001$.

suggests that ER alone or in combination with a limited panel of markers may be used to identify the site of origin of SPCs (Table 1).

▶ Serous papillary carcinoma (SPC) is a high-grade malignancy that can arise from multiple sites, including the uterus, fallopian tube, ovary, or peritoneum. Regardless of the site of origin, this is an aggressive malignancy and often presents with multiorgan involvement or pelvic carcinomatosis. Morphologic features of uterine SPCs and ovarian SPCs are similar, making the distinction between the 2 impossible based on histology alone. Identifying the site of origin has important implications for staging and prognosis. In this study, the authors sought to determine a unique immunohistochemical profile that would help distinguish uterine SPCs from ovarian SPCs. The authors selected 33 cases of confirmed uterine SPCs and 13 cases of confirmed ovarian SPCs. Immunohistochemical analysis for the following markers was then performed on each specimen: estrogen receptor (ER), WT1, insulin-like growth factor-II mRNA-binding protein 3 (IMP3), p53, and p16. Cases were scored as 0, 1, or 2 based on tumor positivity of 0%, less than 50%, or greater than 50%, respectively. ER was the only single marker that showed statistically different positivity between ovarian and uterine SPCs: 92% of ovarian SPCs were positive, whereas only 30% of uterine SPCs were positive ($P < .001$, Table 1). The remaining markers did not show statistically different expression as sole markers. Positivity in the entire panel of ER, WT1, IMP3, p53, and p16, however, strongly favored an ovarian primary tumor ($P < .001$). This suggests that this or a more limited panel of markers including ER may be useful in determining site of origin when the disease presents with widespread involvement. It is worth noting, however, that although this pattern may favor an ovarian primary, 2 of 33 uterine SPCs did show this pattern, so site of origin cannot be determined with absolute certainty based on immunohistochemistry alone. The authors state that uterine SPC expression of these markers is more varied than ovarian; however, the ovarian sample size is smaller, and with further study the spectrum of ovarian SPC expression may increase. The tumor scoring scale (0—2 based on percentage of tumor cell positivity) was not factored into the analysis in this report. It would be interesting to include these data in the analysis to see if the outcome was affected.

M. C. O'Keefe, MD

Hormone-receptor expression and ovarian cancer survival: an Ovarian Tumor Tissue Analysis consortium study

Sieh W, Köbel M, Longacre TA, et al (Stanford Univ, CA; Univ of Calgary, Alberta, Canada; et al)

Lancet Oncol 14:853-862, 2013

Background.—Few biomarkers of ovarian cancer prognosis have been established, partly because subtype-specific associations might be obscured in studies combining all histopathological subtypes. We examined whether tumour expression of the progesterone receptor (PR) and oestrogen receptor (ER) was associated with subtype-specific survival.

Methods.—12 studies participating in the Ovarian Tumor Tissue Analysis consortium contributed tissue microarray sections and clinical data to our study. Participants included in our analysis had been diagnosed with invasive serous, mucinous, endometrioid, or clear-cell carcinomas of the ovary. For a patient to be eligible, tissue microarrays, clinical follow-up data, age at diagnosis, and tumour grade and stage had to be available. Clinical data were obtained from medical records, cancer registries, death certificates, pathology reports, and review of histological slides. PR and ER statuses were assessed by central immunohistochemistry analysis done by masked pathologists. PR and ER staining was defined as negative (<1% tumour cell nuclei), weak (1 to <50%), or strong (≥50%). Associations with disease-specific survival were assessed.

Findings.—2933 women with invasive epithelial ovarian cancer were included: 1742 with high-grade serous carcinoma, 110 with low-grade serous carcinoma, 207 with mucinous carcinoma, 484 with endometrioid carcinoma, and 390 with clear-cell carcinoma. PR expression was associated with improved disease-specific survival in endometrioid carcinoma (log-rank $p<0 \cdot 0001$) and high-grade serous carcinoma (log-rank $p=0 \cdot 0006$), and ER expression was associated with improved disease-specific survival in endometrioid carcinoma (log-rank $p<0 \cdot 0001$). We recorded no significant associations for mucinous, clear-cell, or low-grade serous carcinoma. Positive hormone-receptor expression (weak or strong staining for PR or ER, or both) was associated with significantly improved disease-specific survival in endometrioid carcinoma compared with negative hormone-receptor expression, independent of study site, age, stage, and grade (hazard ratio 0·33, 95% CI 0·21–0·51; $p<0 \cdot 0001$). Strong PR expression was independently associated with improved disease-specific survival in high-grade serous carcinoma (0·71, 0·55–0·91; $p=0 \cdot 0080$), but weak PR expression was not (1·02, 0·89–1·18; $p=0 \cdot 74$).

Interpretation.—PR and ER are prognostic biomarkers for endometrioid and high-grade serous ovarian cancers. Clinical trials, stratified by subtype and biomarker status, are needed to establish whether hormone-receptor

TABLE 4.—Hormone-Receptor Expression and Disease-Specific Survival By Subtype

	High-Grade Serous Carcinoma		Low-Grade Serous Carcinoma		Mucinous Carcinoma		Endometrioid Carcinoma		Clear-Cell Carcinoma	
	Hazard Ratio	*P* Value	Hazard Ratio	*P* Value	Hazard Ratio	*P* Value	Hazard Ratio	*P* Value	Hazard Ratio	*P* Value
Progesterone-receptor expression										
Weak	1·02 (0·89–1·18)	0·74	0·53 (0·23–1·24)	0·14	0·69 (0·20–2·34)	0·55	0·61 (0·37–0·99)	0·047	0·81 (0·36–1·83)	0·60
Strong	0·71 (0·55–0·91)	0·0080	0·39 (0·18–0·86)	0·019	1·31 (0·50–3·45)	0·58	0·38 (0·22–0·65)	0·0005	1·13 (0·42–3·02)	0·81
Oestrogen-receptor expression										
Weak	1·08 (0·89–1·31)	0·44	1·18 (0··30–4·67)	0·81	1·33 (0·34–5·17)	0·68	0·40 (0·22–0·75)	0·0041	1·94 (0·97–3·88)	0·062
Strong	1·05 (0·89–1·24)	0·56	0·84 (0·24–2·92)	0·78	0·52 (0·23–1·21)	0·13	0·41 (0·26–0·63)	0·0001	1·11 (0·64–1·92)	0·72

Data in parentheses are 95% CI. Negative expression used as the referent value for all. Hazard ratios estimated with Cox regression stratified by site and adjusted for age, age^2, and stage (localised, regional, advanced) at diagnosis. We also adjusted for grade in models for high-grade serous carcinoma (moderately, poorly differentiated) and mucinous carcinoma and endometrioid carcinoma (well, moderately, poorly differentiated).

Editor's Note: Please refer to original journal article for full references.

status predicts response to endocrine treatment, and whether it could guide personalised treatment for ovarian cancer (Table 4).

▶ Ovarian cancer is the most lethal gynecologic malignancy in developed countries, causing more than 140 000 deaths per year. Although there are 5 distinct subtypes of ovarian carcinoma (high-grade serous, low-grade serous, endometrioid, clear cell, and mucinous), the importance of various markers, such as steroid hormone receptors, has been difficult to determine, as most studies combine the different histologic types. This study sought to utilize a large data set (2933 patients) from 12 participating groups to have a sufficient number of cases from each type to draw meaningful conclusions. The authors evaluated expression of estrogen receptor (ER) and progesterone receptor (PR) on microarrays composed of tumors from each type, which had patient information and survival data available. They classified expression as negative (< 1%), weak (1%–50%), or strong (> 50%). The outcome measure was disease-specific survival within 10 years of ovarian cancer diagnosis.

The 2 most striking and clinically useful findings of the study were (1) strong PR expression in high-grade serous carcinomas was associated with improved survival, independent of ER staining or clinical variables (site, age, stage, grade). Weak PR staining and ER staining did not have the same correlation. (2) Hormone receptor–positive endometrioid carcinomas (either weak or strong for either ER or PR) had better survival than those that were negative for both markers (Table 4).

There are multiple strengths to this study, most notably the proof that large-scale international collaborations are possible and lend dramatically increased power to findings. They performed the immunohistochemical analysis centrally, and all samples were evaluated by a blinded group of pathologists to ensure uniformity. Although misclassification of tumor subtype is a potential limitation, most tumors had their histologic type confirmed by a gynecologic pathologist, and ancillary studies done by the authors indicate that misclassification (particularly between high-grade serous and high-grade endometrioid) was unlikely to have affected the overall results. It is not yet known why endometrioid and high-grade serous tumors show improved survival in cases of positive hormone receptor status, although one thought is that these tumors may respond better to treatment. Their findings offer a convincing argument that pathologists confronted by ovarian tumors of either endometrioid or high-grade serous histology should perform ER and PR immunohistochemistry, as the results can have significant impacts on counseling of patients and identify those who might benefit from endocrine therapy. For further reading, see reference list.[1,2]

M. D. Post, MD

References

1. Modugno F, Laskey R, Smith AL, Andersen CL, Haluska P, Oesterreich S. Hormone response in ovarian cancer: time to reconsider as a clinical target? *Endocr Relat Cancer.* 2012;19:R255-R279.
2. Thomas C, Gustafsson JA. The different roles of ER subtypes in cancer biology and therapy. *Nat Rev Cancer.* 2011;11:597-608.

Pathologic Examination of Fetal and Placental Tissue Obtained by Dilation and Evacuation

Ernst LM, Gawron L, Fritsch MK (Northwestern Univ Feinberg School of Medicine, Chicago, IL)

Arch Pathol Lab Med 137:326-337, 2013

Context.—Dilation and evacuation (D&E) is an alternative method to induction of labor for pregnancy termination and intrauterine fetal demise, and it is the most common mode of second-trimester uterine evacuation in the United States. Many D&E specimens are examined in surgical pathology, and there is little information available in surgical pathology textbooks or the literature to assist pathologists in these examinations.

Objective.—To provide an overview of the D&E procedure, discuss related legal issues, provide guidelines for routine pathologic examination of D&E specimens, and demonstrate the importance of careful pathologic examination of D&E specimens.

Data Sources.—Case-derived material and literature review.

Conclusions.—Pathologic examination of D&E specimens has been understudied. However, the available literature and our experience support the fact that careful pathologic examination of D&E specimens can identify significant fetal and placental changes that can confirm clinical diagnoses or provide definitive diagnosis, assist in explaining the cause of intrauterine fetal demise, and identify unexpected anomalies that may provide further clues to a diagnostic syndrome or mechanism of anomaly formation (Tables 4 and 5).

▶ Over the last 4 decades, there has been a shift in the percentage of second trimester fetal specimens generated from the dilation and evacuation (D&E) method, which is utilized for women with cervical incompetence, intrauterine fetal death (IUFD), intrauterine growth restriction, genetic abnormalities, maternal health risk, or elective termination of pregnancy. Compared with 1974 when only 35% of second trimester abortions were managed by D&E, in 2005 this number was 96%. This increase is caused by an increasing number of practitioners trained in and offering D&E as well as women's preference for this over labor induction. Given the increase in D&E procedures, it is essential that surgical pathologists develop a systematic and standardized practice to assess these specimens, as the pathologic examination of D&E fetal and placental tissue can offer valuable information about the cause of IUFD, genetic abnormalities that may impact future childbearing decisions, and documentation or confirmation of abnormalities seen on ultrasound scan.

There is a paucity of information in the literature directly addressing the proper grossing of second trimester D&E specimens, and most of these specimens are dissected in surgical pathology and signed out by pathologists who do not usually perform fetal autopsies. The authors did an institutional chart review of 118 IUFD specimens and compared the findings by a perinatal pathologist with those of general pathologists, noting that significantly more abnormalities were found by the perinatal pathologists, including infection, maternal

TABLE 4.—Confirmation of Clinical Diagnosis by Pathologic Examination of Dilation and Evacuation (D&E) Specimen

Clinical Diagnosis	Possible to Confirm Diagnosis by D&E?	Other Comments
CNS		
Ventriculomegaly/hydrocephalus	Almost never	Look for adducted thumbs.
Holoprosencephaly	Almost never (brain)	Can find facial/midline anomalies that are consistent with diagnosis.
Polymicrogyria	Almost never	Can be seen on some intact brain fragments.
Dandy-Walker malformation	Almost never	
Anencephaly	Usually	
Genitourinary		
Renal agenesis	Usually	No kidneys found on examination is highly suggestive because kidneys are found in more than 90% of cases.
Cystic renal disease	Almost always	Nearly always confirmed and histology can be evaluated for diagnosis; should sample liver to rule out ductal plate malformation.
Lower urinary tract outflow obstruction	Usually	Usually find part of GU tract; if bladder is very large usually find disrupted portion of it and portion of ureters.
Cardiac		
Structural cardiac anomalies	Sometimes	Heart tissue frequently found, but complete examination possible in almost half of cases (44%).
Heterotaxy	Almost never	Situs of organs usually not easily established in D&E. Spleen found routinely in only 35% of cases, therefore when not found difficult to interpret. Heart defect can potentially be characterized.
Skeletal		
Ectrodactyly, polydactyly, other extremity abnormalities	Almost always	
Bone abnormalities/skeletal dysplasia	Usually	Radiographs required.
Neural tube defect	Almost always	Spinal defect almost always seen; characterization of sac usually not possible.
Other		
Cleft lip/palate	Usually	
Cystic hygroma	Sometimes	D2-40 stain may be helpful.
Congenital diaphragmatic hernia	Almost never	
Omphalocele/gastroschisis	Sometimes	
Pulmonary hypoplasia	Sometimes	Fragments identified should be weighed in aggregate.

Abbreviations: CNS, central nervous system; GU, genitourinary.

and fetal vasculopathies, growth restriction, hydrops, anatomic anomalies, and chromosomal abnormalities. This highlights the importance of adequate training in examination of these specimens. Most D&E specimens will be fragmented because of the procedure, so it is critical to have an understanding of what tissue to expect and to submit for histologic examination as well as some of the anomalies the pathologist should expect to identify (Tables 4 and 5). This report offers a comprehensive review of the standard of care for

TABLE 5.—Findings on Dilation and Evacuation (D&E) Examination Suspicious for Specific Genetic Abnormality

Genetic Abnormality	Finding on D&E
Turner sydrome (monosomy X)	Fetal hydrops, prominent dorsal edema of hands and feet, aortic coarctation
Trisomy 18	Overlapping fingers, rocker-bottom feet, polydactyly
Trisomy 13	Severe craniofacial anomalies, holoprosencephaly, midline cleft lip, abnormal skull base, polydactyly, splenopancreatic fusion, heart defects
Trisomy 21	Wide space between first and second toes, clinodactyly, single palmar crease, heart defects, duodenal atresia
Triploidy	3–4 syndactyly

examination of these specimens, including findings to seek on the pathologic examination, fetal tissues most commonly identified, findings suspicious for genetic abnormalities, and a sample D&E template for gross examination. The authors cite a 1995 study in which 37 D&E for fetal indication specimens were examined and major pathologic findings identified in up to 92% of the cases. A careful and systematic approach to D&E specimens will contribute to the clinical care of patients by offering information that may influence future family planning, contribute to genetic counseling, and offer answers to questions about IUFD. For additional reading, see reference list.[1,2]

M. E. Quinn, MD

References

1. Gamble SB, Strauss LT, Parker WY, Cook DA, Zane SB, Hamdan S. Abortion surveillance—United States, 2005. *MMWR Surveill Summ.* 2008;57:1-32.
2. Klatt EC. Pathologic examination of fetal specimens from dilation and evacuation procedures. *Am J Clin Pathol.* 1995;103:415-418.

8 Kidney

Epithelioid angiomyolipoma of the kidney: pathological features and clinical outcome in a series of consecutively resected tumors

He W, Cheville JC, Sadow PM, et al (Memorial Sloan-Kettering Cancer Ctr, NY; Mayo Clinic, Rochester, MN; Massachusetts General Hosp, Boston)

Mod Pathol 26:1355-1364, 2013

The 2004 World Health Organization classification of tumors defines epithelioid angiomyolipoma of kidney as a potentially malignant mesenchymal neoplasm with reported metastasis in approximately one-third of the cases. However, this conclusion was based primarily on individual case reports and small retrospective series. More recently reported larger series have shown varying results. We reviewed 437 consecutive renal angiomyolipomas with primary resection at three tertiary-care institutions with high nephrectomy volumes. Only tumors showing >80% epithelioid histology were included in this study. Tumors resected elsewhere and reviewed in consultation were not included. Twenty of these 437 (4.6%) were classified as epithelioid angiomyolipoma. The female to male ratio was 11:9, mean age 49.7 (range, 30–80) years, and mean tumor size 8.7 (range, 1–25) cm. Microscopic tumor necrosis was present in 10 (50%) tumors and mitotic activity (range, <1–5/10 high power fields) in 8 (40%); atypical mitoses were seen in only 1 (5%) tumor. Pleomorphic ganglion-like or multinucleated giant cells were seen in 18 (90%) tumors. With a mean follow-up of 82.5 (range, 1–356) months, seventeen patients were alive with no-evidence-of-disease at the time of last follow-up; two patients died of unrelated causes with no-evidence-of-disease, and one patient (5%) developed distant metastases. Our data, based on consecutively resected angiomyolipomas with long clinical follow-up, suggests that epithelioid angiomyolipomas constitute a small proportion of all angiomyolipomas, and the rate of aggressive behavior among epithelioid angiomyolipomas, even when showing morphologic features previously reported to portend aggressive clinical behavior, is very low.

► The goal of this study was to document the true incidence of epithelioid angiomyolipomas as well as comment on the potential correlation between adverse histologic features and aggressive clinical behavior. One of the unique aspects of this study was the use of 3 separate institutions to generate a high number of consecutively resected renal angiomyolipomas (N = 437). It should be highlighted that the cases represented primary resections, and any consultation material was not included in this review. One of the striking findings is the low overall incidence of true epithelioid angiomyolipoma accounting for less than 5% of all angiomyolipomas resected. Although there were numerous tumors that showed histologic features previously reported to be associated with aggressive clinical behavior, only a single case of the 20 identified actually behaved in an aggressive fashion. Given the results of this study, there are insufficient data at this time to make a correlation between adverse histologic features and clinical outcome. Thus, it may not be prudent to comment on these features, unless widespread, within surgical pathology reports.

For additional investigation, I refer the reader to Aydin et al.[1]

M. L. Smith, MD

Reference

1. Aydin H, Magi-Galluzzi C, Lane BR, et al. Renal angiomyolipoma: clinicopathologic study of 194 cases with emphasis on the epithelioid histology and tuberous sclerosis association. *Am J Surg Pathol.* 2009;33:289-297.

Synovial Sarcoma of the Kidney: A Clinicopathologic, Immunohistochemical, and Molecular Genetic Study of 16 Cases

Schoolmeester JK, Cheville JC, Folpe AL (Mayo Clinic, Rochester, MN)
Am J Surg Pathol 38:60-65, 2014

We report the clinicopathologic and immunohistochemical features of 16 cases of genetically confirmed primary synovial sarcoma of the kidney. The cases occurred in 9 men and 7 women ranging in age from 17 to 78 years (mean, 46 y). The tumors were grossly large, solid, and variably cystic (2.2 to 19.0 cm; mean 8.6 cm). Microscopically, all tumors were of the monophasic type and diffusely immunoreactive for TLE1 and BCL-2. Focal pankeratin positivity was found in just under half. Ten cases carried an *SS18-SSX2* fusion transcript, and 5 cases showed an *SS18-SSX1* transcript by reverse transcription polymerase chain reaction. The remaining case demonstrated *SS18* rearrangement by fluorescence in situ hybridization. Clinical follow-up information was available for 12 patients (range, 1 to 77 mo; mean, 32.5 mo). Fourteen patients underwent radical nephrectomy, and 3 patients had lung metastases at presentation. Six patients died of disease within 1 to 58 months (mean, 31 mo) of their diagnosis. Five patients were alive without evidence of disease 12 to 77 months (mean, 39 mos) after surgery. A single patient was alive with metastases to the spine 11 months after surgery. We conclude that renal synovial sarcoma is an aggressive tumor, with adverse patient outcome in >50% of cases. Synovial sarcoma must be distinguished from morphologically similar lesions of the kidney.

► This is the largest single-center study of primary synovial sarcomas of the kidney to date, as most of the past literature is based on single case reports. One of the stronger aspects of this investigation is the confirmation of the abnormal fusion transcript considered to be specific for the diagnosis of synovial sarcoma.

It is surprising that less than half of the cases showed focal pankeratin positivity. In this setting, you are dealing with a primary spindle cell neoplasm of the kidney, which is keratin negative, and, thus, there is a fairly broad differential diagnosis including solitary fibrous tumor, primitive neuroectodermal tumor, and sarcomatoid renal cell carcinoma, which often may also lose its keratin reactivity. One of the take-home messages from this article is that synovial sarcoma should be considered in the differential diagnosis for any spindle cell lesion of the kidney, even in the absence of keratin reactivity and molecular studies, as the translocation should be considered as part of the workup. The other benefit of this study is the presence of outcome data on 12 patients, which suggests primary renal synovial sarcomas are fairly aggressive tumors with a fairly poor prognosis.

For additional investigation see Iacovelli et al.[1]

M. L. Smith, MD

Reference

1. Iacovelli R, Altavilla A, Ciardi A, et al. Clinical and pathological features of primary renal synovial sarcoma: analysis of 64 cases from 11 years of medical literature. *BJU Int.* 2012;110:1449-1454.

Banff Initiative for Quality Assurance in Transplantation (BIFQUIT): Reproducibility of C4d Immunohistochemistry in Kidney Allografts

Mengel M, Chan S, Climenhaga J, et al (Univ of Alberta, Edmonton, Canada; et al)

Am J Transplant 13:1235-1245, 2013

Detection of C4d is crucial for diagnosing antibody-mediated-rejection. We conducted a multicenter trial to assess the reproducibility for C4d immunohistochemistry on paraffin tissue. Unstained slides from a tissue microarray (TMA) comprising 44 kidney allograft specimens representing a full analytical spectrum for C4d were distributed to 73 institutions. Participants stained TMA slides using local protocols and evaluated their slides following the Banff C4d schema. Local staining details and evaluation scores were collected online. Stained slides were returned for centralized panel re-evaluation. Kappa statistics were used to determine reproducibility. Poor interinstitutional reproducibility was observed (kappa 0.17), which was equally due to limitations in interobserver (kappa 0.44) and interlaboratory reproducibility (kappa 0.46). Depending on the cut-off, reproducibility could be improved by omitting C4d grading and only considering ± calls. Heat-induced epitope recovery (pH 6–7, 20–30 min, citrate buffer) with polyclonal antibody incubation (<1:80, >40 min) appeared as best practice. The BIFQUIT trial results indicated that C4d staining on paraffin sections varies considerably between laboratories. Refinement of the current Banff C4d scoring schema and harmonization of tissue processing and staining protocols is necessary to achieve acceptable reproducibility (Fig 4,Table 4).

▶ This is an important study, as it highlights the poor interobserver and interlaboratory reproducibility with respect to C4d immunohistochemical staining.

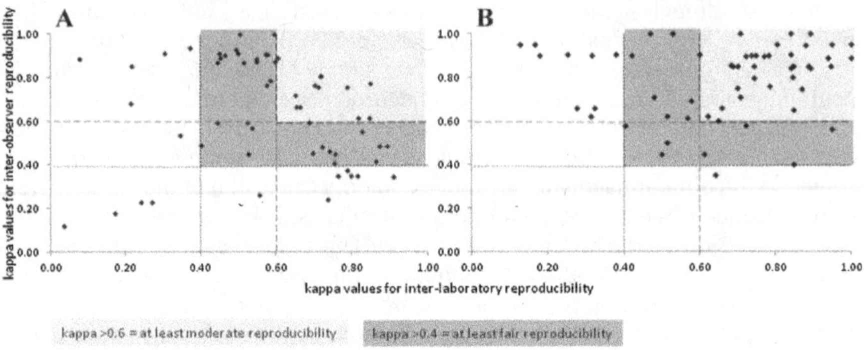

FIGURE 4.—Scatter plots showing the interlaboratory and interobserver reproducibility for each individual participant/participating laboratory using the Banff C4d schema (A) or positive versus negative calls (B; C4d0 vs. C4d ≥ 1). (Reprinted from Mengel M, Chan S, Climenhaga J, et al. Banff initiative for quality assurance in transplantation (BIFQUIT): reproducibility of C4d immunohistochemistry in kidney allografts. *Am J Transplant*. 2013;13:1235-1245, with permission from American Journal of Transplantation and John Wiley and Sons, www.interscience.wiley.com.)

TABLE 4.—Recommendations for C4d Immunohistochemistry on Paraffin Sections

Avoid under-fixation (<1 h) and/or ethanol fixation of tissue specimen
Use heat induced epitope recovery with citrate buffer at pH 6–7
At least incubate polyclonal anti-C4d antibody at a dilution of <1:80 for >40 min
Better results were observed with harsher pre-treatment (e.g. autoclave epitope recovery), higher polyclonal anti-C4d antibody concentrations (1:10), and longer incubation times for the polyclonal anti-C4d antibody (over night/12–16 h)
Refinement of the 2007 Banff C4d grading schema has potential to improve interobserver reproducibility

As for pre-analytical issues related to C4d immunohistochemistry, both a low fixation time (less than 1 hour) and ethanol-based fixation were significantly associated with poor reproducibility. Based on the protocols reportedly being used by the participating institutions, a summary of C4d immunohistochemistry recommendations on paraffin sections is given in Table 4. All pathologists who are involved in reading C4d by immunohistochemistry in kidney allograft specimens should compare their current protocol with the recommended protocol. Fig 4 highlights the improved κ values (>0.6 vs >0,4) when C4ds are evaluated as simply positive or negative vs C4d 0 compared with C4d ≥ 1. These findings help justify a potential refinement of the 2007 Banff C4d grading schema. C4d as an immunohistochemical marker is different than most immunohistochemical markers general surgical pathologists use in that it has the potential to directly impact medical therapy in the patients, similar to HER2/neu immunohistochemistry in mammary carcinoma. Although most pathologists are not in favor of more intensive regulations, it would not be unreasonable to at least have laboratories performing C4d by immunohistochemistry to be involved in some sort of external quality assurance program to be sure their stains are performing adequately. It should also be noted that these issues are not relegated solely to the kidney transplant population but also to the cardiac, pancreas, lung, and liver transplant cohorts.

M. L. Smith, MD

What do we know about adenovirus in renal transplantation?

Florescu MC, Miles CD, Florescu DF (Univ of Nebraska Med Ctr, Omaha)

Nephrol Dial Transplant 28:2003-2010, 2013

Adenoviruses are common pathogens that have the potential to cause opportunistic infections with significant morbidity and mortality in immunocompromised hosts. The significance of adenoviral infection and disease is incompletely known in the setting of kidney transplantation. Reported adenovirus infections in renal transplant recipients have typically manifested as hemorrhagic cystitis and tubulointerstitial nephritis, less severe diseases than often seen in other solid organ transplant recipients (i.e. pneumonia, hepatitis and enteritis). The prevalent adenovirus subgroups associated with cystitis and nephritis are B1 and B2 with the serotypes 7, 11, 34, 35. However, disseminated or severe adenovirus infections, including fatal cases, have been described in renal transplant recipients. There is uncertainty regarding monitoring of and treatment of this virus. Although not supported by randomized clinical trials, cidofovir is used for the treatment of adenovirus disease not responding to reduction of immunosuppression (Fig 1).

► It is very important to remember adenovirus in the differential diagnosis of tubulointerstitial nephritis in the renal transplant setting. Although productive adenovirus infection within renal allografts is rare, the infectious etiology and histologic overlap with acute cellular rejection makes it important to direct treatment toward antiviral medications as opposed to increased immunosuppression. In our

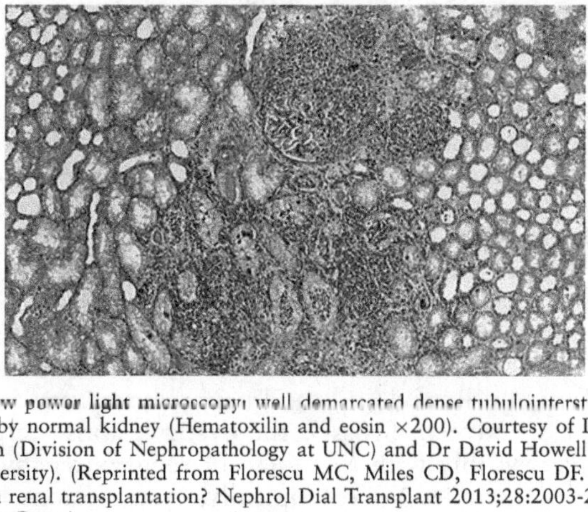

FIGURE 1. Low power light microscopy: well demarcated dense tubulointerstitial nephritis in the center, surrounded by normal kidney (Hematoxilin and eosin ×200). Courtesy of Dr Volker Nickeleit, Dr Harsharan Singh (Division of Nephropathology at UNC) and Dr David Howell (Pathology Department at Duke University). (Reprinted from Florescu MC, Miles CD, Florescu DF. What do we know about adenovirus in renal transplantation? Nephrol Dial Transplant 2013;28:2003-2010, by permission of Oxford University Press.)

experience, productive adenovirus infection within the renal allografts shows relatively distinct low-power morphology of exquisitely tubulocentric-based inflammation with excessive necrosis of the tubular epithelial cells, bordering on granulomatous inflammation (Fig 1). It is the tubulocentric inflammation and necrosis that helps separate this type of tubulointerstitial inflammation from acute cellular rejection. Other potential entities in the differential diagnosis include other viral infections, such as polyomavirus infection and fungal infections, and potentially an adverse drug reaction. Plasma cells and neutrophils are more commonly seen in polyomavirus infection, and necrosis is rare.

For additional investigation, I refer the reader to Ison et al.[1]

M. L. Smith, MD

Reference

1. Ison MG, Green M, AST Infectious Diseases Community of Practice. AST infectious diseases community of practice. adenovirus in solid organ transplant recipients. *Am J Transplant.* 2009;9:S161-S165.

Localized Cystic Disease of the Kidney: Distinction from Cystic Neoplasms and Hereditary Polycystic Diseases

Ding Y, Chen L, Deng F-M, et al (New York Univ Langone Med Ctr; Cleveland Clinic, OH; et al)

Am J Surg Pathol 37:506-513, 2013

Cystic changes are common in both neoplastic and non-neoplastic kidney diseases. The most important diagnostic consideration is to rule out cystic neoplasms and hereditary polycystic kidney disease for patient management. Localized cystic disease of the kidney is a rare, nongenetic and nonprogressive cystic disease that may mimic cystic neoplasms or hereditary polycystic disease. However, reports in the literature on its pathologic characteristics are scarce, and most surgical pathologists are unfamiliar with this entity. We report the clinicopathologic characteristics of 9 such cases that mimicked renal neoplasms and were treated surgically. Nine patients, including 5 men and 4 women, had a mean age of 33.3 years (range, 18 to 56 y) at diagnosis. Two patients presented with gross hematuria. In the remaining 7 patients, localized cystic disease was discovered incidentally. None had a personal history of cystic disease of the kidney or other organs or a family history of cystic renal disease. On imaging studies, solitary multilocular cystic lesions were identified in all patients with a mean size of 2.9 cm (range, 0.8 to 6 cm). Of 7 patients with documented Bosniak classification, 4 lesions were class III, and 3 lesions were class II. Follow-up was available in 5 patients, with a mean follow-up time of 14.6 months (range, 5 to 31 mo). No cysts were observed in the ipsilateral and contralateral kidneys during follow-up. Partial and total nephrectomy was performed in 8 and 1 patient, respectively. Grossly, the cystic lesions were not discrete and merged imperceptibly with the adjacent renal parenchyma without a discrete margin or capsule. Microscopically, cystic lesions involved renal

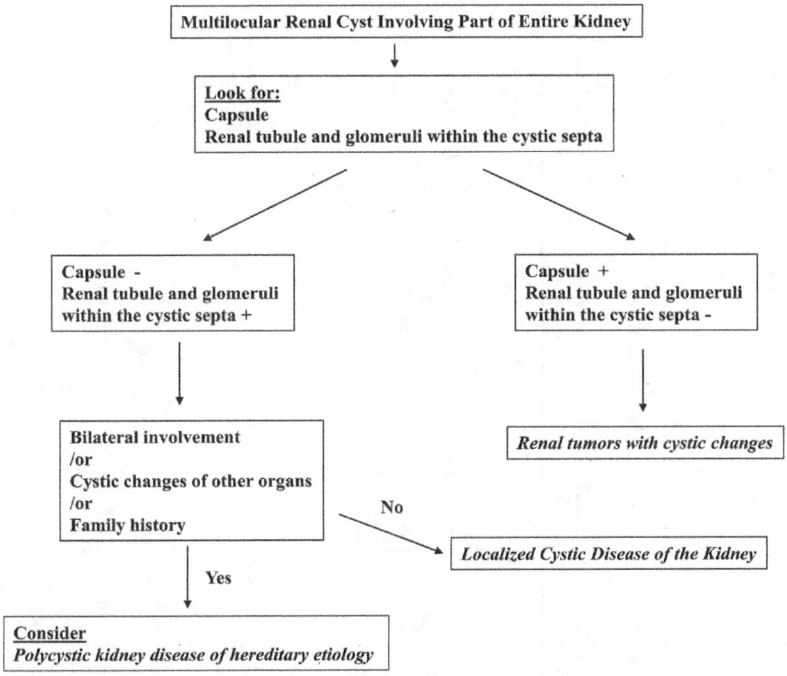

FIGURE 3.—A practical algorithm for diagnosing multilocular cystic renal diseases. (Reprinted from Ding Y, Chen L, Deng F-M, et al. Localized cystic disease of the kidney: distinction from cystic neoplasms and hereditary polycystic diseases. *Am J Surg Pathol.* 2013;37:506-513, with permission from Lippincott Williams & Wilkins.)

papillae in all cases, and the cystic space was continuous with dilated collecting ducts. Cysts were lined with cuboidal or flat epithelial cells identical to those lining the collecting ducts. Significant inflammation was absent. The surrounding renal parenchyma was normal. With this study, we hope to raise awareness among surgical pathologists of this rare cystic lesion in order to avoid potential misdiagnosis of this lesion as a cystic neoplasm or hereditary polycystic disease. We also presented a diagnostic algorithm for working up the renal cystic lesions (Fig 3, Table 2).

▶ Although most surgical pathologists are fairly comfortable with polycystic kidney disease and cystic renal cell carcinoma, there is a spectrum of cystic disease ranging from benign to neoplastic and malignant that is included when encountering cystic renal lesions. This retrospective descriptive study highlights the variety of entities within the differential diagnosis. Two of the most important histologic features to evaluate include looking for a capsule around the cystic lesion and the presence of renal tubules and glomeruli within the septae of the cyst. Based on these findings, the authors present an algorithm (Fig 3) that may prove useful in the evaluation of cystic renal lesions. Unfortunately, one of the challenges with these lesions is that they relatively infrequently come across the desk of the practicing surgical pathologist. In this study, which included several

TABLE 2.—Differential Diagnosis of Renal Lesions With Prominent Cystic Component

	LCD	ADPKD	Medullary Sponge Kidney	Multilocular Cystic Nephroma	Multilocular Cystic RCC	Tubulocystic Carcinoma	Cystic Partially Differentiated Nephroblastoma
Presentation age	Mean 33.3 y	Newborn to 5th decade	> 30 y	> 30 y	Mean 51 y	Mean 55 y	< 5 y old; majority < 2 y
M:F ratio	5:4	1.1-1.6:1	F > M	1:8	2-3:1	6-7:1	M > F
Symptoms	Incidental finding	Hematuria, proteinuria, chronic flank pain	Nephrolithiasis, urinary tract infection, hematuria	Abdominal mass, abdominal pain or hematuria	Abdominal mass or abdominal tenderness; may have hematuria and hypertension	Abdominal mass, abdominal pain, or hematuria	Palpable abdominal mass
Extrarenal manifestations	None	Intracranial berry aneurysms, hypertension, colonic diverticula, extrarenal cysts, cardiac valve abnormalities	None	None	None	None	10% associated with dysmorphic syndromes (WAGR syndrome, Denys-Drash syndrome; Beckwith-Wiedemann syndrome; familial nephroblastoma)
Hereditary	None	Autosomal dominant	Congenital, nonhereditary	None	None	None	None
Tumor capsule	None	None	None	Encapsulated, thin walled	Well circumscribed with fibrous capsule	Well circumscribed	Well circumscribed with fibrous pseudocapsule
Cysts	Multilocular	Numerous involving entire kidney	Ectatic collecting ducts involving 1 or more pyramids	Multilocular, focal hemorrhage often seen	Multilocular	"Spider-web" appearance	Multilocular

Cyst location	Unilateral, renal papillae with occasional cortical involvement	Bilateral cortex and medulla	Unilateral or bilateral, involving medulla	Unilateral	Unilateral	Unilateral	Unilateral
Cystic content	Serous	Proteinaceous, calcified deposits often seen	Serous	Serous	Serous or hemorrhagic fluid	Serous	Serous
Cystic lining	Cuboidal or flat epithelial cells	Single layer of flat to cuboidal epithelial cells	Transitional, columnar, or occasionally squamous epithelial cells	Single layer of flat, cuboidal, or hobnail cells	Single or a few layers of tumor cells with clear cytoplasm	Single layer of flat, cuboidal, or hobnail cells with abundant eosinophilic cytoplasm with prominent nucleoli	Flat, cuboidal, or hobnail epithelium or lack lining
Stromal septa	Fibrous with remnants of compressed and atrophic renal parenchyma	Interstitial fibrosis, lymphocytic infiltrate, tubular atrophy, and glomerular and vascular sclerosis	Small foci of interstitial fibrosis and chronic inflammation may be seen	Dense hyalinized or cellular stroma resembling ovarian stroma. No renal nephron elements within stroma	Fibrous tissue, variable in thickness; contains aggregates of clear cells with grade I nuclei	Dense fibrotic	Blastema, nephroblastomatous epithelial elements, and differentiated and/or undifferentiated mesenchymal elements (skeletal muscle, cartilage, fat or myxoid mesenchyme)

ADPKD indicates adult onset polycystic kidney disease; F, female; LCD, localized cystic disease of the kidney; M, male; RCC, renal cell carcinoma.

reference institutions, only 9 such cases were identified. Table 2 also gives a nice clinicopathologic correlation table, including all of the lesions with a prominent cystic component within the kidney.

For additional investigation, I direct the reader to Bisceglia et al.[1]

M. L. Smith, MD

Reference

1. Bisceglia M, Galliani CA, Senger C, Stallone C, Sessa A. Renal cystic diseases: a review. *Adv Anat Pathol.* 2006;13:26-56.

Validation of the new classification of pauci-immune glomerulonephritis in a United States cohort and its correlation with renal outcome

Ellis CL, Manno RL, Havill JP, et al (The Johns Hopkins Hosp and School of Medicine, Baltimore, MD)

BMC Nephrol 14:210, 2013

Background.—Renal biopsies provide important diagnostic and prognostic information in ANCA associated glomerulonephritis. A new classification for prognostication of pauci-immune glomerulonephritis (GN) based on four categories (Mixed, Crescentic, Sclerotic and Focal) was proposed by an international working group of renal pathologists (IWGRP). The goal of our study was to apply the proposed classification system to a United States cohort of vasculitis patients and determine the association of IWGRP class with estimated glomerular filtration rate (eGFR) at one year.

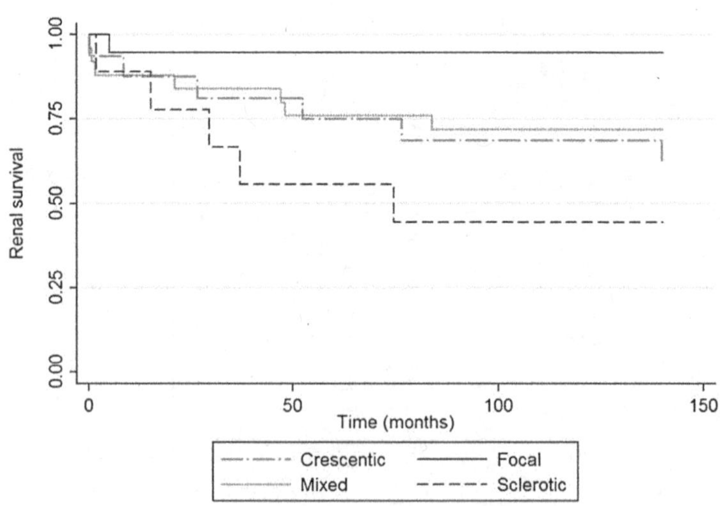

FIGURE 1.—Renal survival is depicted by Kaplan Meier survival estimates as time (in months) to the development of ESRD (defined by need for renal replacement therapy by dialysis or transplant). (Reprinted from Ellis CL, Manno RL, Havill JP, et al. Validation of the new classification of pauci-immune glomerulonephritis in a United States cohort and its correlation with renal outcome. *BMC Nephrol.* 2013;14:210, with permission from licensee BioMed Central Ltd.)

Methods.—Seventy-six cases of pauci-immune glomerulonephritis diagnosed from 1995 to 2011 from a single center were identified for this retrospective study. Clinical data were collected by abstraction from medical records. Histology was reviewed by a pathologist and classified according to the new classification. MDRD formula was used to calculate eGFR. We correlated IWGRP class to renal function at presentation and at one year. x^2, ANOVA, and linear regression analysis were performed as appropriate.

Results.—Renal biopsies were categorized as focal: n = 20, crescentic: n = 18, mixed: n = 27, sclerotic: n = 11. The baseline e-GFR was lowest in the crescentic class and highest in the focal class. In linear regression analysis investigating e-GFR at 1 year age and baseline e-GFR were independent predictors of e-GFR at 1 year.

Conclusions.—The e-GFR at diagnosis and age were predictors of e-GFR at 1 year. Pathologic class at diagnosis may also be a helpful tool in risk stratification at diagnosis (Fig 1).

► All classification schemas require validation to prove their clinical or prognostic usefulness. In 2010 a working group of expert renal pathologists introduced a proposed classification system for antineutrophil cytoplasmic antibody (ANCA)-associated glomerulonephritis.[1] A few European studies have already found prognostic usefulness of the proposed classification system, with the most impressive data coming from the focal category, which showed very good renal survival outcomes. The main finding of this study is shown in Fig 1, which correlates the proposed classification system to renal survival. For those unfamiliar, the focal category shows greater than 50% normal glomeruli, crescentic with greater than 50% showing cellular crescents, mixed category with less than 50% normal, less than 50% crescentic, and less than 50% globally sclerotic. The sclerotic category shows greater than 50% globally sclerotic glomeruli. The findings of this study support those of previous studies from Europe and also support the use of the ANCA-associated glomerulonephritis classification system that has been proposed. However, this study is limited in its retrospective design and small sample size (76). Further prospective studies to definitively define the usefulness of the classification system are needed.

M. L. Smith, MD

Reference

1. Berden AE, Ferrario F, Hagen EC, et al. Histopathologic classification of ANCA-associated glomerulonephritis. *J Am Soc Nephrol.* 2010;21:1628-1636.

Glomerular tip adhesions predict the progression of IgA nephropathy

Maeda K, Kikuchi S, Miura N, et al (Aichi Med Univ School of Medicine, Japan)

BMC Nephrol 14:272, 2013

Background.—Focal segmental glomerulosclerosis-like lesions have been proposed to be predictive factors for IgA nephropathy. This single center, retrospective cohort study was designed to clarify which clinical and

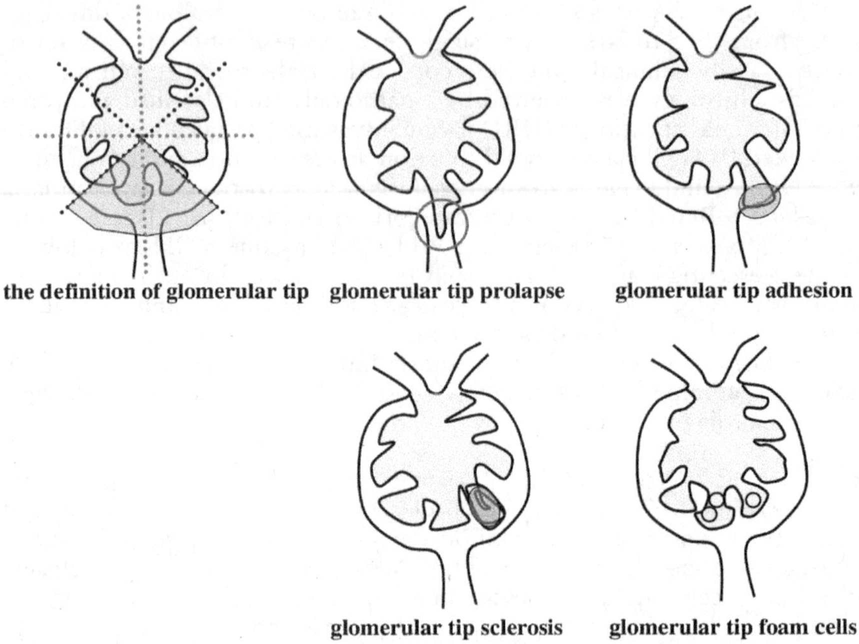

FIGURE 2.—Definition of glomerular tip and types of glomerular tip lesions. The glomerular tip is defined as the outer 25% of the tuft next to the origin of the proximal tubule, based on the Columbia Classification. Glomerular tip prolapse means that some component of the glomerulus, such as the basement membrane or the mesangial cells, is prolapsing into the proximal tubules. Glomerular tip adhesion is defined as a continuity of the extracellular matrix between the glomerular tuft and Bowman's capsule in the tip domain. Glomerular tip sclerosis is defined as segmental sclerosis in a portion of the glomerular tip. Glomerular tip foam cells refer to the presence of foam cells in a portion of the glomerular tip. (Reprinted from Maeda K, Kikuchi S, Miura N, et al. Glomerular tip adhesions predict the progression of IgA nephropathy. *BMC Nephrol.* 2013;14:272, with permission from Maeda et al.; licensee BioMed Central Ltd.)

TABLE 1.—Six Clinicopathologic Parameters Associated With Progression of IgA Nephropathy Identified Through Multiple Linear Regression Analysis With Backward Elimination

	Decrease in eGFR Multiple linear regression $F(6.50) = 4.202565$, $P = 0.001692$, $R^2 = 0.335242$	
	β	*p* value
Serum albumin	−0.23405	0.1380
Diastolic blood pressure	0.292789	0.0244
Initial eGFR	0.633544	0.0002
Global sclerosis	0.310904	0.0190
Total glomerular adhesion	−0.22385	0.1419
Glomerular tip adhesion	0.398646	0.0043

eGFR; estimated glomerular filtration rate (ml/minute per 1.73 m^2).
Total glomerular adhesion: glomerular tip adhesion plus adhesions in other parts of the glomerulus.

pathological factors are predictive of decreased estimated glomerular filtration rate (eGFR) at 5 and 10 years in IgA nephropathy patients.

Methods.—Of the 229 patients with IgA nephropathy who were admitted to Aichi Medical University Hospital between 1986 and 2010, 57 were included in this study during the 5 to 10 years after renal biopsy. Clinical, laboratory, and pathological parameters were analyzed by multiple linear regression analysis with backward elimination to determine independent risk factors. After identifying such factors, we compared patients with and without each factor using the Student's t test, Wilcoxon test, or Mann–Whitney U test.

Results.—Four variables were identified as predictive factors for progression of IgA nephropathy: initial eGFR ($p = 0.0002$), glomerular tip adhesion ($p = 0.004$), global sclerosis ($p = 0.019$), and diastolic blood pressure ($p = 0.024$). The annual decrease in eGFR of patients with ($n = 9$) or without glomerular tip adhesions ($n = 48$) was 4.13 ± 3.58 and 1.49 ± 2.89 ml/min/1.73 m2, respectively ($p = 0.015$). Serum total cholesterol levels were 231 ± 45 mg/dl and 196 ± 42 mg/dl, respectively (two-sided $p = 0.064$; one-sided $p = 0.032$).

Conclusions.—The presence of glomerular tip adhesions predicts the progression of IgA nephropathy. High levels of serum total cholesterol may affect glomerular tip adhesions (Fig 2, Table 1).

► In the coming era of health care reform, pathologists will be expected to continually add value without significantly increasing cost. One way to add value is to identify novel histopathologic features that can help predict progression in various diseases. This article shows how tip lesions, classically thought of as lesions associated with focal segmental glomerulosclerosis, seen in the setting of immunoglobulin A (IgA) nephropathy are associated with progression, defined by changes in estimated glomerular filtration rate (GFR). Fig 2 highlights the 5 different tip lesions described within the article. Table 1 shows the 6 clinical and pathologic parameters associated with progression of IgA nephropathy. It is not necessarily surprising that patients who develop tip lesions in the setting of the different disease process, in this case IgA nephropathy, might progress over time. These lesions likely do represent the beginning of focal segmental glomerular scarring, which would in this setting be secondary focal segmental glomerulosclerosis. This indicates hyperfiltration and a progression of the disease from typical IgA nephropathy to a focal segmental scarring process. Each loss of nephron owing to scarring will result in decreased GFR. One of the limitations associated with this report is the identification of only 9 patients who showed glomerular tip adhesions, despite the evaluation of 230 with IgA nephropathy over the course of more than 20 years. This study should be repeated in other institutions to evaluate for reproducibility.

For additional investigation, I refer the reader to El Karoui et al.[1]

M. L. Smith, MD

Reference

1. El Karoui K, Hill GS, Karras A, et al. Focal segmental glomerulosclerosis plays a major role in the progression of IgA nephropathy. II. Light microscopic and clinical studies. *Kidney Int.* 2011;79:643-654.

C3 glomerulopathy: consensus report

Pickering MC, D'Agati VD, Nester CM, et al (Imperial College London, UK; Columbia Univ Med Ctr and the New York Presbyterian Hosp; Univ of Iowa, Iowa City; et al)

Kidney Int 84:1079-1089, 2013

C3 glomerulopathy is a recently introduced pathological entity whose original definition was glomerular pathology characterized by C3 accumulation with absent or scanty immunoglobulin deposition. In August 2012, an invited group of experts (comprising the authors of this document) in renal pathology, nephrology, complement biology, and complement therapeutics met to discuss C3 glomerulopathy in the first C3 Glomerulopathy Meeting. The objectives were to reach a consensus on: the definition of C3 glomerulopathy, appropriate complement investigations that should be

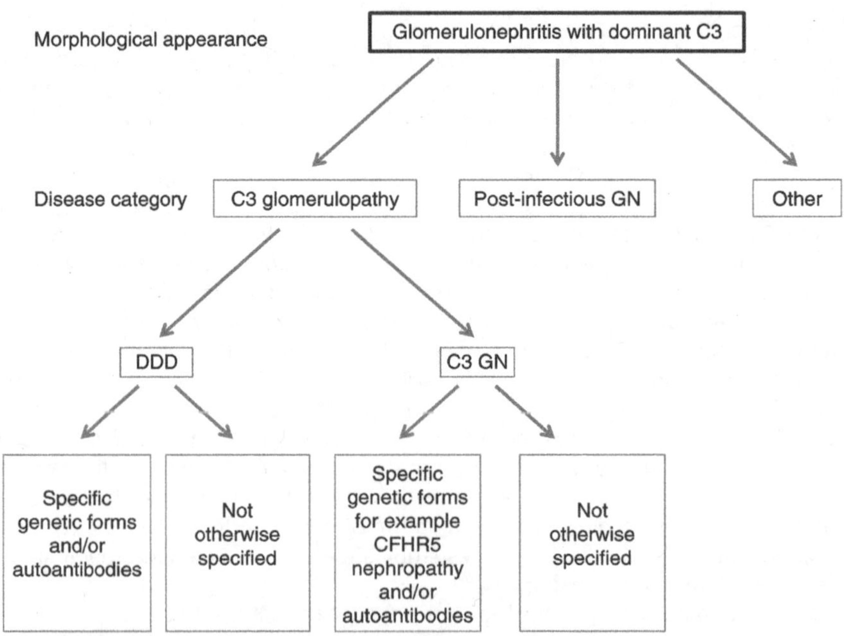

FIGURE 4.—A schematic diagram showing an approach to the classification of disease in a biopsy showing the morphological changes of a glomerulonephritis with dominant C3. DDD, dense deposit disease; Post-infectious GN, post-infectious glomerulonephritis. (Reprinted with permission from Macmillan Publishers Ltd: Kidney International. Pickering MC, D'Agati VD, Nester CM, et al. C3 glomerulopathy: consensus report. *Kidney Int.* 2013;84:1079-1089, Copyright 2013, with permission from International Society of Nephrology.)

TABLE 1.—Complement investigations in C3 glomerulopathy

Tests recommended in all patients	Comment
Measurement of serum C3 and C4	Low C3 with normal C4 indicates alternative pathway activation
Measurement of C3 nephritic factor	C3 nephritic factors are associated with C3 glomerulopathy; their correlation with disease course is unclear
Measurement of serum factor H	Factor H deficiency is associated with C3 glomerulopathy and is invariably associated with reduction in serum C3
Serum paraprotein detection	Paraproteinemia associated with C3 glomerulopathy, specialist tests required to determine whether paraprotein is a cause of uncontrolled C3 activation
Screening for CFHR5 mutation	CFHR5 nephropathy is a well-characterized cause of C3 glomerulopathy,[3,21] and thus screening for this mutation is clinically informative
Tests that should be considered on a case-by-case basis as they require expert interpretation and/or clinical validation	**Comment**
Measurement of serum factor B	Uncontrolled alternative pathway activation may be associated with reduced factor B levels
Measurement of serum C5	May be reduced in terminal pathway activation and could indicate group most likely to benefit from therapeutic C5 inhibition
Measurement of markers of C3 activation, e.g., C3d, C3c, C3adesArg	Activated C3 components are more sensitive markers of C3 activation than antigenic levels of intact C3
Measurement of markers of C5 activation, e.g., C5adesArg, soluble C5b-9	Activated C5 components are more sensitive markers of C5 activation than antigenic levels of intact C5
Measurement of anti-factor H autoantibodies	Anti-factor H autoantibodies are associated with C3 glomerulopathy; correlation with disease course is unclear; especially important to measure in patients with low C3 and negative C3 nephritic factor
Anti-factor B autoantibodies	Anti-factor B autoantibodies are associated with C3 glomerulopathy; correlation with disease course is unclear
Mutation screening of complement regulatory genes (e.g., *CFH, CFI, CD46*), activation protein genes (*C3, CFB*) and assessment of copy number variation across the *CFH-CFHR* locus	Mutations in these genes associated with C3 glomerulopathy; especially important to screen for *CFH* mutations in patients with low C3 and negative C3 nephritic factor

Editor's Note: Please refer to original journal article for full references.

performed in these patients, and how complement therapeutics should be explored in the condition. This meeting report represents the current consensus view of the group (Fig 4, Table 1).

▶ This is an excellent consensus review that summarizes the current status of C3 glomerulopathy as a pathologic entity. Several important concepts and suggestions are made. Fig 4 shows a schematic approach to the diagnosis of C3 glomerulopathy and C3 glomerulonephritis. It is recommended that C3 glomerulopathy be used to define the specific disease process, and, for the time being, cases that show a glomerulonephritis with dominant C3 by immunofluorescence should be designated "glomerulonephritis with dominant C3." This of course is a morphologic description and includes several diseases, including postinfectious glomerulonephritis and other forms of C3 glomerulopathy. It is suggested that C3 dominance be defined by a greater than 2-fold difference between C3 and any immunoglobulin (Ig) staining. A caveat was made that IgM is more likely to be nonspecific and may show some 1+ staining; therefore it is the background staining of IgA and IgG that is most important. Currently, some cases of postinfectious glomerulonephritis may show dominant C3 by immunofluorescence and, therefore, cannot be definitively distinguished. A diagnosis of dense deposit disease can be made only when characteristic very dense osmophilic deposits are identified by electron microscopy. There are no specific light microscopy findings for C3 glomerulonephritis, and a spectrum of findings has been reported ranging from normal to mesangial proliferative to membranoproliferative to crescentic. The real goal of the pathologic examination is to identify cases of C3 predominance and, thus, activate additional complement investigation within these patients. Table 1 highlights the recommended and other complement tests that should be considered in these patients. Sufficient treatment data are not available to make a firm recommendation.

For additional investigation on this topic, I refer the reader to Fakhouri et al.[1]

M. L. Smith, MD

Reference

1. Fakhouri F, Frémeaux-Bacchi V, Noël LH, Cook HT, Pickering MC. C3 glomerulopathy: a new classification. *Nat Rev Nephrol.* 2010;6:494-499.

The reproducibility and predictive value on outcome of renal biopsies from expanded criteria donors

Antonieta Azancot M, Moreso F, Salcedo M, et al (Universitat Autònoma Barcelona, Spain)

Kidney Int 2013 [Epub ahead of print]

Reproducibility and predictive value on outcome are the main criteria to evaluate the utility of histological scores. Here we analyze the reproducibility of donor biopsy assessment by different on-call pathologists and the retrospective evaluation by a single renal pathologist blinded to clinical outcomes. We also evaluate the predictive value on graft outcome of both evaluations. A biopsy was performed in donors with any of the following: age ≥55 years, hypertension, diabetes, creatinine >1.5 mg/dl, or stroke. Glomerulosclerosis, interstitial fibrosis, tubular atrophy, intimal thickening, and arteriolar hyalinosis evaluated according to the Banff criteria were added to obtain a chronic score. Biopsies were classified as mild (≥3), intermediate (4–5), or advanced (6–7) damage, and unacceptable (≥8) for transplantation of 127 kidneys biopsied. Weighted κ value between both readings was 0.41 (95% CI: 0.28-0.54). Evaluation of biopsies by the renal pathologist was significantly and independently associated with

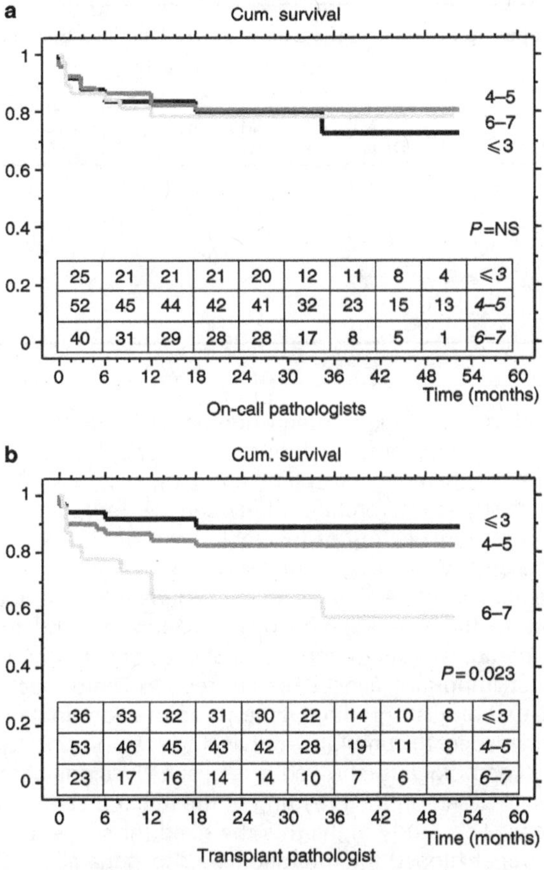

FIGURE 2.—Kaplan–Meier survival curves for the composite outcome variable. Kaplan–Meier survival curves for the composite outcome variable according to donor damage score evaluated by (**a**) on-call pathologists and (**b**) renal pathologist. The number of patients at risk at each time period is shown in the table. (Reprinted from Antonieta Azancot M, Moreso F, Salcedo M, et al. The reproducibility and predictive value on outcome of renal biopsies from expanded criteria donors. *Kidney Int* 2013 [Epub ahead of print], with permission from International Society of Nephrology.)

estimated 12-month glomerular filtration rate and a significant composite outcome variable, including death-censored graft survival and time to reach an estimated glomerular filtration rate <30 ml/min per 1.73 m^2. Thus, there was no association between readings of on-call pathologists and outcome. The lack of association between histological scores obtained by the on-call pathologists and graft outcome suggests that a specific training on renal pathology is recommended to optimize the use of kidneys retrieved from expanded criteria donors (Fig 2, Table 1).

▶ This report generates some startling data for any pathologist involved in the interpretation of preimplantation potential kidney donor biopsies. This was a

TABLE 1.—Relationship Between Donor Biopsy Scores Obtained by On-call Pathologists and the Renal Pathologist (MS)

Renal Pathologist	Total	On-call Pathologist Mild Damage ≤3	Moderate Damage 4–5	Advanced Damage 6–7	Unacceptable ≥8
Mild damage ≤3	36	17	15	4	0
Moderate damage 4–5	53	3	31	19	0
Advanced damage 6–7	25	3	4	16	2
Unacceptable ≥8	8	0	0	0	8
Total	122	23	50	39	10

P-value < 0.001 (χ^2).

retrospective study of expanded criteria donors and sought to investigate the association between preimplantation biopsy scores and outcome in on-call pathologists compared with renal transplant pathologists. Table 1 highlights the differences in pathologic interpretation between the renal pathologist and on-call pathologist. Close inspection of this table highlights a tendency of the on-call pathologist to overcall the degree of damage. I think this tendency to overcall the degree of damage is interesting, as, in my experience, pathologists without a lot of experience in the interpretation of renal biopsies tend to undercall the chronic lesions, particularly the chronic vascular lesions. Fig 2 highlights, in my opinion, the most important aspect of this report. There was no association between on-call pathologists grading of the chronic lesions in these preimplantation biopsies with respect to cumulative survival with a 5-year follow-up. Alternatively, transplant pathologists showed a statistically significant difference in cumulative survival based on their reading of the initial preimplantation biopsies for chronic lesions. This study highlights the need for some specific training in preimplantation renal biopsy interpretation by the general surgical pathology community. I find it interesting that in most academic centers in the United States this duty is left for the on-call general surgical pathology fellows. The general pathology community should strive to improve this practice for the transplant patients and services.

M. L. Smith, MD

Long-term Kidney Disease Outcomes in Fibrillary Glomerulonephritis: A Case Series of 27 Patients

Javaugue V, Karras A, Glowacki F, et al (Université de Poitiers, France; Université Paris Descartes, France; Université Lille 2, France; et al)

Am J Kidney Dis 62:679-690, 2013

Background.—Fibrillary glomerulonephritis (GN) is a rare disorder with poor renal prognosis. Therapeutic strategies, particularly the use of immunosuppressive drugs, are debated.

Study Design.—Case series.

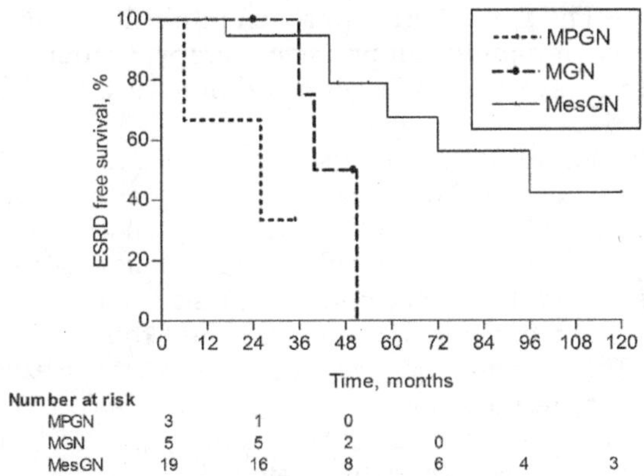

FIGURE 3.—Kaplan-Meier survival analysis in nonamyloid fibrillary glomerulonephritis according to the light microscopic pattern of glomerular lesions. Membranoproliferative glomerulonephritis (MPGN) versus mesangial glomerulonephritis (MesGN; $P = 0.001$); MGN vs membranous glomerulonephritis (MGN; $P = 0.03$), MPGN vs MGN ($P = 0.06$). Abbreviation: ESRD, endstage renal disease. (Reprinted from Javaugue V, Karras A, Glowacki F, et al. Long-term kidney disease outcomes in fibrillary glomerulonephritis: a case series of 27 patients. *Am J Kidney Dis*. 2013;62:679-690, Copyright 2013, with permission from the National Kidney Foundation.)

Setting & Participants.—27 adults with fibrillary GN referred to 15 nephrology departments in France between 1990 and 2011 were included. All patients were given renin-angiotensin system blockers and 13 received immunosuppressive therapy, including rituximab (7 patients) and cyclophosphamide (3 patients).

Outcomes & Measurements.—Clinical and histologic features of patients and kidney disease outcome. Renal response was defined as a >50% decrease in 24-hour proteinuria with <15% decline in estimated glomerular filtration rate (eGFR).

Results.—All patients presented with proteinuria, associated with nephrotic syndrome (41%), hematuria (73%), and hypertension (70%). Baseline median eGFR was 49 mL/min/1.73 m^2. Eight patients had a history of autoimmune disease and none had evidence of hematologic malignancy during follow-up. Light microscopic studies showed mesangial GN (70%), predominant pattern of membranous GN (19%), or membranoproliferative GN (11%). By immunofluorescence, immunoglobulin G (IgG) deposits (IgG4, 15/15; IgG1, 9/15) were polyclonal in 25 cases. Serum IgG subclass distribution was normal in the 6 patients tested. After a median 46-month follow-up, renal response occurred in 6 of 13 patients who received immunosuppressive therapy with rituximab (5 patients) or cyclophosphamide (1 patient). Of these, 5 had a mesangial or membranous light microscopic pattern, and median eGFR before therapy was 76 mL/min/1.73 m^2. In contrast, chronic kidney disease progressed in 12 of 14 patients who were not given immunosuppressive therapy, 10 of whom reached end-stage renal disease.

Limitations.—Number of patients, retrospective study, use of multiple immunosuppressive regimens.

Conclusions.—The therapeutic approach in fibrillary GN remains challenging. The place of immunosuppressive therapy, particularly anti–B-cell agents, needs to be assessed in larger collaborative studies (Fig 3).

► This article attempts to characterize the outcome of patients with fibrillary glomerulonephritis (immunotactoid glomerulonephritis was excluded based on the electron micrograph findings). Unfortunately, the low number of patients in this retrospective study makes the interpretation of the results challenging. Nevertheless, the results do show a fairly poor prognosis for patients with fibrillary glomerulonephritis, a prognosis that is generally well known in the renal pathology community. They defined a complete response as protein excretion less than 0.5 g/dL with an estimated glomerular filtration rate (GFR) of greater than 60, and a partial response was defined as a 50% decrease in 24-hour proteinuria with a less than 15% decrease in estimated GFR compared with baseline. A little less than half of the patients that received immunosuppressive therapy showed a renal response, but a large proportion (5 of 6) received rituximab. Although the number of subjects involved in this study make it woefully underpowered, these data are fairly intriguing and suggest some multicenter prospective trials involving the use of rituximab for fibrillary glomerulonephritis are necessary. Fig 3 highlights the importance of the different pathologic patterns of presentation in cases of fibrillary glomerulonephritis with respect to patient outcomes.

For further investigation of this topic, I refer the reader to Collins et al.[1]

M. L. Smith, MD

Reference

1. Collins M, Navaneethan SD, Chung M, et al. Rituximab treatment of fibrillary glomerulonephritis. *Am J Kidney Dis.* 2008;52:1158-1162.

IgG subclass staining in renal biopsies with membranous glomerulonephritis indicates subclass switch during disease progression

Huang CC, Lehman A, Albawardi A, et al (The Ohio State Univ, Columbus)
Mod Pathol 26:799-805, 2013

Recent breakthrough findings revealed that most patients with idiopathic (primary) membranous glomerulonephritis have IgG4 antibodies to the phospholipase A2 receptor (PLA2R). These IgG4 antibodies can be detected in the glomerular immune complexes and they colocalize with PLA2R. In secondary forms of membranous glomerulonephritis, such IgG4 antibodies are absent or less prevalent. There are no studies addressing the IgG subclass distribution across different stages of membranous glomerulonephritis. During a 25-month period, we identified 157 consecutive biopsies with membranous glomerulonephritis with adequate tissue for light, immunofluorescence and electron microscopy. Of the 157 membranous glomerulonephritis cases, 114 were primary membranous glomerulonephritis and 43 were secondary membranous glomerulonephritis. We

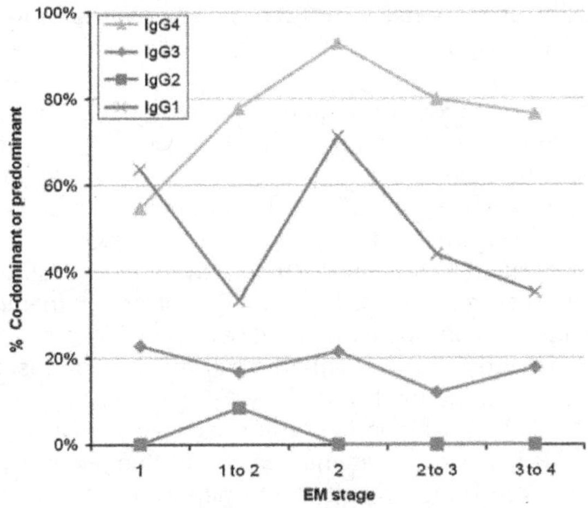

FIGURE 3.—IgG subclass predominance or codominance in different stages of primary membranous glomerulonephritis. (Reprinted by permission from Macmillan Publishers Ltd: Modern Pathology. Huang CC, Lehman A, Albawardi A, et al. IgG subclass staining in renal biopsies with membranous glomerulonephritis indicates subclass switch during disease progression. *Mod Pathol.* 2013;26:799-805, Copyright 2013, by USCAP, Inc, http://www.nature.com/modpathol.)

TABLE 1.—IgG Predominance/Codominance in Primary and Secondary Membranous Glomerulonephritis

IgG Subclass	N (%) Predominance/Codominance Primary (n = 114)	Secondary (n = 43)	*P*-value
IgG1	53 (46%)	26 (60%)	0.1184
IgG2	3 (3%)	2 (5%)	0.6151
IgG3	20 (18%)	10 (23%)	0.4169
IgG4	86 (75%)	21 (49%)	0.0018

compared the intensity of IgG subclass staining (on a semiquantitative scale of 0 to 3+) and the IgG subclass dominance between primary and secondary membranous glomerulonephritis and between the different stages of membranous glomerulonephritis. In primary membranous glomerulonephritis most (76% of cases) were IgG4 dominant. In contrast, in secondary membranous glomerulonephritis IgG1 was dominant in 60% of biopsies ($P = 0.0018$). Interestingly, in early stage (stage 1) primary membranous glomerulonephritis, IgG1 was the dominant IgG subclass (64% of cases); in all later stages IgG4 dominated ($P = 0.0493$). It appears that there is an inverse relationship between the intensity of glomerular capillary IgG4 and C1q staining. In secondary forms of membranous glomerulonephritis (heterogeneous group with low case numbers), we did not find such associations. Our data indicate that in early stage membranous glomerulonephritis, antibody response is different from later stages, with IgG1 dominant deposits. It is possible that early on, antigens other than PLA2R have an important role. Alternately, there may be an IgG subclass switch in the antibody response with IgG4 taking over later as the dominant immunoglobulin (Fig 3, Table 1).

▶ This interesting study sheds considerable light on the topic of immunoglobulin G (IgG) subclass in primary and secondary membranous nephropathy. It also generates more questions than answers. Most renal pathologists at this point are aware of the association between idiopathic or primary membranous glomerulonephritis and IgG4-predominant antibodies to phospholipase A2 receptor. Although this association has been documented in several different studies, a comparison of the presence of IgG4 dominance or codominance over various stages of membranous nephropathy has not been investigated, and this was the primary goal of the study. Fig 3 highlights the main study results and that in early membranous nephropathy it is actually IgG1 that is the most dominant or codominant IgG subclass. This is important, as many renal pathologists have begun to incorporate IgG subclass staining into their standard practice for the designation of primary vs secondary membranous nephropathy. It should be noted as well that IgG4 predominant subclass staining, although more common in primary membranous glomerulonephritis, was actually dominant or codominant in almost 50% of secondary membranous cases (Table 1). Therefore, caution should be used when interpreting IgG subclasses for the designation of primary vs secondary membranous glomerulonephritis. Other findings including mesangial changes, mesangial hypercellularity, and clinical features should also be used for the final determination of primary vs secondary membranous glomerulonephritis.

For further investigation of this topic, I refer the reader to Beck et al[1] and Qin et al.[2]

M. L. Smith, MD

References

1. Beck LH Jr, Bonegio RG, Lambeau G, et al. M-type phospholipase A2 receptor as target antigen in idiopathic membranous nephropathy. *N Engl J Med.* 2009;361: 11-21.
2. Qin W, Beck LH Jr, Zeng C, et al. Anti-phospholipase A2 receptor antibody in membranous nephrhopathy. *J Am Soc Nephrol.* 2011;22:1137-1143.

Nonneoplastic Renal Cortical Scarring at Tumor Nephrectomy Predicts Decline in Kidney Function

Salvatore SP, Cha EK, Rosoff JS, et al (Weill Cornell Med College, NY)
Arch Pathol Lab Med 137:531-540, 2013

Context.—Evaluating nontumor portions of tumor nephrectomies is useful to diagnose nonneoplastic renal disease.

Objective.—To determine the medical renal disease frequency and to assess the prognostic significance of the various renal pathologic variables with long-term follow-up in tumor nephrectomy patients.

Design.—We reviewed nonneoplastic kidney sections of 456 consecutive cases from 1998 to 2008. Seventy-five cases were excluded (19 tumor compression, 25 no nonneoplastic tissue, 22 embolized kidneys, 9 end stage).

TABLE 1.—Nonneoplastic Diagnoses Made in Tumor Nephrectomy Specimens

Diagnosis	No.
Diabetic nephropathy[a]	28
Hypertensive nephropathy	11
Focal segmental glomerulosclerosis[b]	7
Collapsing glomerulopathy[c]	2
Granulomatous tubulointerstitial nephritis[d]	2
Acute pyelonephritis	1
Thrombotic microangiopathy	1
Atheroembolic disease	1
Reflux nephropathy[e]	1
Proliferative glomerulonephritis[f]	1
Membranous glomerulonephritis[g]	1
Amyloidosis	1

[a]All patients had clinical diabetes. Proteinuria was present in 9 of 15 urine studies on record (range, 0–10.6 g/24 h) and creatinine levels ranged from 0.7 to 4.5 mg/dL (mean 1.5 mg/dL) (to convert mg/dL to μmol/L, multiply by 88.4).

[b]Five patients with additional clinical information all had proteinuria: 1 in the nephrotic range, 1 at 1.5 g/24 h, and the other 3 spot proteins only.

[c]One patient with additional information had 1.3 g/24 h proteinuria.

[d]One patient had a history of ulcerative colitis and the second had documented fungal forms within the granulomas.

[e]The patient had documented reflux.

[f]Patient with newly diagnosed multiple myeloma and immunoglobulin G-κ mesangial deposits.

[g]Proteinuria was recorded at 9.4 g/24 h.

Special staining, immunofluorescence, and/or electron microscopy was performed where appropriate. Vascular sclerosis was scored from mild to severe; interstitial fibrosis/tubular atrophy and global glomerulosclerosis (GS) were expressed as percentages. Follow-up, minimum 12 months, was evaluated in 156 cases. All renal pathologic variables were compared with regard to change in creatinine level from preoperative assessment to follow-up.

Results.—Of 381 cases, 57 had additional medical renal disease (15%), most frequently diabetic nephropathy (28) and hypertensive nephropathy (11). Postoperative creatinine levels increased significantly in patients with severe arteriosclerosis or arteriolosclerosis, >5% GS, and >10% interstitial fibrosis/tubular atrophy. Seventy-four percent of cases with additional nonneoplastic diagnoses showed severe arteriolosclerosis. Higher corresponding GS was seen in the more affected vascular cases: mean, 5.56% GS for mild versus 23% GS for severe. Three patients progressed to renal failure 1 to 4 years after nephrectomy, 2 with hypertensive nephrosclerosis and 1 with diabetic nephropathy.

Conclusions.—Medical renal disease was identified in 15% of tumor nephrectomy specimens. The degrees of vascular sclerosis, GS, and interstitial fibrosis/tubular atrophy are predictive of elevated creatinine levels in postnephrectomy patients. Prognostic implications of the nontumor pathology are important in nephrectomized patients (Table 1).

► In the last few years an increased emphasis has been put on the evaluation of the nonneoplastic renal cortical parenchyma in nephrectomy specimens for tumor. Although obviously the correct classification/subclassification and staging of the primary renal neoplasm are of paramount importance, recent data suggest that most general surgical pathologists give the nonneoplastic renal cortical parenchyma little to no attention. The goal of this study was to identify any histopathologic findings that could predict decreases in renal function after radical nephrectomy for neoplastic disease. Not surprisingly, as with most other similar studies, the most commonly identified background renal cortical nonneoplastic diseases were diabetic nephropathy and hypertensive-related nephropathy. However, Table 1 shows the variety of other pathologic diagnoses rendered in this study set. Not surprisingly, the degree of interstitial fibrosis, tubular atrophy, and arteriolosclerosis correlated with declines in kidney function after radical nephrectomy. Although these data may not be immediately useful to either the urologist or oncologist treating the patient, they become critically important for the nephrologist when the patient has renal insufficiency. In our practice, all radical nephrectomy specimens are screened with a section of renal cortex away from the primary neoplasm in a hematoxylin and eosin (H&E)-stained slide cut at normal thickness (5 μm). If there are any suspicious findings on the screening H&E section, the block can then be subjected to a typical renal biopsy protocol, which includes thin 2-μm sections as well as periodic acid—Schiff (PAS), Jones silver, and trichrome stains for complete analysis. Although immunofluorescence is not possible after formalin fixation, several electron microscopy laboratories can do a fairly good job with deparaffinization electron microscopy.

For a nice review on the diagnosis of nonneoplastic renal disease in nephrectomy specimens, I refer the reader to Henriksen et al.[1]

M. L. Smith, MD

Reference

1. Henriksen KJ, Meehan S, Chang A. Nonneoplastic kidney diseases in adult tumor nephrectomy and nephroureterectomy specimens: common, harmful, yet underappreciated. *Arch Pathol Lab Med.* 2009;133:1012-1025.

9 Head and Neck

Human Papillomavirus–related Carcinoma With Adenoid Cystic–like Features: A Peculiar Variant of Head and Neck Cancer Restricted to the Sinonasal Tract

Bishop JA, Ogawa T, Stelow EB, et al (The Johns Hopkins Med Institutions, Baltimore, MD; Univ of Virginia, Charlottesville)

Am J Surg Pathol 37:836-844, 2013

Human papillomavirus (HPV)-related carcinomas of the head and neck are characterized by a predilection for the oropharynx, a nonkeratinizing squamous morphology, and infection with the HPV 16 type; but comprehensive HPV testing across all head and neck sites has shown that the pathologic features of HPV-related carcinoma may be more wide ranging than initially anticipated. In particular, a subset of sinonasal carcinomas are HPV positive, and these include a variant that is histologically similar to adenoid cystic carcinoma (ACC). Cases were identified by retrospective and prospective analyses of head and neck carcinomas with ACC features. HPV analysis was performed using p16 immunohistochemistry and high-risk HPV in situ hybridization. HPV-positive cases were confirmed and typed using HPV type-specific quantitative polymerase chain reaction and further characterized on the basis of their immunohistochemical profile and *MYB* gene status. HPV was detected in 8 carcinomas of the sinonasal tract, but it was not detected in any ACCs arising outside of the sinonasal tract. The HPV types were 33 ($n = 6$), 35 ($n = 1$), and indeterminate ($n = 1$). Six patients were women, and 2 were men, ranging in age from 40 to 73 years (mean 55 y). The carcinomas were characterized by a nested growth, a prominent basaloid component showing myoepithelial differentiation and forming microcystic spaces, and a minor epithelial component with ductal structures. Squamous differentiation, when present, was restricted to the surface epithelium. The carcinomas were not associated with the *MYB* gene rearrangement that characterizes a subset of ACCs. These cases draw attention to an unusual variant of HPV-related carcinoma that has a predilection for the sinonasal tract. Despite significant morphologic overlap with ACC, it is distinct in several respects including an association with surface squamous dysplasia, absence of the *MYB* gene rearrangement, and an association with HPV, particularly type 33. As HPV positivity confers distinct clinicopathologic characteristics when encountered in the oropharynx, a more comprehensive analysis of risk

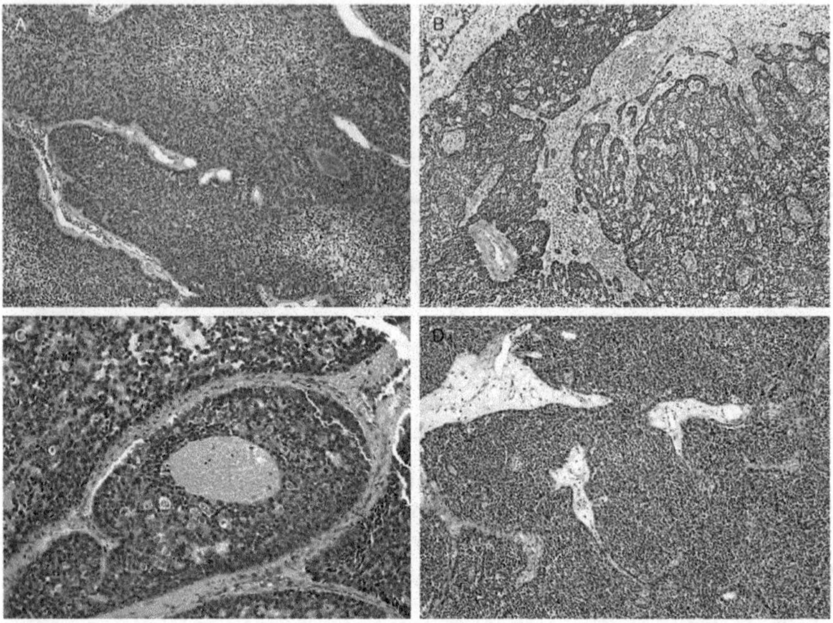

FIGURE 1.—HPV-related carcinomas with ACC-like features exhibit a consistent lobular pattern of growth. All 4 of these cases (A–D) show a proliferation of basaloid cells that are compacted into nests and lobules separated by a fibrous stroma. (Reprinted from Bishop JA, Ogawa T, Stelow EB, et al. Human papillomavirus–related carcinoma with adenoid cystic–like features: a peculiar variant of head and neck cancer restricted to the sinonasal tract. *Am J Surg Pathol.* 2013;37:836-844, with permission from Lippincott Williams & Wilkins.)

factors, response to therapy, and clinical outcomes is warranted for HPV-related carcinomas of the sinonasal tract (Figs 1 and 2).

▶ This is a nice study on a morphologic variant of a human papillomavirus (HPV)-related carcinoma of the sinonasal tract. Interestingly, this cancer not only shows features similar to adenoid cystic carcinoma (ACC) but also to the basaloid variant of squamous cell carcinoma. In spite of the similarity to ACC, the main point of differentiation was the absent relationship to HPV in ACCs arising outside the sinonasal tract, absence of *MYB-NFIB* gene fusion, and association with squamous metaplasia. The authors theorize that the presence of squamous dysplasia with these tumors may be caused by HPV-induced changes targeting the ductal system of minor salivary glands near its transition with the surface epithelium. The tumor also has myoepithelial and ductal components similar to those of the usual adenoid cystic carcinomas. Certainly, we need to know more about that tumor and whether the nomenclature of "ACC-like carcinoma" holds distinctly from the usual ACC, or is it truly a distinct subtype of ACC that

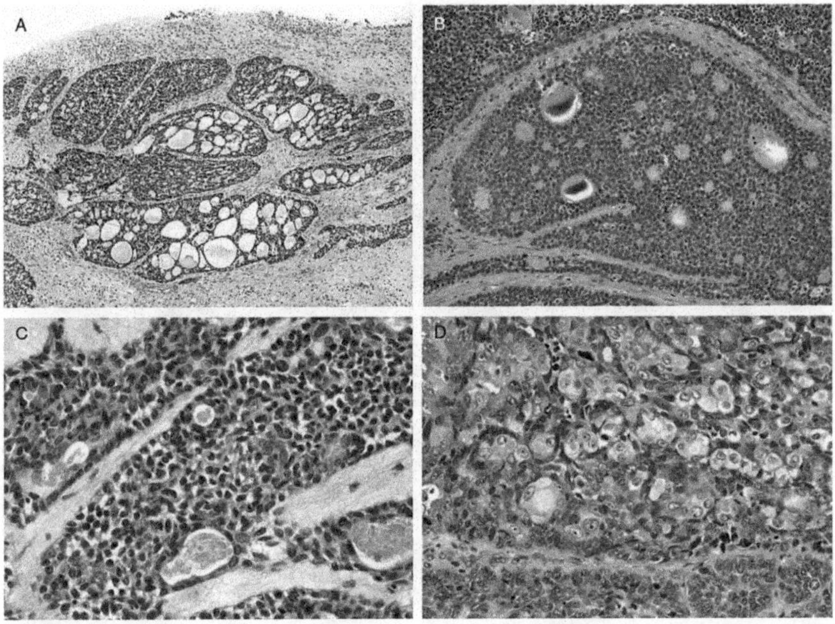

FIGURE 2.—Unlike basaloid variants of squamous cell carcinoma, HPV-related carcinomas with ACC often exhibited cribriform structures (A and B) and true ductal formations (C and D). (Reprinted from Bishop JA, Ogawa T, Stelow EB, et al. Human papillomavirus—related carcinoma with adenoid cystic—like features: a peculiar variant of head and neck cancer restricted to the sinonasal tract. *Am J Surg Pathol.* 2013;37:836-844, with permission from Lippincott Williams & Wilkins.)

occurs in the nasal cavity on exposure to HPV 33? What prognostic implications, especially according to the authors' clinical follow-up, were limited?

M. Sherif Said, MD, PhD

Human Papillomavirus-related Carcinomas of the Sinonasal Tract

Bishop JA, Guo TW, Smith DF, et al (The Johns Hopkins Med Institutions, Baltimore, MD)

Am J Surg Pathol 37:185-192, 2013

High-risk human papillomavirus (HPV) is an established cause of head and neck carcinomas arising in the oropharynx. The presence of HPV has also been reported in some carcinomas arising in the sinonasal tract, but little is known about their overall incidence or their clinicopathologic profile. The surgical pathology archives of The Johns Hopkins Hospital were searched for all carcinomas arising in the sinonasal tract from 1995 to 2011, and tissue microarrays were constructed. p16 immunohistochemical analysis and DNA in situ hybridization for high-risk types of HPV were performed. Demographic and clinical outcome data were extracted from patient medical records. Of 161 sinonasal carcinomas, 34 (21%) were positive for high-risk HPV DNA, including type 16 (82%), type 31/33 (12%),

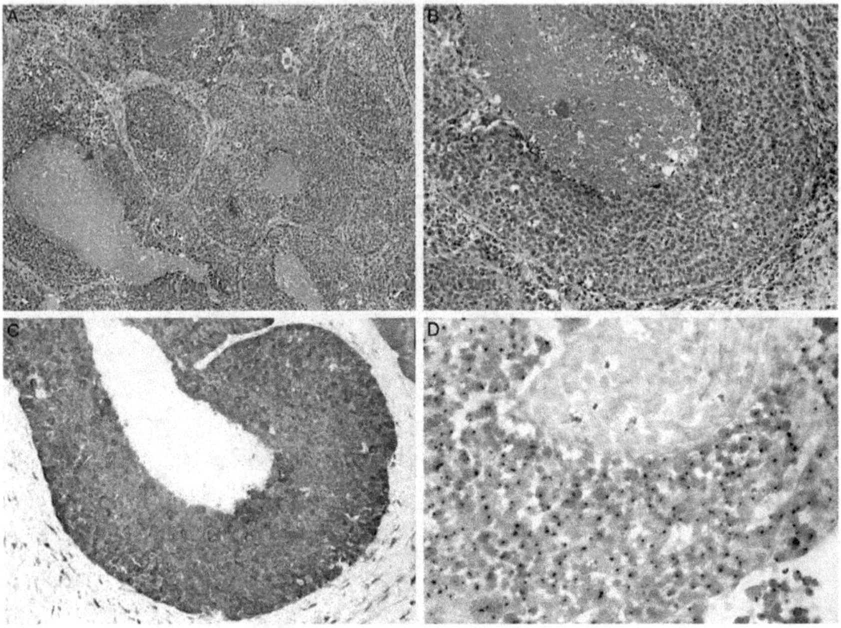

FIGURE 1.—HPV-related sinonasal carcinomas. A and B, Most of the HPV-related sinonasal squamous cell carcinomas were morphologically identical to HPV-related oropharyngeal carcinomas, exhibiting little or no keratinization, tumor infiltration by lymphocytes, and limited desmoplastic stromal reaction (A and B, hematoxylin and eosin). C, All but 1 of the HPV-positive cases was diffusely positive for p16 in a nuclear and cytoplasmic distribution (p16 immunohistochemistry). D, HPV positivity was defined by the presence of dot-like in situ hybridization signals in tumor nuclei (high-risk HPV in situ hybridization). (Reprinted from Bishop JA, Guo TW, Smith DF, et al. Human papillomavirus-related carcinomas of the sinonasal tract. *Am J Surg Pathol.* 2013;37:185-192, with permission from Lippincott Williams & Wilkins.)

and type 18 (6%). HPV-positive carcinomas consisted of 28 squamous cell carcinomas and variants (15 nonkeratinizing or partially keratinizing, 4 papillary, 5 adenosquamous, 4 basaloid), 1 small cell carcinoma, 1 sinonasal undifferentiated carcinoma, and 4 carcinomas that were difficult to classify but exhibited adenoid cystic carcinoma-like features. Immunohistochemistry for p16 was positive in 59/161 (37%) cases, and p16 expression strongly correlated with the presence of HPV DNA: 33 of 34 (97%) HPV-positive tumors exhibited high p16 expression, whereas only 26 of 127 (20%) HPV-negative tumors were p16 positive ($P < 0.0001$). The HPV-related carcinomas occurred in 19 men and 15 women ranging in age from 33 to 87 years (mean, 54 y). A trend toward improved survival was observed in the HPV-positive group (hazard ratio = 0.58, 95% confidence interval [0.26, 1.28]). The presence of high-risk HPV in 21% of sinonasal carcinomas confirms HPV as an important oncologic agent of carcinomas arising in the sinonasal tract. Although nonkeratinizing squamous cell carcinoma is the most common histologic type, there is a wide morphologic spectrum of HPV-related disease that includes a variant that resembles adenoid cystic carcinoma. The distinctiveness of these

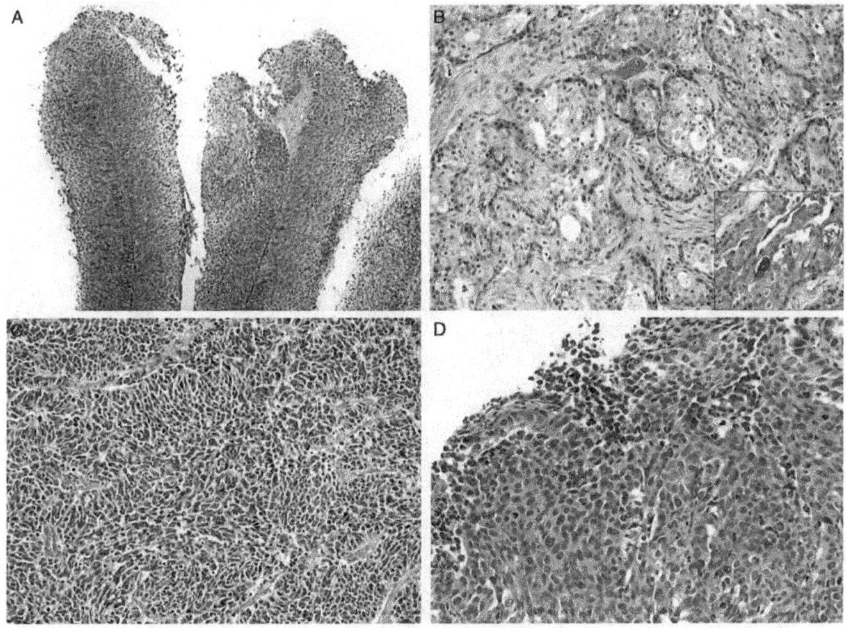

FIGURE 2.—HPV-related sinonasal carcinomas. Histologic variants of HPV-related sinonasal carcinomas included: (A) 5 papillary squamous cell carcinomas (hematoxylin and eosin); (B) 5 adenosquamous carcinomas [hematoxylin and eosin and mucicarmine (inset)]; (C) 1 small cell carcinoma (hematoxylin and eosin); and (D) 1 sinonasal undifferentiated carcinoma (hematoxylin and eosin). (Reprinted from Bishop JA, Guo TW, Smith DF, et al. Human papillomavirus-related carcinomas of the sinonasal tract. *Am J Surg Pathol.* 2013;37:185-192, with permission from Lippincott Williams & Wilkins.)

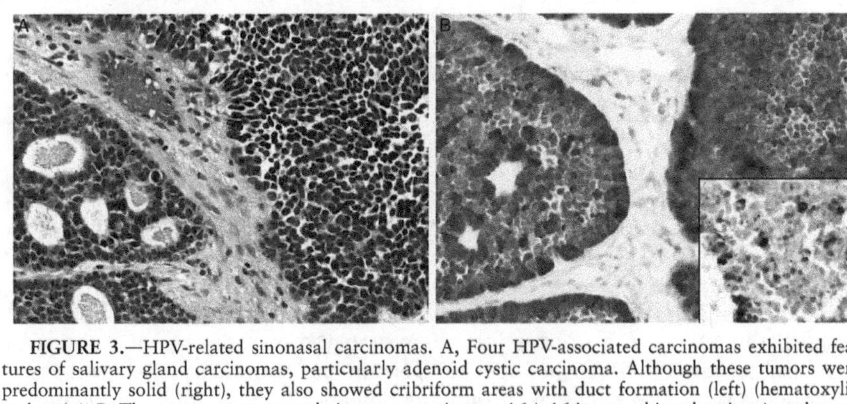

FIGURE 3.—HPV-related sinonasal carcinomas. A, Four HPV-associated carcinomas exhibited features of salivary gland carcinomas, particularly adenoid cystic carcinoma. Although these tumors were predominantly solid (right), they also showed cribriform areas with duct formation (left) (hematoxylin and eosin). B, The tumors were strongly immunoreactive to p16 (p16 immunohistochemistry), and punctate hybridization signals were seen in tumor nuclei on HPV in situ hybridization (inset, high-risk HPV in situ hybridization). (Reprinted from Bishop JA, Guo TW, Smith DF, et al. Human papillomavirus-related carcinomas of the sinonasal tract. *Am J Surg Pathol.* 2013;37:185-192, with permission from Lippincott Williams & Wilkins.)

TABLE 1.—HPV Status of Sinonasal Carcinomas by Tumor Type

		HPV DNA In Situ Hybridization (%)				
Tumor Type	p16 IHC (%)	Type 16	Type 18	Type 31/33	High-Risk Cocktail	Total
Squamous cell carcinoma	42/91 (46)	24/91 (26)	2/91 (2)	2/91 (2)	24/91 (26)	28/91 (31)
Keratinizing	3/25 (12)	0/25 (0)	0/25 (0)	0/25 (0)	0/25 (0)	0/25 (0)
Non/partially keratinizing	24/44 (55)	14/44 (32)	1/44 (2)	0/44 (0)	12/44 (27)	15/44 (34)
Basaloid squamous	5/8 (63)	3/8 (38)	0/8 (0)	1/8 (13)	4/8 (50)	4/8 (50)
Papillary	5/5 (100)	2/5 (40)	1/5 (20)	1/5 (20)	3/5 (60)	4/5 (80)
Adenosquamous	5/6 (83)	5/6 (83)	0/6 (0)	0/6 (0)	5/6 (83)	5/6 (83)
Sarcomatoid	0/3 (0)	0/3 (0)	0/3 (0)	0/3 (0)	0/3 (0)	0/3 (0)
Adenoid cystic-like carcinomas	4/4 (100)	2/4 (50)	0/4 (0)	2/4 (50)	4/4 (100)	4/4 (100)
Salivary gland carcinoma	4/34 (12)	0/34 (0)	0/34 (0)	0/34 (0)	0/34 (0)	0/34 (0)
Adenoid cystic	3/26 (12)	0/26 (0)	0/26 (0)	0/26 (0)	0/26 (0)	0/26 (0)
Myoepithelial	0/3 (0)	0/3 (0)	0/3 (0)	0/3 (0)	0/3 (0)	0/3 (0)
Mucoepidermoid	1/2 (50)	0/2 (0)	0/2 (0)	0/2 (0)	0/2 (0)	0/2 (0)
Acinic cell	0/1 (0)	0/1 (0)	0/1 (0)	0/1 (0)	0/1 (0)	0/1 (0)
Epithelial-myoepithelial	0/1 (0)	0/1 (0)	0/1 (0)	0/1 (0)	0/1 (0)	0/1 (0)
Adenocarcinoma, NOS	0/1 (0)	0/1 (0)	0/1 (0)	0/1 (0)	0/1 (0)	0/1 (0)
Sinonasal adenocarcinoma	2/7 (29)	0/7 (0)	0/7 (0)	0/7 (0)	0/7 (0)	0/7 (0)
Intestinal type	0/1 (0)	0/1 (0)	0/1 (0)	0/1 (0)	0/1 (0)	0/1 (0)
Nonintestinal type, low grade	0/4 (0)	0/4 (0)	0/4 (0)	0/4 (0)	0/4 (0)	0/4 (0)
Nonintestinal type, high grade	2/2 (100)	0/2 (0)	0/2 (0)	0/2 (0)	0/2 (0)	0/2 (0)
Small cell carcinoma	4/6 (67)	1/6 (17)	0/6 (0)	0/6 (0)	1/6 (17)	1/6 (17)
SNUC	4/16 (25)	1/16 (6)	0/16 (0)	0/16 (0)	0/16 (0)	1/16 (6)
NUT midline carcinoma	0/3 (0)	0/3 (0)	0/3 (0)	0/3 (0)	0/3 (0)	0/3 (0)
Total	60/161 (37)	28/161 (17)	2/161 (1)	4/161 (2)	30/161 (19)	34/161 (21)

IHC indicates immunohistochemistry; NOS, not otherwise specified; NUT, nuclear protein in testis; SNUC, sinonasal undifferentiated carcinoma.

HPV-related carcinomas of the sinonasal tract with respect to risk factors, clinical behavior, and response to therapy remains to be clarified (Figs 1-3, Table 1).

▶ Because human papillomavirus (HPV) is implicated more in head and neck cancers, this article is a good effort examining the relationship of a series of sinonasal tumors to HPV using specific DNA in situ hybridization—based studies coupled with P16 levels expression as detected by immunohistochemistry. The complete results of these studies are shown in Table 1 and their histologic features shown in Figs 1-3. In addition to oropharyngeal cancers and their relationship to HPV, other studies have found evidence to suggest no relationship between salivary gland tumors and HPV. This study shows that almost all of the cancers of the sinonasal tract possibly related to HPV squamous cell carcinoma with its variants are the most closely related, whereas those of minor salivary gland origin or the adenocarcinoma type cancers do not show such relationship, findings which corroborate other evidence in the literature.[1] Interestingly, those sinonasal-positive HPV cancers, like their oropharyngeal counterparts, showed a trend to improved survival rates as mentioned in the abstract. No doubt that more studies are required to further establish and define the role of HPV in sinonasal carcinomas in a larger cohort of patients with similar demographic and clinicopathologic backgrounds, a stance that the authors also advocate.

M. S. Said, MD, PhD

Reference

1. El-Mofty SK, Lu DW. Prevalence of high-risk human papillomavirus DNA in nonkeratinizing (cylindrical cell) carcinoma of the sinonasal tract: a distinct clinicopathologic and molecular disease entity. *Am J Surg Pathol.* 2005;29:1367-1372.

Molecular profiling of sinonasal undifferentiated carcinoma

Gelbard A, Hale KS, Takahashi Y, et al (The Univ of Texas MD Anderson Cancer Ctr, Houston)

Head Neck 2013 [Epub ahead of print]

Background.—Sinonasal undifferentiated carcinoma (SNUC) remains a poorly characterized malignancy at both the clinical and molecular level, and, consequently, the optimal treatment strategy remains undefined.

Methods.—We used a mass spectroscopy–based approach (Sequenom) to evaluate 95 hallmark single nucleotide variations (SNVs) within 12 oncogenes or tumor suppressor genes (AKT, BRAF, CDK4, Beta-catenin, epidermal growth factor receptor [EGFR], FBXW7, JAK2, c-KIT, KRAS, PDGFR, PI3K, and vascular endothelial growth factor [VEGF]) in 13 histologically confirmed SNUC cases.

Results.—None of the samples demonstrated activating mutations in any of the 95 SNVs.

Conclusion.—Select clinically relevant activating genomic mutations were not identified in the 13 patient samples. However, polymorphisms were noted within the promoter region of VEGF. These may merit future studies as predictive biomarkers for treatment response or overall survival. Additionally, future studies focusing on larger tumor sets and utilizing whole genome or exome sequencing may help define genetic aberrations in SNUC that can be clinically targeted with available or emerging biological agents (Figs 1 and 4, Table 2).

► Sinonasal undifferentiated carcinoma (SNUC) is a rare malignancy with often unfavorable outcome and characteristic histologic appearance (Fig 1). Many series, current[1] and past, have consistently shown poor survival outcomes regardless of the modalities of treatment used (chemoradiation or surgery followed by adjuvant therapy). This article is one of the early attempts at molecular characterization of this tumor, and although clinically relevant genomic mutations were not

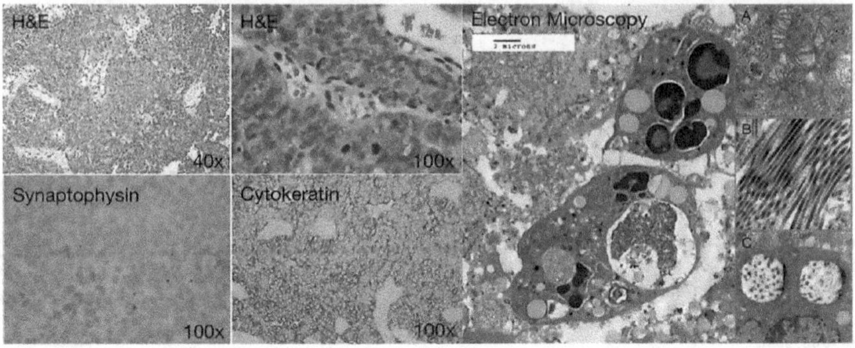

FIGURE 1.—Histological examination of sinonasal undifferentiated carcinoma (SNUC) after hematoxylin-eosin staining reveals characteristic hypercellular proliferation with a trabecular growth pattern, medium to large pleomorphic and hyperchromatic nuclei, inconspicuous to prominent nucleoli, varying amount of eosinophilic cytoplasm, and high nuclear-to-cytoplasmic ratio. Immunohistochemistry is negative for synaptophysin, positive for pancytokeratin, negative for lymphoid markers (not shown), S100 (not shown), and HMB45 (not shown). Electron microscopy demonstrates undifferentiated polygonal cells with sparse intracellular membrane structures and numerous polyribosomes, mitochondria (A), and abundant lipid-filled vacuoles. Occasional tonofilaments and microtubules (B) are visible along with membrane-bound, dense-core, neurosecretory granules (C). (Reprinted from Gelbard A, Hale KS, Takahashi Y, et al. Molecular profiling of sinonasal undifferentiated carcinoma. *Head Neck*. 2013 [Epub ahead of print], with permission from Head & Neck and John Wiley and Sons, www.interscience.wiley.com.)

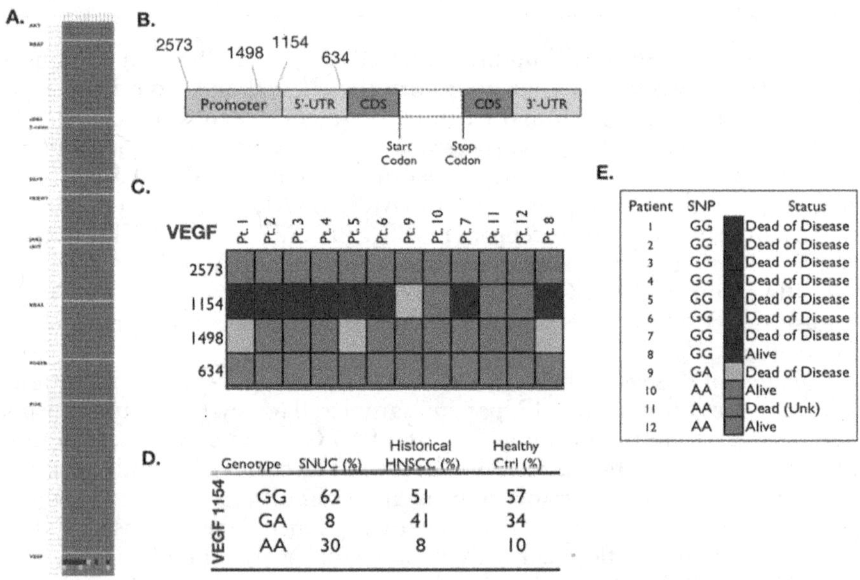

FIGURE 4.—None of the 13 samples demonstrated known activating mutations in any of the 95 single nucleotide variations (SNVs) (A). Structure of vascular endothelial growth factor (VEGF) gene and position of single nucleotide polymorphisms (SNPs) relative to translation start site, dashed lines indicate the region consisting of coding sequence (CDS) and 7 introns, untranslated region (UTR) (B). Polymorphisms were noted in genotype 1154 and 1498 of VEGF (C). VEGF 1154 genotype frequencies of patients with sinonasal undifferentiated carcinoma (SNUC) contrasted with a group of 100 patients with head and neck squamous cell carcinoma (HNSCC) and healthy controls (D). VEGF 1154 SNP genotypes and survival of 12 patients with SNUC (E). Of the 3 patients alive at last contact, 2 possessed the historically protective AA genotype. (Reprinted from Gelbard A, Hale KS, Takahashi Y, et al. Molecular profiling of sinonasal undifferentiated carcinoma. *Head Neck*. 2013 [Epub ahead of print], with permission from Head & Neck and John Wiley and Sons, www.interscience.wiley.com.)

TABLE 2.—Genes

BRAF	**EGFR**	**PI3K**
BRAF_D594_1781A	EGFR_G719_G2155	PIK3CA_A1046V
BRAF_E586K_1756GA_Slp	EGFR_L858R_TG	PIK3CA_C420R
BRAF_G464_1391G	EGFR_T790M_C2369T_Spl	PIK3CA_E110K
BRAF_G466_1397G	**VEGF**	PIK3CA_E418K
BRAF_G466R_1396_GC	VEGF_5_1154_GA_ref	PIK3CA_E453K
BRAF_G469_1407A	VEGF_5_1498_CT	PIK3CA_E542_1624G
BRAF_K601E_AG	VEGF_5_2573_CA	PIK3CA_E545_1633G
BRAF_K601N_A	VEGF_5_634_GC_ref	PIK3CA_E545_1634A
BRAF_L597R_1790TG	**c-KIT**	PIK3CA_E545_1635G
BRAF_V600_1798G_1	KIT_D816H_GC	PIK3CA_F909L
BRAF_V600_1799T_1	KIT_D816V_AT	PIK3CA_G1049R
BRAF_V600_1799T_2	KIT_K642E_AG	PIK3CA_H1047
BRAF_V600_1800G	KIT_L576P_TC	PIK3CA_H1047_1
KRAS	KIT_N556D_AG	PIK3CA_H1047Y
KRAS_A146_436	KIT_R634W_CT	PIK3CA_H701P
KRAS_G12_34G	KIT_V559_T	PIK3CA_K111N
KRAS_G12_35G	KIT_V560D_TA_SPLICE	PIK3CA_M1043V
KRAS_G12_36T	KIT_V825A_TC	PIK3CA_N345K
KRAS_G13_37G	KIT_Y553N_TA	PIK3CA_P539R
KRAS_G13_38G	**PDGFR A**	PIK3CA_Q060K
KRAS_G13_39	PDGFRA_D842_A2525T	PIK3CA_Q546_1636C
KRAS_Q61_181C	PDGFRA_D842_G2524	PIK3CA_Q546_1637A
KRAS_Q61_182A	PDGFRA_E996K_G2986	PIK3CA_R088Q
KRAS_Q61_183A	PDGFRA_N659K_C1977A	PIK3CA_S405F
Beta-catenin	PDGFRA_N659Y_A1975T	PIK3CA_T1025_3073A
CTNNB1_D32_94G	PDGFRA_V561D_T1682A	PIK3CA_Y1021_3061T
CTNNB1_D32_95A	PDGFRA_V824L_G2470C	PIK3CA_Y1021C_3062
CTNNB1_G34_101G	**FBXW7**	**AKT**
CTNNB1_S33_97T	FBWX7_R465C_C1393T	AKT1_E17K_G49A
CTNNB1_S37_109T	FBWX7_R465H_G1394A	AKT2_E17K_G49A
CTNNB1_S37_110C	FBWX7_R479_G1436	AKT3_E17K_G49K
CTNNB1_S45_133T	FBWX7_R505_G1514	**JAK2**
CTNNB1_S45_134C	FBWX7_R505C_C1513T	JAK2_V617F_G1849T
CTNNB1_T41_121A	FBWX7_S582L_C1745T	**CDK4**
	FBXW7_H460R_A1379G	CDK4_R24C_C70T

Single nucleotide variations (SNVs) in 95 hallmark mutations within 12 oncogenes or tumor suppressor genes (AKT, BRAF, CDK4, Beta-catenin, epidermal growth factor receptor [EGFR], FBXW7, JAK2, c-KIT, KRAS, PDGFRA, PI3K, and vascular endothelial growth factor [VEGF]) probed in this experiment.

identified in the examined samples (Table 2), it remains important to know in the beginning of that road. However, polymorphisms in the *VEGF* gene promotor regions (induce proliferation, differentiation, and migration of vascular endothelial cells) were found in the 1154 or 1498 locations (Fig 4). As the authors mention, *VEGF* gene overexpression in head and neck cancers has been associated with head and neck squamous cell carcinoma and with metastasis, recurrence, and poor prognosis, which puts it as a potential target for treatment strategy in SNUC. The authors also point out the work by Takahashi et al[2] in establishing a SNUC cell line, which will help future efforts in further characterizing the molecular parameters of SNUC.

M. S. Said, MD, PhD

References

1. Xu CC, Dziegielewski PT, McGaw WT, Seikaly H. Sinonasal undifferentiated carcinoma (SNUC): the Alberta experience and literature review. *J Otolaryngol Head Neck Surg*. 2013;42:1-6.
2. Takahashi Y, Kupferman ME, Bell D, et al. Establishment and characterization of novel cell lines from sinonasal undifferentiated carcinoma. *Clin Cancer Res*. 2012; 18:6178-6187.

Sinonasal mucosal melanomas: The prognostic value of tumor classifications

Michel J, Perret-Court A, Fakhry N, et al (Aix-Marseille Univ, Marseille cedex, France)

Head Neck 2013 [Epub ahead of print]

Background.—The purpose of this study was to assess the prognostic value of the 3 staging systems found in the literature for sinonasal mucosal melanomas tumors: the Ballantyne staging system modified by Prasad (Ballantyne/Prasad staging system), the American Joint Committee on Cancer (AJCC) TNM classification for mucosal melanomas (mmTNM), and the 2009 AJCC TNM classification for carcinomas of the nasal cavity and sinuses (carTNM).

Methods.—A retrospective study of 35 patients treated between 1995 and 2010 was conducted for this study. Each patient was retrospectively staged using the Ballantyne/Prasad staging system, mmTNM, and carTNM.

Results.—There were 20 women (57.1%) and 15 men (42.9%). Only carTNM was significantly correlated with overall survival ($p = .012$) and disease-free survival ($p = .041$). The other 2 classifications were not correlated with survival except for metastatic patients whose overall survival was lower ($p = .032$).

TABLE 1.—Ballantyne, Ballantyne/Prasad and American Joint Committee on Cancer Staging Mucosal Melanoma of the Head and Neck (TNM classification for mucosal melanomas) Staging Systems

Stage	Ballantyne 1970	Ballantyne/Prasad 2004	Mucosal Melanoma TNM 2009	Stage
I	Any T N0M0			
		Level 1: in situ	T3: epithelium/submucosal	III
		Level 2: invasion up to lamina propria		T3N0
		Level 3: deep tissue invasion	T4a: deep soft tissue, cartilage, bone	IVa
			T4b: brain, dura, skull base	T4aN0
				T3/T4a N1
II	Any T N+M0			IVb
				T4b
III	Any T any N M1			IVc
				M1

TABLE 2.—American Joint Committee on Cancer Sinonasal Tracts Carcinoma TNM

carTNM	Maxillary Sinus (MS)	Nasal Cavity and Ethmoid Sinus
T1	Limited to maxillary sinus	One subsite
T2	Hard palate, middle nasal meatus except posterior wall of MS	Two subsites in a single region or extending to involve an adjacent region
T3	Bone of posterior wall of MS, subcutaneous tissues, orbit, pterygoid fossa, ethmoid sinus	Medial floor of the orbit, maxillary sinus, palate, cribriform plate
T4a	Orbital content, skin, pterygoid plates, cribriform plate	Anterior orbital content, skin, minimal extension to cranial fossa, pterygoid, plates, sphenoid, or frontal sinus
T4b	Orbital apex, dura, brain. . .	Orbital apex, dura, brain. . .

Staging: Stage 0 Tis, N0, M0; Stage I T1, N0, M0; Stage II T2, N0, M0; Stage III T3, N0, M0 - T1–T2, N1, M0; Stage IVA T4a, N0/N1, M0 - T1–T4a, N2, M0; Stage IVB T4b, any N, M0 - Any T, N3, M0; Stage IVC Any T, Any N, M1.

Used with the permission of the American Joint Committee on Cancer (AJCC), Chicago, Illinois. The original source for this material is the AJCC Cancer Staging Manual, Seventh Edition (2010) published by Springer Science and Business Media LLC, http://www.springerlink.com/.

TABLE 4.—Head and Neck Mucosal Melanomas: 5-year Disease-free Survival and 5-year Overall Survival Reported in the Literature and in Our Series

Authors	No. of Patients	5-year Disease-free Survival, %	5-year Overall Survival, %	% Of Postoperative Radiotherapy
Prasad et al.[2] (2004)	61	42.8	30.8	22
Patel et al.[3] (2001)	35	–	47	–
Dauer et al.[4] (2008)	61	–	22	28
Temam et al.[6] (2004)	69	–	20	57
Bridger et al.[8] (2005)	27	14.54	43	52
Cheng et al.[9] (2007)	22	–	15.65	41
Manolidis et al.[13] (1997)	14	–	14.3	14.2
Huang et al.[14] (2007)	15	–	33	77
Narasimhan et al.[15] (2009)	18	–	34	56
Jethanamest et al.[16] (2011)	815	32.4	25.2	–
Our series	19	17.8	34.1	42

Editor's Note: Please refer to original journal article for full references.

Conclusion.—On the basis of these findings, we believe that carTNM should be the primary staging system for patients with mucosal melanomas of the sinonasal tract (Tables 1, 2 and 4).

▶ Sinonasal mucosal melanoma is a serious condition with guarded prognosis and low survival rate (Table 4). From my personal experience and probably the experience of many pathologists who see a considerable number of head and neck entities, classification of these tumors is variable depending on the classification system used and that the usual cutaneous parameters (eg, Clark index or Breslow score) are not useful in these types of melanomas, as most of them, unfortunately, present past the in situ stage. Additionally, the complexity of the sinonasal anatomy makes the use of these parameters difficult. I find this an interesting article comparing the commonly used systems (as presented in Tables 1 and 2) to indicate which is most useful when considering the patient prognosis and overall survival. The authors also critically evaluated the different systems and pointed out some weaknesses from their perspective, which others may disagree with. For example, they found that one of the drawbacks of the Ballantyne/Prasad system was that it devoted an entire stage (stage II) for lymph node involvement; however, they noted that this type of involvement is seldom detected (only in 5% to 10% of cases) at the onset of diagnosis of these tumors. They also noted that the American Joint Committee on Cancer TNM classification for mucosal melanomas associated data from the Ballantyne/Prasad system with data from the carcinomas of the nasal cavity and sinuses TNM system and observed that it correlated weakly with the survival in their series of patients. As interesting as this finding is and as the authors themselves recommended, larger prospective, multicenter studies are needed to evaluate this finding.

M. S. Said, MD, PhD

Epithelial salivary gland tumors in children: A twenty-five-year experience of 122 patients

Fang Q-G, Shi S, Li Z-N, et al (China Med Univ, Shenyang, Liaoning)
Int J Pediatr Otorhinolaryngol 77:1252-1254, 2013

Objective.—The purpose of this study was to evaluate our 25-year experience of pediatric salivary tumors.

Methods.—Patients less than 19 years old with a diagnosis of salivary tumor were identified at Oral-maxillofacial Head and Neck Tumor Center, China Medical University from 1987 to 2011.

Results.—122 patients were included in our study, 105 tumors were benign and 17 were malignant. The most common involved site was parotid gland, pleomorphic adenoma represented 91.4% in benign group, and mucoepidermoid carcinoma represented 47.1% in malignant group. All tumors in submandibular gland were benign. Warthin's tumor was diagnosed in one patient. In our follow-up, no regional recurrences occurred in patients without neck dissection. The 5- and 10-year overall survival rates of patients with malignant salivary tumors were 81.8% and 66.7% respectively.

Conclusions.—Epithelial salivary tumor was rare, parotid gland was most common involved site, pleomorphic adenoma and mucoepidermoid carcinoma were the most common benign and malignant tumor respectively. The prognosis of patients with malignant salivary tumors was not very favorable (Table 1).

▶ Salivary gland tumors in children are rare entities, with few series in the existing literature shedding light on their frequency or prevalence, so it was interesting in 2013 to see this article and another from China[1] dealing with this subject in a total of 241 children and adding to the existing series in the world literature. All the existing series overwhelmingly put pleomorphic adenoma as the most common tumor and mucoepidermoid carcinoma as a distant second in prevalence in the pediatric population, and it seems that this fact still holds in the

TABLE 1.—Tumor Distribution in Salivary Glands

Histotype	Number	Parotid	Site Submandibular Gland	Sublingual Gland	Others
Pleomorphic adenoma	96	66	21	1	8
Warthin tumor	1	1	0	0	0
Myoepithelioma	5	3	0	0	2
Basel cell adenoma	3	3	0	0	0
Mucoepidermoid carcinoma	8	8	0	0	0
Cystadenocarcinoma	1	1	0	0	0
Basal cell adenocarcinoma	1	1	0	0	0
Duct carcinoma	1	1	0	0	0
Acinic cell carcinoma	4	4	0	0	0
Adenoid cystic carcinoma	2	0	0	1	1

findings of these 2 series. It is also of interest to see that like some older series, acinic cell carcinoma remains the second most common malignant salivary gland tumor in these 2 series, in spite of its relative rarity as a malignant salivary gland tumor in general. As in the adult population and previous pediatric series the parotid gland also overwhelmingly remains the most common site of these tumors. This current series mentions that the prognosis of malignant tumors in their pediatric population was worse than that of some of the published series and attributed that to the smaller number of their cases; however, it was not clear from the article if these patients presented to treatment early after the onset of the mass appearing or after considerable delay because of other factors including social factors and regional variations of availability of health care, which may have made the tumors more established, and it seems from what is mentioned that adjuvant therapy was limited only to one patient in the above series. In any event, these 2 reports supply an additional glimpse into pediatric salivary gland tumors in that part of the world.

M. S. Said, MD, PhD

Reference

1. Deng R, Huang X, Hao J, Ding J, Hu Q. Salivary gland neoplasms in children. *J Craniofac Surg*. 2013;24:511-513.

Cytomegalovirus-induced salivary gland pathology: AREG, FGF8, TNF-α, and IL-6 signal dysregulation and neoplasia

Melnick M, Deluca KA, Sedghizadeh PP, et al (USC, Los Angeles, CA)
Exp Mol Pathol 94:386-397, 2013

Mucoepidermoid carcinoma (MEC) is the most common malignant tumor originating in major and minor salivary glands (SGs). Although the precise multifactorial etiology of human SG-MEC is largely unknown, we have recently shown that cytomegalovirus (CMV) is an important component of MEC tumorigenesis. Despite the well-documented overexpression of the EGFR → ERK signaling pathway in SG-MEC, there has been limited

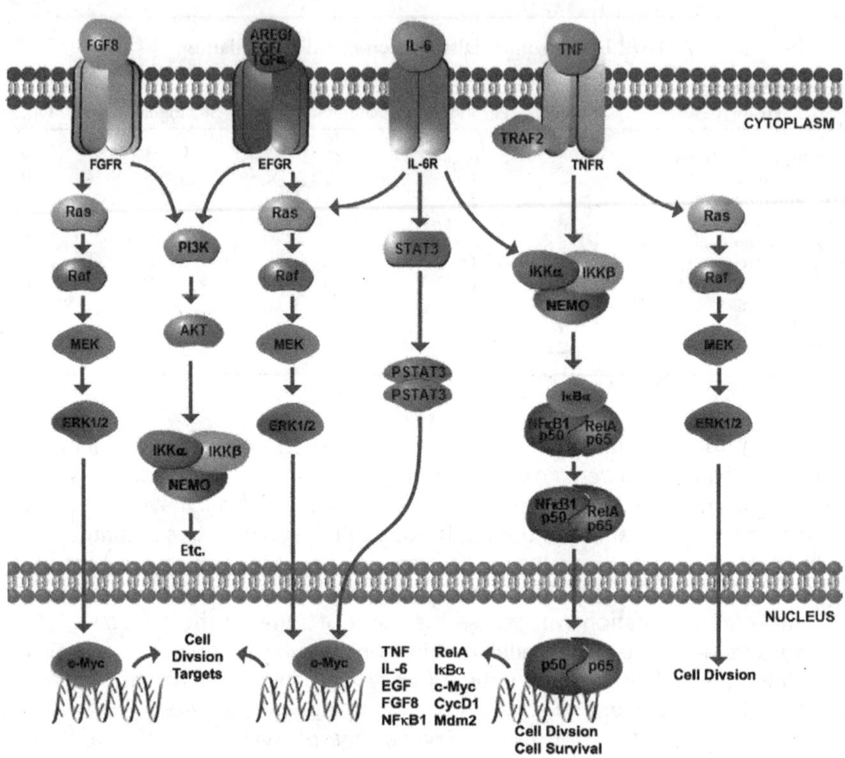

FIGURE 3.—Subcircuit map: a relational model that postulates how signaling events likely propagate during SMG pathogenesis; a conceptionally simple subcircuit for subsequent network modeling that is experimentally constrained and computationally accessible. This subcircuit is composed of 4 signaling pathways that are known to be critical to SMG ontogeny and share post-activation downstream targets (see text). (Reprinted from Melnick M, Deluca KA, Sedghizadeh PP, et al. Cytomegalovirus-induced salivary gland pathology: AREG, FGF8, TNF-α, and IL-6 signal dysregulation and neoplasia. *Exp Mol Pathol.* 2013;94:386-397, with permission from Elsevier.)

to no clinical success with inhibition of this pathway. Using our previously characterized mouse model of CMV-induced SG dysplasia/neoplasia, we report that inhibitors of the EGFR → ERK pathway do not ameliorate or rescue well-established pathology, either singly or in combination, but they do inhibit the evolution of progressive pathogenesis ("disease tolerance") in the face of mounting CMV burden. Failure to rescue SG pathology, suggested a possible increase in the ligand levels of alternative pathways that share cell proliferation and survival effectors (e.g. ERK and PI3K). Here we present evidence of a highly significant upregulation of ligands for the EGFR, FGFR, IL-6R, and TNFR signaling pathways, all of which converge upon the Raf/MEK/ERK amplifier module. This explains our finding that even in the presence of the highest nontoxic dose of an ERK phosphorylation inhibitor, pERK is undiminished. Given the considerable pathway crosstalk, a deep understanding of subversion and dysregulation of the SG interactome by CMV is a priori quite daunting. Circumventing this dilemma, we present evidence that concurrent inhibition of ERK phosphorylation (U0126) and CMV replication (acyclovir) obviates progressive pathogenesis and results in complete SG rescue (tumor regression). These findings provide a mechanistic foundation for potential clinical trials that utilize similar concurrent treatment with extant FDA-approved drugs (Fig 3).

▶ This report as well as previous reports[1,2] discussed the important relationship of cytomegalovirus (CMV) induction of mucoepidermoid carcinoma in an attempt to define the various pathways of the CMV-induced changes. Overall, through these studies using a mouse model, it was found that CMV induces mesenchymal to epithelial transformation; epithelial and mesenchymal hyperplasia, dysplasia, and neoplasia; loss of basement membrane zone components with reduced expression of epithelial-specific adherent junction proteins (E-cadherine); expression of CRTC1 protein found in mucoepidermoid carcinoma; and upregulation of activated COX/AREG/EGFR/ERK. In this report they added evidence of upregulation for epidermal growth factor receptor, interleukin-6R, and tumor necrosis factor receptor signaling pathway that converges on RAF/MEK/ERK pathway amplifier module (Fig 3). This study provides useful insight into CMV and mucoepidermoid carcinoma development as more evidence of virus-induced neoplasia. Such findings are of great importance in preventing these tumors and in treating patients, particularly when neoadjuvant therapy is recommended.

M. S. Said, MD, PhD

References

1. Melnick M, Sedghizadeh PP, Allen CM, Jaskoll T. Human cytomegalovirus and mucoepidermoid carcinoma of salivary glands: cell-specific localization of active viral and oncogenic signal proteins is confirmatory of a causal relationship. *Exp Mol Pathol.* 2012;92:118-125.
2. Melnick M, Abichaker G, Htet K, Sedghizadeh P, Jaskoll T. Small molecule inhibitors of the host cell COX/AREG/EGFR/ERK pathway attenuate cytomegalovirus-induced pathogenesis. *Exp Mol Pathol.* 2011;91:400-410.

Lipomatous Salivary Gland Tumors: A Series of 31 Cases Spanning Their Morphologic Spectrum With Emphasis on Sialolipoma and Oncocytic Lipoadenoma

Agaimy A, Ihrler S, Märkl B, et al (Univ Hosp, Erlangen, Germany; Laboratory for Dermatohistology and Oral Pathology, Munich, Germany; Klinikum Augsburg, Germany; et al)

Am J Surg Pathol 37:128-137, 2013

Lipomatous neoplasms of the salivary glands are rare. Their wide histologic spectrum has not been sufficiently studied. We collected 31 fat-containing salivary gland lesions excluding pleomorphic adenoma and myoepithelioma with lipometaplasia. There were 19 male and 12 female patients aged 7 to 89 years (mean, 53 y). Tumors originated in the parotid (n = 29) and the submandibular (n = 2) gland. On the basis of the proportion

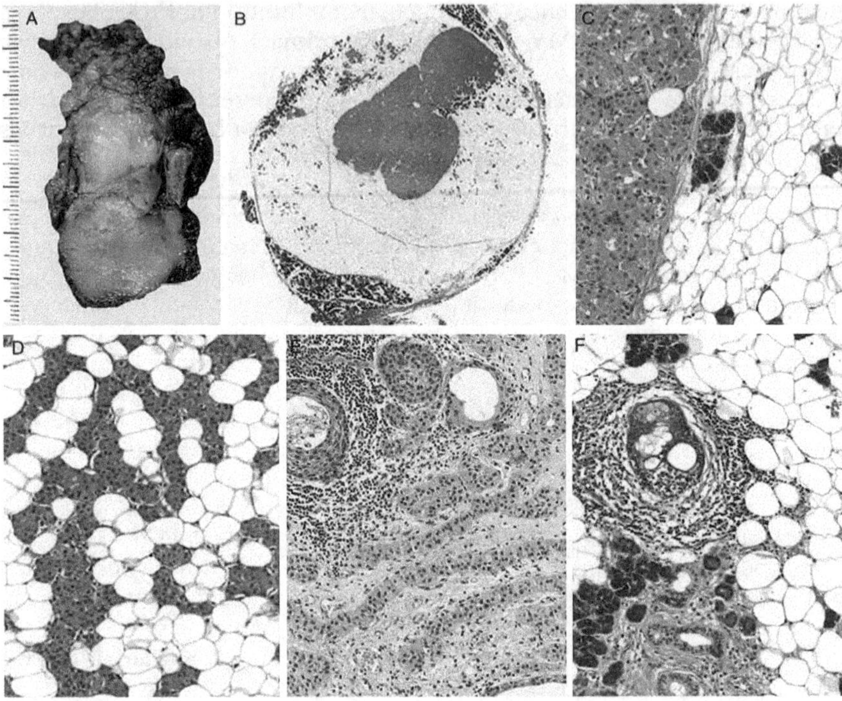

FIGURE 2.—Images showing oncocytic lipoadenoma of the parotid gland. A, Gross specimen (case 22) showed typical lobulation with yellowish fat-rich (upper) and brown oncocyte-dominated areas (lower). B, This lesion showed a biphasic pattern with well-circumscribed oncocytic epithelial component within the adipocytic background imparting a "nodule-in-nodule" pattern. Note variation in the fat content of the tumor lobules and the presence of sialolipoma-like lobules at the periphery. C, Closely juxtaposed fat-poor oncocytic lobule (left) and fat-rich lobule containing normal serous acini (right). D, This lobule showed equal amount of fat and oncocytic epithelium. E, Another case showed trabecular epithelial arrangement; note squamous foci surrounded by dense lymphocytic aggregates. F, A small focus of sebaceous metaplasia was surrounded by lymphocytic aggregates,fat, and serous acini closely mimicking sialolipoma. (Reprinted from Agaimy A, Ihrler S, Märkl B, et al. Lipomatous Salivary gland tumors: a series of 31 cases spanning their morphologic spectrum with emphasis on sialolipoma and oncocytic lipoadenoma. *Am J Surg Pathol.* 2013;37:128-137, with permission from Lippincott Williams & Wilkins.)

and distribution of adipose tissue and the epithelial type, tumors could be categorized into 3 main groups: ordinary lipoma (n = 20) identical to soft tissue lipoma but located within the salivary gland, oncocytic lipoadenoma (n = 6) composed predominantly of oncocytes with variable fatty component, nononcocytic sialolipoma (n = 4) composed of lobular fatty tissue (≥70%) with evenly distributed normal salivary tissue recapitulating the composition of normal salivary glands and microcystic lipoadenoma (n = 1) composed of cystic ducts admixed with adipose tissue. The mean tumor size was 3.3, 3.8, and 2.9 cm for lipoma, oncocytic lipoadenoma, and nononcocytic sialolipoma, respectively. Associated diseases included Madelung disease with bilateral atypical lipomatous tumors of the neck and bilateral parotid lipoma (1), oncocytic lipoadenoma after irradiation for sinonasal adenocarcinoma (1), and periparotideal lipoma excised years

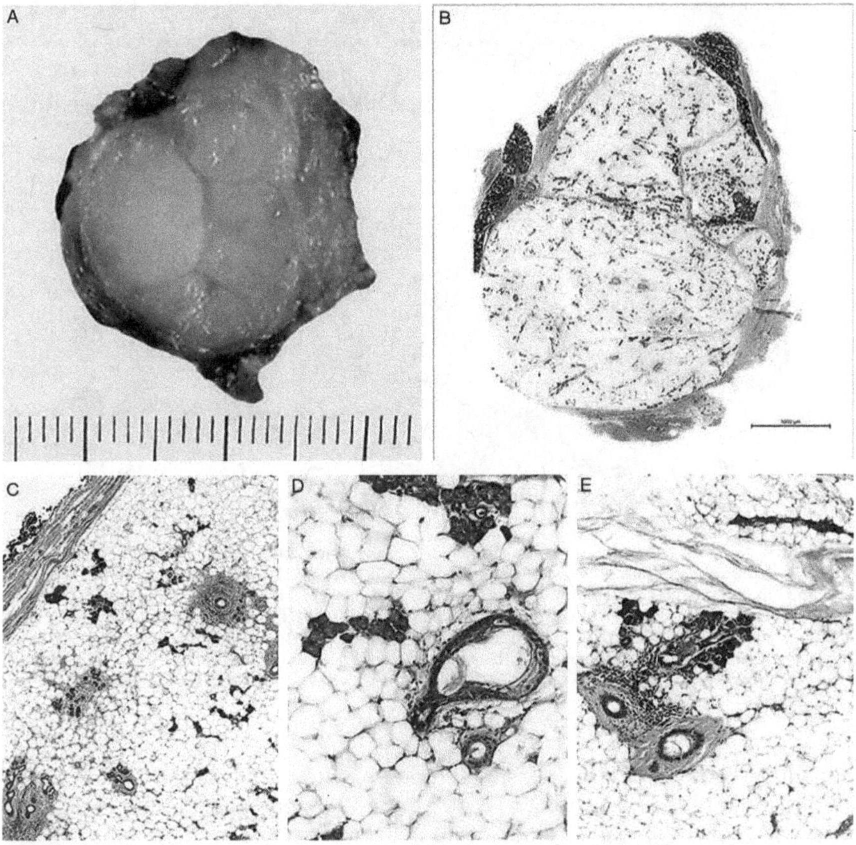

FIGURE 3.—Examples of nononcocytic sialolipoma. A, Gross specimen displaying typical lobulation and yellowish appearance due to fat predominance (case 27). B, Whole-mount section showing the characteristic lobulation with evenly distributed salivary gland structures in an adipocytic background. C, Close resemblance to normal salivary gland was evident in this image; note periductal inflammation/fibrosis and encapsulation. D, Dilated duct with sebaceous metaplasia and a small adjacent striated duct. E, Higher magnification of (C). (Reprinted from Agaimy A, Ihrler S, Märkl B, et al. Lipomatous Salivary gland tumors: a series of 31 cases spanning their morphologic spectrum with emphasis on sialolipoma and oncocytic lipoadenoma. *Am J Surg Pathol.* 2013;37:128-137, with permission from Lippincott Williams & Wilkins.)

before oncocytic lipoadenoma (1) and nononcocytic sialolipoma (1). No recurrence was recorded at a mean follow-up of 72 months (range, 6 to 184 mo). Sebaceous islands were seen in 5/6 oncocytic lipoadenomas and in 2/4 sialolipomas. Periductal inflammation/ fibrosis was common in sialolipoma and oncocytic lipoadenoma. This study demonstrates the wide morphologic spectrum of fatty salivary gland lesions. Oncocytic lipoadenoma is an epithelial-predominant tumor that is distinct from the fat-dominated nononcocytic sialolipoma, but the 2 types seem to merge in some cases (Figs 2-4).

▶ In 2013, this article and another by Starkman et al[1] reviewed lipomatous salivary gland tumors in 101 cases. These are two interesting articles for an entity

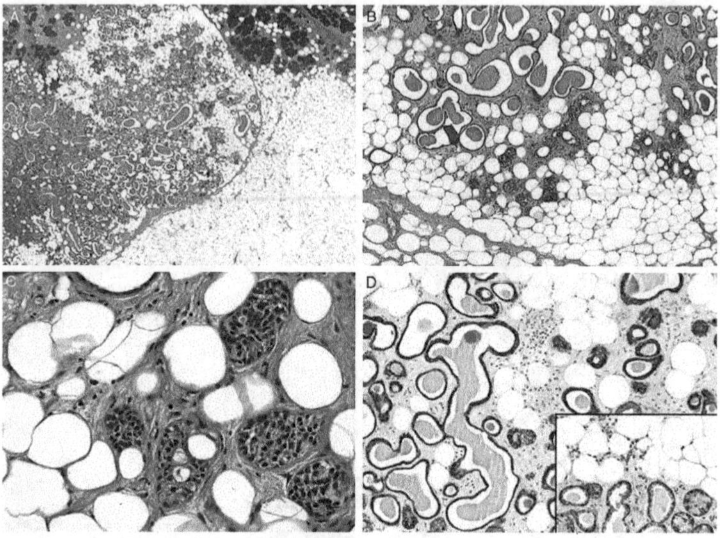

FIGURE 4.—This unusual case of lipoepithelial lesion showed an admixture of microcystic glands filled with hyaline secretion and interspersed adipose tissue (A). B, At higher magnification, the glands were lined by flat atrophic epithelium. C, Small foci showed basal cell hyperplasia imparting a cribriform pattern to some glands. D, Cytokeratin immunostaining confirmed the luminal-basal bilayered glands (main image: CK7; inset: CK5). (Reprinted from Agaimy A, Ihrler S, Märkl B, et al. Lipomatous Salivary gland tumors: a series of 31 cases spanning their morphologic spectrum with emphasis on sialolipoma and oncocytic lipoadenoma. *Am J Surg Pathol.* 2013;37:128-137, with permission from Lippincott Williams & Wilkins.)

with limited emphasis in the existing literature. Although ordinary lipomas constituted most of the cases in both reports, the Starkman et al[1] report included a description of the usual varieties of lipoma (sialolipoma, angiolipoma, fibrolipoma) and one case of liposarcoma. Agaimy et al, however, added more descriptive criteria to characterize the lipomatous lesions, including nononcocytic sialolipoma, oncocytic lipoadenoma, and microcystic lipoadenoma, which they termed *biphasic lipoepithelial lesions* with oncocytic or nononcocytic categories. Most of these tumors occurred in the parotid glands, although some occurred in the submandibular gland (only ordinary lipomas). It will be interesting to see if this wide spectrum of lipomatous lesions can gradually fall into universal acceptance in the pathologist's description of these rare lesions.

M. S. Said, MD, PhD

Reference

1. Starkman S, Olsen S, Lewis J, Olsen KD, Sabri A. Lipomatous lesions of the parotid gland: analysis of 70 cases. *Laryngoscope.* 2013;123:651-656.

Human papillomaviruses are not involved in the etiopathogenesis of salivary gland tumors

Skalova A, Kašpírková J, Andrle P, et al (Faculty of Medicine in Pilsen, Czech Republic; Molecular Biology Laboratory, Pilsen, Czech Republic)

Cesk Patol 49:72-75, 2013

Background.—Tumor-related high risk human papillomaviruses (HPV) 16 and 18 have been repeatedly detected in head and neck cancers, particularly, they are well known risk factors in squamous cell carcinoma of the oropharyngeal and tonsillar region. Little is known, however, about the possible role of HPV in salivary gland tumors.

Methods.—Fifty-five cases of benign and malignant salivary gland tumors were tested using p16 immunohistochemistry followed by HPV DNA polymerase chain reaction (PCR) using SPF, CPSGB, GP5+/GP6+ primers, and type specific primers for HPV 16, 18, 31, 33, 35, 45 in the cases with strong immunohistochemical expression for p16 protein (score 3+).

Results.—Only 5 tumors of 55 (9%) were completely devoid of any p16 staining, and in 10 cases (18%), less than 25% of tumor cells stained (score 1+). In the majority of cases (35 of 55; 64%) there was a patchy nuclear and cytoplasmic strong staining in 26 to 50% of tumor cells (score 2+). In five cases (9%), strong nuclear and cytoplasmic staining in more than 51% of tumor cells was detected (score 3+). However, none of the p16-positive cases showed any evidence of high-risk HPV by PCR.

Conclusions.—The results of the study indicate that HPV, in particular oncogenic types 16 and 18, are not involved in the etiology of benign and malignant epithelial tumors of salivary glands. Therefore, it is likely that salivary gland tumors belong to the category of tissues in which the p16 positive immunohistochemistry is not biologically relevant to the oncogenic role of HPV infection (Fig 2).

▶ As more efforts are made to further define the effect of human papillomavirus (HPV) in head and neck cancers, mainly squamous cell carcinoma, this report offers an interesting study on the relationship of HPV to salivary gland tumors. The types of tumors tested were varied and included benign (pleomorphic adenoma, Warthin's tumor, myoepithelioma, oncocytoma, cystadenoma, and basal cell adenoma) and malignant tumors (polymorphous low-grade adenocarcinoma, cribriform carcinoma of the tongue, adenoid cystic carcinoma, salivary duct carcinoma, mucoepidermoid carcinoma, acinic cell carcinoma, hyalinizing clear cell carcinoma, and carcinosarcoma ex pleomorphic adenoma [Fig 2]). The report also mentions previous similar studies that offered opposing results. Atula et al[1,2] did not detect the presence of HPV in 38 benign and malignant salivary glands and Vageli et al[3] detected them in 7 of 9 cases of parotid gland tumors. The study so far is the largest, with 55 cases, adding to 11 previously tested cases of lymphadenomas of salivary glands in which none were found to be positive for HPV. This is a study that some of the authors of the current study previously shared.[4] The authors used detection methods of combined immunohistochemistry for P16 followed by polymerase chain reaction for the

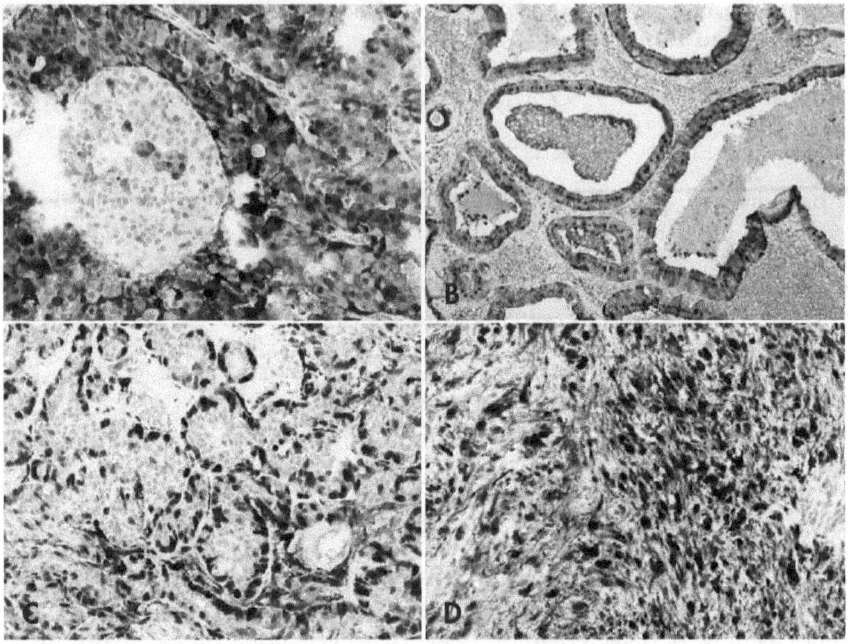

FIGURE 2.—p16 immunostaining in a variety of salivary gland tumors. **A:** Diffuse strong staining in oncocytoma of parotid gland (score 2+). Immunohistochemistry, 400x. **B:** Diffuse p16 staining in epithelial cell of benign Warthin tumor (score 3+). Immunohistochemistry, 200x. **C:** Strong patchy nuclear and cytoplasmic staining limited to abluminal cells of basal cell adenoma (score 2+). Immunohistochemistry, 200x. **D:** Diffuse staining in cellular pleomorphic adenoma of tongue (score 3+). Immunohistochemistry, 200x. (Reprinted from Skalova A, Kašpírková J, Andrle P, et al. Human papillomaviruses are not involved in the etiopathogenesis of salivary gland tumors. *Cesk Patol.* 2013;49: 72-75.)

P16-positive cases using primers similar to those of Vageli et al[3] but failed to show a relationship in spite of the P16 positivity, hence the conclusions mentioned in the above abstract. As the authors noted in their discussion, recent evidence suggests that the most appropriate way is the measurement of E6/E7 HPV expression.[5] Although this study definitely supports the contention of Atula et al[1,2] so far, further studies, probably using even more sensitive methods similar to those the authors mentioned, may further support or overturn the contention of this study. Additionally, it will be probably interesting to test cases of primary squamous cell carcinomas of salivary glands, which are unfortunately rare, to see if this relationship exists like it does for cervical cancer and a subset of squamous cell carcinomas of the head and neck.

M. S. Said, MD, PhD

References

1. Atula T, Grenam R, Klemi P, Syranen S. Human papillomavirus and Epstein-Barr virus in salivary gland tumors. *Clinc Otolaryngologol.* 1998;23:471-472.
2. Atula T, Grenam R, Klemi P, Syranen S. Human papillomavirus, Epstein-Barr virus, human herpesvirus 8 and human cytomegalovirus involvement in salivary gland tumors. *Oral Oncol.* 1998;34:391-395.

3. Vageli D, Sourvinos G, Loannou M, Koukoulis GK, Spandidos DA. High-risk human papillomavirus (HPV) in parotid lesions. *Int J Biol Markers.* 2007;22: 239-244.
4. Seethala RR, Thompson LDR, Gnepp DR, et al. Lymphadenoma of the salivary gland: clinicopathological and immunohistochemical analysis of 33 tumors. *Mod Pahol.* 2012;25:26-35.
5. Smeets SJ, Hesselink AT, Speel EJ, et al. A novel algorithm for reliable detection of human papillomavirus in paraffin embedded head and neck cancer specimen. *Int J Cancer.* 2007;121:2465-2472.

Primary Inner Ear Schwannomas: A Case Series and Systematic Review of the Literature

Van Abel KM, Carlson ML, Link MJ, et al (Mayo Clinic School of Medicine, Rochester, MN)

Laryngoscope 123:1957-1966, 2013

Objectives/Hypothesis.—To describe the natural history of primary inner ear schwannomas (PIES) and evaluate management outcomes and relationship between PIES location, clinical presentation, and time to diagnosis.

Study Design.—Retrospective chart review and systematic review of the literature.

Methods.—Vestibular schwannoma confined to or arising from the inner ear were included. PIES classification was based on anatomic subsite(s) involved. Detailed clinical history and outcomes were recorded.

Results.—In a systematic review (1933–2011), including 14 patients from the authors' institution (1999–2009), a total of 72 studies comprising 234 patients were evaluated. Mean follow-up was 32.8 ± 39.1 months (range, 0–183 months). The cochlea was the most commonly involved subsite (51%). Hearing loss was the most frequent presenting symptom (99%). Vertigo and abnormal balance were more common among tumors involving the vestibular system ($P < .01$). Average delay between symptom onset and diagnosis was 7.0 ± 8.0 years (median, 5 years; range, 0–40 years). Recent onset hearing loss was more likely to elicit an earlier diagnosis ($P = .01$). The majority of patients were observed without treatment (53%). Tumor progression was seen in 52% of patients.

Conclusions.—PIES are rare tumors and most commonly involve the cochlea. Tumor location is often associated with clinical presentation and correlates with delay between symptom onset and diagnosis. A watch-and-scan approach is the management strategy of choice in the absence of intractable vertigo or extensive tumor growth. The majority of patients report stable or improved symptoms over time, regardless of treatment (Fig 1).

► Schwannoma is a very common pathologic diagnosis made by pathologists every day, and most schwannomas reported in relation to the ear involve acoustic neuromas (vestibular type) in the cerebellopontine angle and internal auditory canal. This report represents a series of patients collected from over 80 years with schwannomas involving the inner ear itself as the primary location and

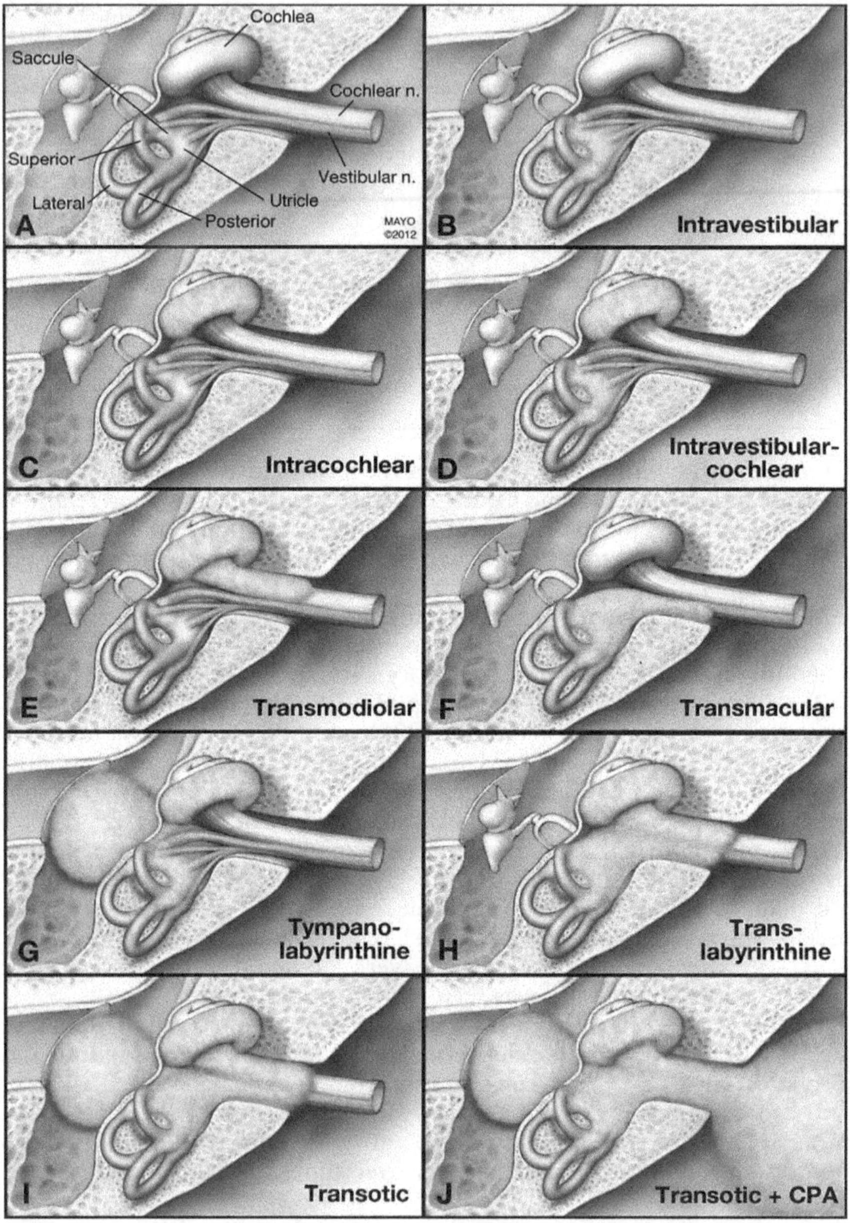

FIGURE 1.—Modified Kennedy classification[4] system for primary inner ear schwannomas. Schematic drawing demonstrating the modified Kennedy classification describing primary inner ear schwannoma location. (A) Anatomy of the inner ear and adjacent structures. (B–J) Extent of tumor involvement for each subtype is depicted in yellow. [Color figure can be viewed in the online issue, which is available at wileyonlinelibrary.com] *Editor's Note*: Please refer to original journal article for full references. (Reprinted from Van Abel KM, Carlson ML, Link MJ, et al. Primary inner ear schwannomas: a case series and systematic review of the literature. *Laryngoscope*. 2013;123:1957-1966, with permission from Laryngoscope and John Wiley and Sons, www.interscience.wiley.com.)

offers a new classification system (Fig 1) modifying the one proposed by Kennedy et al in 2004.[1] It is intriguing to know that this entity, for a long time, was not diagnosed clearly and was only discovered sporadically and incidentally during surgery or in an autopsy setting. Doyle and Brackmann in 1994 described the first preoperatively diagnosed series using magnetic resonance imaging,[2] which helped expedite the diagnosis and localization of these tumors. This report is probably of importance to pathologists (although it does not add to histologic findings in any unique way) who need to be aware of the presence of these tumors in this inner ear location and their proper classification when submitting their diagnosis. The authors also noted the management strategies for these tumors, including primary microsurgical resection, stereotactic radiosurgery, or chemical labyrinthectomy.

M. S. Said, MD, PhD

References

1. Kennedy RJ, Shelton C, Salzman KL, Davidson HC, Harnsberger HR. Intralabyrinthine schwannomas: diagnosis, management, and a new classification system. *Otol Neurotol.* 2004;25:160-167.
2. Doyle KJ, Brackmann DE. Intralabyrinthine schwannomas. *Otolaryngol Head Neck Surg.* 1994;110:517-523.

Follicular epithelial dysplasia of the thyroid: morphological and immunohistochemical characterization of a putative preneoplastic lesion to papillary thyroid carcinoma in chronic lymphocytic thyroiditis

Chui MH, Cassol CA, Asa SL, et al (Univ Health Network, Toronto, Ontario, Canada)

Virchows Arch 462:557-563, 2013

In chronic lymphocytic thyroiditis (CLT), the follicular epithelial cells display cytological atypia resembling papillary thyroid carcinoma (PTC), and epidemiological studies have suggested an increased risk of PTC in patients with this condition. While reactive atypia is observed diffusely in CLT-affected thyroid parenchyma, it is not unusual to find microscopic foci morphologically distinct from the surrounding parenchyma, exhibiting more pronounced cytological and architectural atypia. These small atypical lesions, which we term "follicular epithelial dysplasia" (FED), are particularly prominent in cases of severe CLT, yet lack invasive growth, papillary architecture, or intranuclear pseudoinclusions. To gain further insight into their biological significance, we constructed a tissue microarray of 70 cases of CLT, comprised of morphologically normal thyroid, thyroid with reactive atypia, FED, follicular nodular disease (nodular hyperplasia or follicular adenoma), and PTC. Immunohistochemical staining was performed for a marker panel including PTC (HBME-1, cytokeratin 19, galectin-3, and cyclin-D1) as well as TTF-1, thyroglobulin, and p63. Slides were digitally scanned and immunohistochemical staining evaluated using automated image analysis software. FED lesions were positive for TTF-1 and thyroglobulin (50/50, 100%), though some (13/50, 26%) also expressed

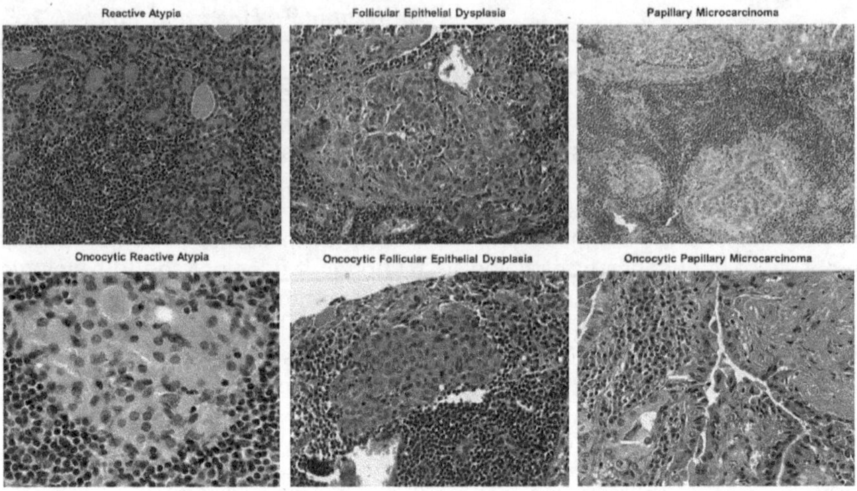

FIGURE 2.—The spectrum of atypical follicular epithelial lesions in chronic lymphocytic thyroiditis. There are regions where the follicular epithelium exhibits nuclear atypia in a diffuse distribution, likely reflective of a reactive process. In contrast, "follicular epithelial dysplasia" (FED) refers to discrete microscopic foci (<0.1 cm) of atypical follicular cells morphologically distinct from the surrounding parenchyma and often closely associated with severe chronic inflammation. Unlike papillary microcarcinomas, they lack invasive growth, stromal desmoplasia, papillary architecture, or intranuclear pseudoinclusions. (With kind permission from Springer Science+Business Media. Chui MH, Cassol CA, Asa SL, et al. Follicular epithelial dysplasia of the thyroid: morphological and immunohistochemical characterization of a putative preneoplastic lesion to papillary thyroid carcinoma in chronic lymphocytic thyroiditis. *Virchows Arch.* 2013;462:557-563.)

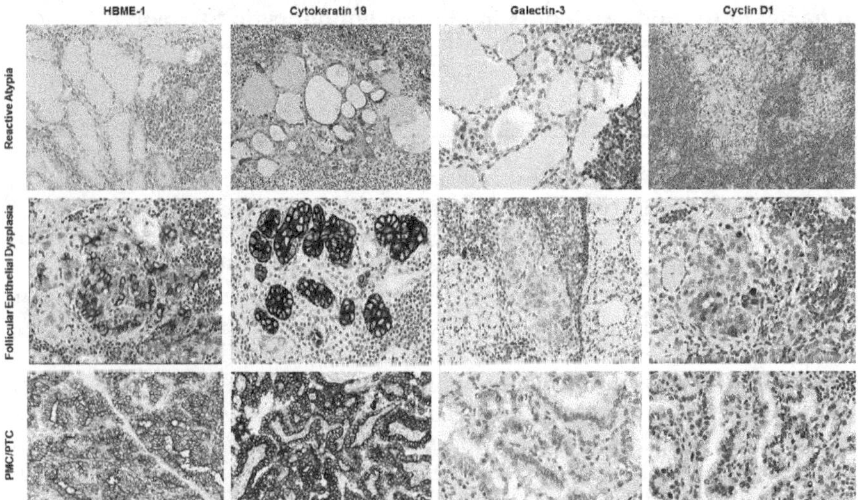

FIGURE 3.—Immunoprofile of atypical follicular epithelial lesions in chronic lymphocytic thyroiditis. The majority of FED lesions show diffuse strong immunoreactivity for HBME-1, galectin-3, cytokeratin 19, and cyclin D1, similar to the immunoprofile of papillary (micro)carcinomas. In contrast, lesions designated as reactive atypia are negative for all markers, though focal weak positivity, especially for cytokeratin 19, is observed areas with severe chronic inflammation. (With kind permission from Springer Science+Business Media. Chui MH, Cassol CA, Asa SL, et al. Follicular epithelial dysplasia of the thyroid: morphological and immunohistochemical characterization of a putative preneoplastic lesion to papillary thyroid carcinoma in chronic lymphocytic thyroiditis. *Virchows Arch.* 2013;462:557-563.)

TABLE 1.—Histological Features of Follicular Epithelial Lesions in CLT

Histologic Feature	Reactive Atypia	FED	Papillary Microcarcinoma
Nuclei Size and shape	Mildly enlarged with round shape or subtle nuclear membrane irregularities	Mild to moderate enlargement and nuclear membrane irregularities resulting in loss of nuclear roundness	Marked enlargement and nuclear membrane irregularities resulting in loss of nuclear roundness
Optical clearing/ chromatin margination	Often present	Often present	Often present and marked
Grooves	Rare	Present, variable extent	Easily identifiable
Crowding/ overlapping	Mild	Mild to moderate	Moderate to severe
Pseudoinclusions	Absent	Absent	Rare but diagnostic
Architecture	Follicles with mild variation in size and shape, no papillary architecture	Irregularly shaped follicles, trabecular, solid, nests, no papillary architecture	Papillary, follicular, solid
Distinct transition from surrounding parenchyma[a]	No	Yes	Yes
Sclerosis/fibrotic stroma	None or minimal	None or minimal	Often present, may be prominent
Chronic inflammation	Often abundant lymphocyte predominant	Often abundant lymphocyte predominant	Not frequent except Warthin-like variant
Infiltrative growth	No	No	May be present
Size	n/a	<1.0 mm	n/a

CLT Chronic lymphocytic thyroiditis, *FED* Follicular epithelial dysplasia
[a]Important diagnostic feature—a combination of cytologic and architectural changes.

p63. Similar to PTC, strong diffuse staining was observed for HBME-1 (43/50, 86%), cytokeratin 19 (48/50, 96%), galectin-3 (20/50, 40%) and cyclin-D1 (38/50, 76%). In contrast, normal thyroid, reactive atypia, and follicular nodular disease were negative, or at most, exhibited focal weak staining for HBME-1, cytokeratin 19, and galectin-3. The results of this study demonstrate the presence of atypical microscopic lesions in CLT with an immunohistochemical profile similar to PTC, supporting the concept of a premalignant lesion preceding PTC, arising in the context of severe chronic inflammation (Figs 2 and 3, Table 1).

▶ This is an interesting effort that discusses the morphologic criteria to subclassify the range of atypia observed in chronic lymphocytic thyroiditis—associated follicular lesions (Figs 2 and 3, Table 1) and introduces the concept of premalignant/dysplastic category into the interpretation of thyroid lesions. Previous work by Prasad et al[1] 2004, although in agreement with current findings, as the authors note, did not fully address the histomorphologic aspects. It is interesting to see that they could also introduce distinct immunohistochemical parameters to support that. Further studies to investigate the reproducibility of their morphologic and immunohistochemical findings probably will be the ultimate test for further validation of these findings and whether this study will eventually stand out. It will be informative if the authors follow that study with molecular tests of the lesions to determine points of similarity or difference with papillary thyroid carcinoma, which they mentioned was not included in this study. This study opens the way for more questions, such as: How many of these follicular epithelial dysplasia lesions are likely to transform to full-blown papillary carcinoma? Is the frequency of these lesions in an excised gland indicative of its future potential to full malignant transformation? If a hemilobectomy showed these lesions, is that an indication for complete thyroidectomy? At the end of the day, good studies open the door for further questions.

M. S. Said, MD, PhD

Reference

1. Prasad ML, Huang Y, Pellegata NS, de la Chapelle A, Kloos RT. Hashimoto's thyroiditis with papillary thyroid carcinoma (PTC)-like nuclear alterations express molecular markers of PTC. *Histopathology.* 2004;45:39-46.

Aggressive variants of follicular cell derived thyroid carcinoma; the so called 'Real Thyroid Carcinomas'

Baloch Z, Livolsi VA, Tondon R (Perelman School of Medicine, Philadelphia, PA; Univ of Pennsylvania, Philadelphia)

J Clin Pathol 2013 [Epub ahead of print]

The pathological diagnoses and classification schemes for thyroid carcinoma have changed over the past 20 years and continue to do so. New entities have been described and molecular analyses have suggested better characterisation and grouping of certain tumours. Because some of the lesions have been named differently by different authors, clinicians and patients may be confused as to what a specific patient's lesion represents. In this review, we discuss the thyroid tumours of follicular origin which are clinically unusual but important to recognise as their behaviour may be aggressive, they may not respond to radioiodine treatment and they may cause significant mortality. This paper describes these important but rare lesions, their pathological features, important clinicopathological correlations, molecular correlates and prognostic implications (Figs 1-5).

▶ This is an interesting review article that lists the recognized aggressive variants of thyroid cancer and discusses their histologic features and briefly recounts the most recent molecular findings. These include the following variants of papillary carcinoma: tall cell variant (Fig 1), columnar cell variant (Fig 2), diffuse sclerosing variant (Fig 3), solid variant (Fig 4), and hobnail variant (Fig 5) in addition to poorly differentiated and anaplastic carcinoma. The hobnail variant is a particularly interesting new addition to the known aggressive variants of papillary carcinoma.[1] The article also provides a concise review of the different molecular profiles of these aggressive types of thyroid cancer that have been investigated so far and are proving important in the diagnosis and treatment of these tumors.

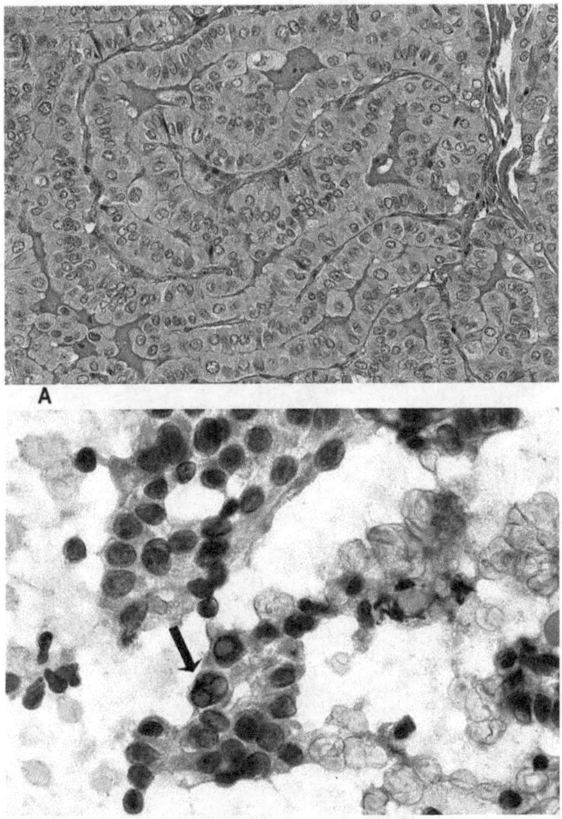

FIGURE 1.—Tall cell variant. Papillary formations are lined by tumour cells with eosinophilic cytoplasm and cell height 2–3 times the width (A— H&E stain, 60×). Fine needle aspiration of tall cell variant of papillary thyroid carcinoma demonstrating 'soap bubble intranuclear inclusions' (arrow) (B—Papanicolaou stain, 100×). (Reprinted from Baloch Z, Livolsi VA, Tondon R. Aggressive variants of follicular cell derived thyroid carcinoma; the so called 'Real Thyroid Carcinomas'. *J Clin Pathol*, with permission from the BMJ Publishing Group Ltd. 2013 [Epub ahead of print.])

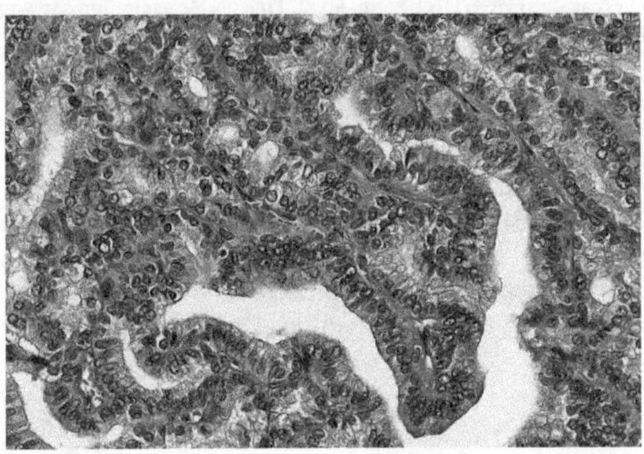

FIGURE 2.—Columnar cell variant. Papillary formation, hyperchromatic elongated nuclei and prominent nuclear pseudostratification (H&E stain, 60×). (Reprinted from Baloch Z, Livolsi VA, Tondon R. Aggressive variants of follicular cell derived thyroid carcinoma; the so called 'Real Thyroid Carcinomas'. *J Clin Pathol*, with permission from the BMJ Publishing Group Ltd. 2013 [Epub ahead of print.])

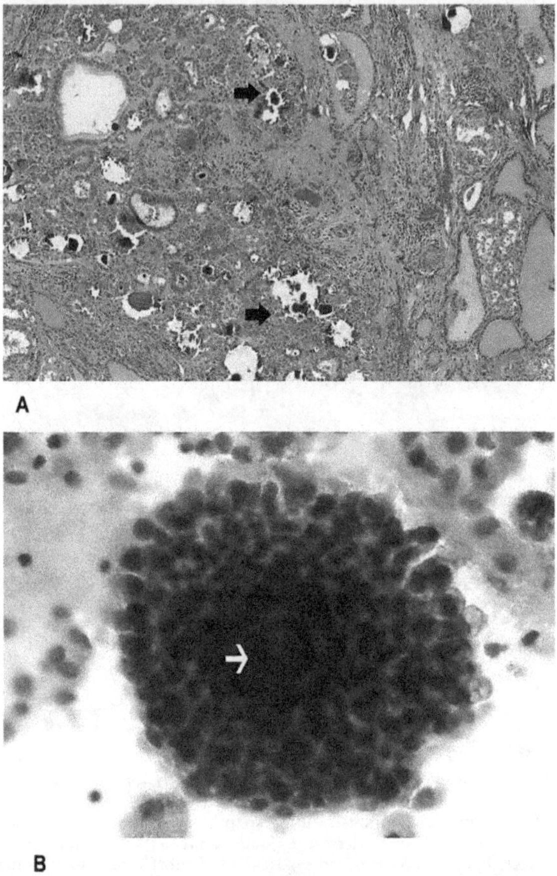

FIGURE 3.—Diffuse sclerosis variant. Low power showing an infiltrating tumour containing numerous psammoma bodies (arrows) (A— H&E stain, 40×). Fine needle aspiration showing a nest of tumour cells containing a psammoma body (arrow) (B—Papanicolaou stain, 100×). (Reprinted from Baloch Z, Livolsi VA, Tondon R. Aggressive variants of follicular cell derived thyroid carcinoma; the so called 'Real Thyroid Carcinomas'. *J Clin Pathol*, with permission from the BMJ Publishing Group Ltd. 2013 [Epub ahead of print.])

These aggressive forms of thyroid cancer do not usually respond favorably to the traditional thyroid cancer treatment with surgery and radioactive iodine ablation. Recognition of these variants is an important requirement in the diagnostic aspects of thyroid cancer at the moment and influences the patient prognostic and treatment aspects.

M. S. Said, MD, PhD

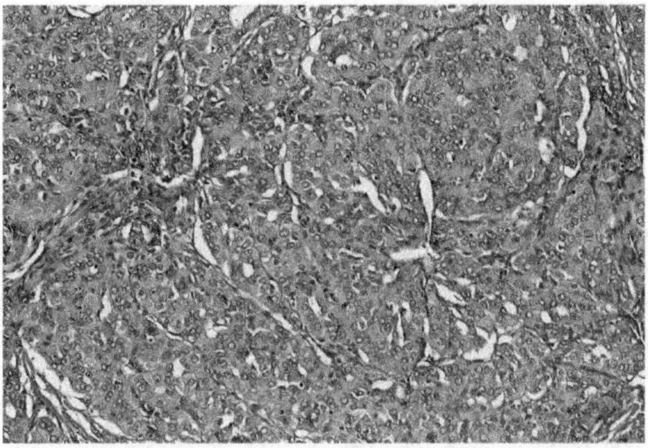

FIGURE 4.—Solid variant: Solid nests of tumour cells showing nuclear features of papillary thyroid carcinoma (H&E stain, 40×). (Reprinted from Baloch Z, Livolsi VA, Tondon R. Aggressive variants of follicular cell derived thyroid carcinoma; the so called 'Real Thyroid Carcinomas'. *J Clin Pathol*, with permission from the BMJ Publishing Group Ltd. 2013 [Epub ahead of print.])

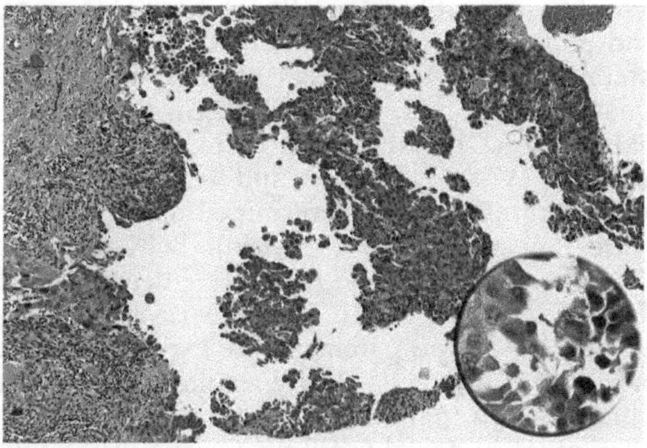

FIGURE 5.—Hobnail variant: Tumour with papillary growth pattern; the inset shows some of the tumour cell nuclei are eccentrically placed causing bulging of the nuclei at the tip of the cell imparting the so-called 'hobnail' appearance to the cells (H&E Stain, 20× and 60×). (Reprinted from Baloch Z, Livolsi VA, Tondon R. Aggressive variants of follicular cell derived thyroid carcinoma; the so called 'Real Thyroid Carcinomas'. *J Clin Pathol*, with permission from the BMJ Publishing Group Ltd. 2013 [Epub ahead of print.])

Reference

1. Aisoli S, Erickson LA, Sebo TJ, et al. Papillary thyroid carcinoma with prominent hobnail features: a new aggressive variant of moderately differentiated papillary carcinoma. A clinicopathologic, immunohistochemical, and molecular study of 8 cases. *Am J Surg Pathol.* 2010;34:44-52.

Biomarkers of Parathyroid Carcinoma

Erovic BM, Harris L, Jamali M, et al (Wharton Head and Neck Program, Toronto, Ontario, Canada; Univ Health Network, Toronto, Ontario, Canada)
Endocr Pathol 23:221-231, 2012

The diagnosis of parathyroid carcinoma can be challenging, and adjuvant therapies such as radiotherapy and chemotherapy are not particularly beneficial in the management of this disease, creating a challenge when dealing with unresectable recurrent and metastatic malignancy. We investigated the expression profile of biomarkers that represent potential markers of malignancy or targets for novel therapies in this disease. We constructed a tissue microarray of parathyroid carcinomas from 10 patients as well as parathyroid adenomas from 25 patients and stained the slides for 34 proteins involved in angiogenesis (platelet-derived growth factor receptor (PDGFR)-α, PDGFR-β, vascular endothelial growth factor receptor-2 (VEGFR-2), and epidermal growth factor receptor (EGFR)), inflammation (cyclooxygenase (COX)-1 and COX-2), cell adhesion (matrix metalloproteinase (MMP)-1, CD9, and keratin 7), cell cycle (Cdc2p34, cyclin D1, retinoblastoma (Rb), p27, p21, parafibromin, Bmi-1, 14-3-3σ, and p53), and apoptosis (Bcl-2a, Mcl-1, Bcl-xL, and glutathione-*S*-transferase-isoenzyme π (Gst-π)) along with some markers of the sonic hedgehog (Smo, SHH, Gli-1, Gli-2, Gli-3, and patched), mTOR (AKT, mammalian target of rapamycin (mTOR), and Forkhead box O (FoxO)-1), and WNT (Wisp-1, Wisp- 2, and β-catenin) signal transduction pathways. Protein expression was determined using computerized image analysis software (Spectrum Plus©, Aperio). Bcl-2a, parafibromin, Rb, and p27 were significantly decreased to variable degrees in all parathyroid carcinomas. COX-1/2, CD9, MMP-1, FoxO-1, VEGFR-2, PDGFR-α/β, Gst-π, Gli-1, Gli-2, Gli-3, and patched were expressed in the majority of benign and malignant tumor cells. These results indicate that the use of a panel that includes Bcl-2a, parafibromin, Rb, and p27 may be helpful in the assessment of atypical parathyroid neoplasms. Although the majority of other markers studied are also expressed in both benign and malignant parathyroid neoplasms, we have identified several potentially important target proteins related to angiogenesis and cell proliferation along with COX-1/2, Gst-π and members of sonic hedgehog pathway that may be therapeutic targets in parathyroid carcinoma. While these results are preliminary, a successful outcome of a clinical trial directed against these novel targets would provide much needed systemic adjuvant treatment for patients with metastatic parathyroid carcinoma (Fig 3).

► Parathyroid carcinoma has been a concerning topic for pathologists. It is not only rare, but its malignant features can be subtle and, in many instances, the morphologic differentiation from a hypercellular parathyroid tissue (both adenoma or hyperplasia) is minimal and difficult and depends mostly on the demonstration of some features that can also be seen in an adenoma (fibrous bands, increased mitotic activity) or vascular invasion (present only in 10% to

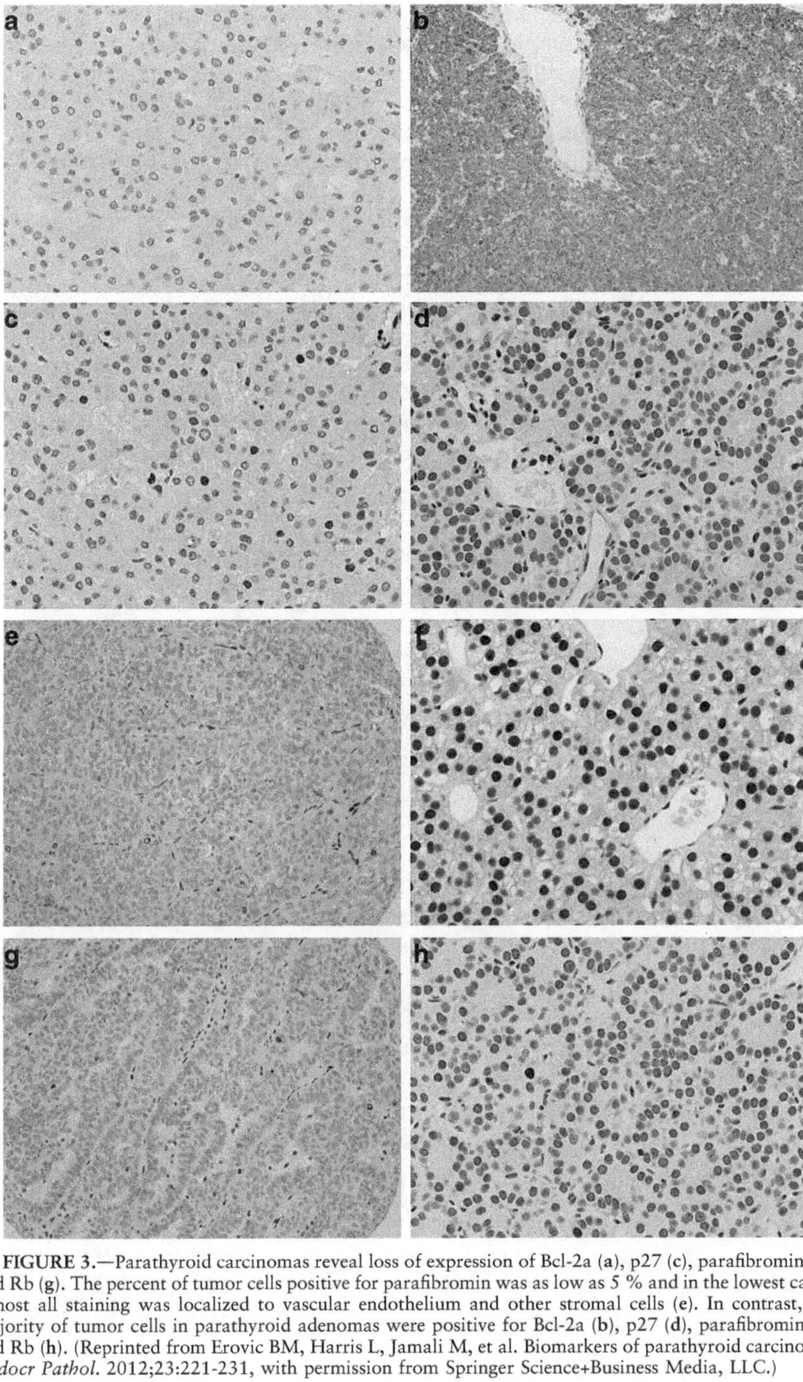

FIGURE 3.—Parathyroid carcinomas reveal loss of expression of Bcl-2a (**a**), p27 (**c**), parafibromin (**e**), and Rb (**g**). The percent of tumor cells positive for parafibromin was as low as 5 % and in the lowest cases, almost all staining was localized to vascular endothelium and other stromal cells (**e**). In contrast, the majority of tumor cells in parathyroid adenomas were positive for Bcl-2a (**b**), p27 (**d**), parafibromin (**f**), and Rb (**h**). (Reprinted from Erovic BM, Harris L, Jamali M, et al. Biomarkers of parathyroid carcinoma. *Endocr Pathol.* 2012;23:221-231, with permission from Springer Science+Business Media, LLC.)

15% of cases), perineural invasion, or capsular invasion with infiltrating to the surrounding tissue. Sometimes it is only recognized after the onset of metastasis. This article is a good effort aimed at finding a biomarker for parathyroid carcinoma that exceeds the classical teaching that in parathyroid carcinoma the serum calcium level is elevated (in excess of 14 mg/dL) with marked elevation of the parathyroid hormone. The authors explored a gamut of markers as mentioned in their abstract and found a panel for parathyroid carcinoma that may prove helpful in assessing a parathyroid carcinoma (BCL-2a, parafibromin, RB, and P27) that showed decreased expression in the carcinoma cases. Many of these markers are available and can be used by practicing pathologists. It would be interesting to see if other similar studies can duplicate the findings of these authors as a preliminary way to find better methods of defining this difficult type of cancer. The authors also showed (Fig 3) that the hedgehog pathway proteins and COX1/2 have been expressed in both benign and malignant parathyroid neoplasms, which also may be helpful, particularly in the adjuvant therapies for metastatic parathyroid carcinomas, which can be difficult to control using available methods of therapy.

M. S. Said, MD, PhD

10 Cytopathology

Cytology of Spontaneous Nipple Discharge—Is It Worth It? Performance of Nipple Discharge Preparations in the College of American Pathologists Interlaboratory Comparison Program in Nongynecologic Cytopathology

Moriarty AT, Schwartz MR, Laucirica R, et al (AmeriPath Indiana, Indianapolis; The Methodist Hosp, Houston, TX; Baylor College of Medicine, Houston, TX; et al)

Arch Pathol Lab Med 137:1039-1042, 2013

Context.—The usefulness of spontaneous nipple discharge analysis is controversial. Nipple discharge preparations are rare in clinical practice and malignant cases are exceptional. The College of American Pathologists Interlaboratory Comparison Program in Nongynecologic Cytopathology has included nipple discharge preparations since its inception.

Objective.—To evaluate participant responses in the College of American Pathologists Interlaboratory Comparison Program in Nongynecologic Cytopathology to assess the accuracy of cytologic interpretation of nipple discharge preparation.

Design.—General diagnostic category (benign, suspicious, malignant), participant type (pathologist, cytotechnologist), stain (Papanicolaou, modified Giemsa), and program year (2005-2009) were analyzed using χ^2 and a nonlinear mixed model for slide factor correlation structure.

Results.—Of 2506 responses, 1280 (51%) were malignant, 171 (7%) were papillary, and 1055 (42%) were benign. There were 222 discordant general category responses with a false-positive/ suspicious rate of 12.8% and a false-negative rate of 3.4%. The most common falsenegative diagnosis was mastitis/abscess (125 of 1272 responses; 9.8%). The most common false-positive response was papillary lesion (26 of 457 responses; 5.7%). There were no differences between stains or years. Cytotechnologists performed better than pathologists; pathologists had a higher false-negative rate than cytotechnologists (15.3% versus 7.9%, $P < .001$).

Conclusions.—There is poor accuracy in evaluating nipple discharge preparation in the College of American Pathologists Interlaboratory Comparison Program in Nongynecologic Cytopathology. If the findings in the program parallel clinical practice, nipple discharge preparations may adversely impact patient care. A benign nipple discharge cytologic diagnosis does not exclude malignancy, and the false-positive/suspicious rate

TABLE 2.—Participant Diagnosis for Reference Diagnosis of Adenocarcinoma

Participant Diagnosis	No.	%
Adenocarcinoma	1045	82.1
Mastitis/abscess/subareolar abscess	125	9.8
Papillary lesion	66	5.2
Fibrocystic changes	19	1.5
Invalid	13	1.0
Normal/reactive	4	0.3
Unsatisfactory	1	0.1
Total	1273	100

requires confirmation of a malignant nipple discharge prior to definitive patient management (Table 2).

▶ The data reported by Moriarty et al indicate that nipple discharge cytopathology specimens have a relatively high false-positive/suspicious rate (Table 2) in this College of American Pathologists interlaboratory comparison program. It is unclear if these data apply to actual practice, as pathologists may use other indeterminate diagnoses, such as atypical. Moriarty et al show some photomicrographs and describe diagnostic criteria, although in actual practice, many pathologists see relatively few nipple discharge specimens, and the application of criteria is challenging. For additional reading, see reference list.[1,2]

S. Raab, MD

References

1. Louie LD, Crowe JP, Dawson AE, et al. Identification of breast cancer in patients with pathologic nipple discharge: does ductoscopy predict malignancy? *Am J Surg*. 2006;192:530-533.
2. Das DK, Al-Ayadhy MT, Ajrawi MT, et al. Cytodiagnosis of nipple discharge: a study of 602 samples from 484 cases. *Diagn Cytopathol*. 2001;25:25-37.

Assessment of Malignancy for Atypia of Undetermined Significance in Thyroid Fine-Needle Aspiration Biopsy Evaluated by Whole-Slide Image Analysis

Collins BT, Collins LE (Washington Univ School of Medicine, St Louis, MO)
Am J Clin Pathol 139:736-745, 2013

Atypia of undetermined significance (AUS) in thyroid fine-needle aspiration (FNA) has a low to intermediate incidence of malignancy, and objective criteria could allow for improved assessment of malignancy. Consecutive thyroid FNA AUS cases with surgical excision were selected. Whole-slide images (WSIs) were evaluated for basic criteria by image analysis, including total groups and nuclear/cytoplasmic (N/C) ratio. The 44 cases encompassed 23 benign and 21 malignant entities. Seventeen (81%) of 21 malignant cases and 11 (48%) of 23 benign cases had an N/C ratio of 0.50 or less. An N/C ratio of 0.50 or less had an odds ratio for malignancy of 4.64 ($P = .03$).

A combined category of an N/C ratio of 0.50 or less and greater than 20 cell groups had an odds ratio for malignancy of 7.0 ($P = .04$). Establishing defined objective WSI criteria has the potential to provide an assessment of malignancy for AUS thyroid FNA cases.

▶ The reason we use the category of atypia of undetermined significance (AUS) in thyroid gland fine-needle aspiration (FNA) is because we cannot definitively separate neoplastic from non-neoplastic entities based on light microscopic evaluation. There are many latent causes of this situation, and the lack of well-defined criteria and patterns and the lack of the application of these criteria to actual practice are 2 causes. I think the challenge is in better defining the criteria and patterns of benign and neoplastic entities, rather than better defining AUS. Collins and Collins initiate this approach by examining the criteria in subsets of AUS with follow-up. It is unclear if image analysis was necessary for this approach and if pathologists alone could make the criteria distinction based on digital image or light microscopy. In addition, an important cause of the inability to make a definitive diagnosis in thyroid gland FNA, which affects the appearance of image criteria and patterns, and the assessment of this quality, should be determined in addition to the re-examination of criteria. For further reading, see reference list.[1,2]

S. Raab, MD

References

1. Bongiovanni M, Krane JF, Cibas ES, Faquin WC. The atypical thyroid fine-needle aspiration: past, present, and future. *Cancer Cytopathol.* 2012;120:73-86.
2. Krane JF, Vanderlaan PA, Faquin WC, Renshaw AA. The atypia of undetermined significance/follicular lesion of undetermined significance: malignant ratio: a proposed performance measure for reporting in The Bethesda System for thyroid cytopathology. *Cancer Cytopathol.* 2012;120:111-116.

The Diagnostic Reliability of Urinary Cytology: A Retrospective Study

Raisi O, Magnani C, Bigiani N, et al (Mirandola's Hosp, Italy; et al)

Diagn Cytopathol 40:608-614, 2012

The aim of this study was twofold. The first aim was to estimate the diagnostic reliability of urinary cytology for detection and management of urothelial neoplasms by using a specific preserving fluid for sample collection, and the liquid-based thin layer method for specimen preparation, the estimate was based on the correlation between the cytological findings of 10,000 non-hospitalized patients, and their histological diagnoses. A second aim was to compare the reliability of two instruments for thinlayer preparation, i.e., TP2000, TP3000, capable of processing the specimens at very different rates. The preservation of cell structure is ameliorated by the procedure of sample collection and treatment here described. This allows a more accurate reading of LBC slides as shown by: (a) the significant concordance between cytological and histological diagnosis (92%); (b) the significant number of low-grade urothelial carcinomas (20.5%) revealed by urinary cytology and validated by histologic diagnosis; (c) the low rate (8%) of misjudgement of cytological diagnosis reached in this study. The quality of performances of the two instruments tested for thin-layer preparation, i.e., TP2000 and TP3000, is statistically comparable. We recommend the procedure that makes use of preserving fluid for sample collection (cytolyt TM) and treatment (preservcyt TM) as here described. We also recommend the use of thin-layer method for specimen preparation since it allows a more uniform distribution of the cells on the support with reduction of overlapping phenomena. Finally, economic considerations suggest the preferential use of Thin Prep 3000.

▶ Although Raisi and colleagues mainly wrote a technology assessment of 2 instruments for producing thin-layer preparations, an important aspect of this article is the evaluation of the ability of these preparations to detect low-grade urothelial carcinomas in outpatient urine samples. Based on diagnoses of malignant or suspicious, the authors concluded that 20.5% of the detected cancers were low grade. The debate in the cytology literature, however, continues, as some authors contest that low-grade lesions cannot be detected in a urine sample. These data show otherwise. The authors do not provide a list of criteria to separate low- from high-grade urothelial carcinoma and simply appear to lump the low-grade lesions with high-grade urothelial carcinomas. This is a limitation, because reinforcing the use of published criteria of low-grade urothelial carcinoma would have strengthened this study. For additional reading, see reference list.[1,2]

S. Raab, MD

References

1. Bastacki S, Ibrahim S, Wilczynski SP, Murphy WM. The accuracy of urinary cytology in daily practice. *Cancer.* 1999;87:118-128.
2. Glatz K, Willi N, Glatz D, et al. An international telecytologic quiz on urinary cytology reveals educational deficits and absence of a commonly used classification system. *Am J Clin Pathol.* 2006;126:294-301.

A simplified economic approach to thyroid FNA cytology and surgical intervention in thyroid nodules

Poller DN, Kandaswamy P (Queen Alexandra Hosp, Cosham, Portsmouth, UK; Natl Inst for Health and Clinical Excellence, Manchester, UK)
J Clin Pathol 66:583-588, 2013

Objective.—Few studies have modelled the economics of thyroid FNA.

Methods.—A simple spreadsheet economic model for delivery of thyroid fine needle aspiration (FNA) cytology is described using the UK Royal College of Pathologists' Classification for thyroid FNA which is based on The Bethesda System for Reporting Thyroid Cytopathology.

Results.—We show an estimated 27.8% cost treatment reduction per patient if low rates of non-diagnostic for cytological diagnosis (Thy 1) and neoplasm possible atypia/non-diagnostic (Thy 3a) are achieved, which require rapid onsite FNA adequacy assessment of aspiration samples. If we assume that the number of thyroid FNAs performed in the UK annually is around 500 per million, and the UK population is 62 million, this could save the UK National Health Service significant sums, as the additional cost per patient treated in this model varies from £781 for a scenario with ultrasound guided FNA and inclinic cell adequacy assessment to £998 where aspirates are taken in conventional fashion without any inclinic adequacy assessment.

Conclusions.—This model makes a strong economic case for the introduction of rapid onsite assessment of thyroid FNA across cancer networks, to improve the diagnostic efficacy of thyroid FNA.

▶ Very few economic analyses have been performed in the field of cytopathology testing service. For thyroid gland fine-needle aspiration, this report indicates that the use of ultrasonography and immediate assessment improves specimen quality, which, in turn, improves the interpretive component. The components of national system redesign to achieve this approach are complex. For additional reading, see reference list.[1,2]

S. Raab, MD

References

1. Borget I, Vielh P, Leboulleux S, et al. Assessment of the cost of fine-needle aspiration cytology as a diagnostic tool in patients with thyroid nodules. *Am J Clin Pathol.* 2008;129:763-771.
2. Eedes CR, Wang HH. Cost-effectiveness of immediate specimen adequacy assessment of thyroid fine-needle aspirations. *Am J Clin Pathol.* 2004;121:64-69.

Interobserver agreement in determining non-small cell lung cancer subtype in specimens acquired by EBUS-TBNA

Steinfort DP, Russell PA, Tsui A, et al (Royal Melbourne Hosp, Parkville, Victoria, Australia; St Vincent's Hosp, Fitzroy, Australia)
Eur Respir J 40:699-705, 2012

Endobronchial ultrasound (EBUS)-guided transbronchial needle aspiration (TBNA) may diagnose suspected lung cancer. Determination of non-small cell lung cancer (NSCLC) subtype may guide therapy in select patients. Small-volume biopsies may be subject to significant interobserver variability in subtype determination.

Three pathologists independently reviewed specimens from 60 patients who underwent EBUS-TBNA for diagnosis/staging of suspected/known NSCLC. Smear, haematoxylin and eosin (H&E) and immunohistochemistry (IHC) specimens were reviewed without reference to other specimen types obtained from the same patient. Final diagnoses, and degree of confidence in the diagnosis, were recorded for each specimen.

Almost perfect agreement was seen for distinguishing between small cell lung cancer and NSCLC for all specimen types. Agreement in determination of NSCLC subtype for smear, H&E and IHC specimens was slight (κ = 0.095, 95% CI −0.164–0.355), fair (κ = 0.278, 95% CI 0.075–0.481) and moderate (κ = 0.564, 95% CI 0.338–0.740), respectively. Perfect agreement was seen when all three observers were confident of diagnoses made on IHC specimens.

Interobserver agreement in interpretation of EBUS-TBNA specimens is moderate for determination of NSCLC subtype. Agreement is highest following examination of IHC specimens. Clinicians should be aware of the degree of pathologist confidence in the tissue diagnosis prior to commencement of subtype-specific therapy for NSCLC.

▶ Steinfort et al report that the interobserver variability of practicing cytopathologists in their interpretation of endobronchial ultrasound–guided transbronchial needle aspiration of non–small cell lung cancer (NSCLC) is low for smears and hematoxylin and eosin–stained sections. The use of immunohistochemistry adds greater precision. Dunnill and Gatter previously reported that only 30% of lung carcinomas are of a single cell type, so the findings in this study are not surprising. Cytopathology smears are excellent in demonstrating the differences in malignant cell types, as the cytoplasm often has easily discernable differences on Pap and rapid stains. Consequently, one may expect high levels of disagreement if cytopathologists are asked to classify specimens based on single malignant cell type. Better agreement probably would be seen if cytopathologists were asked to determine if the NSCLC was homogeneous or heterogeneous. For clinical practice, these data indicate that the cytopathologic diagnosis may best be listed as NSCLC with a further listing of the main cell type or a listing of the different cell types. A standardized immunohistochemical panel could further add value. For further reading, please see reference list.[1,2]

S. Raab, MD

References

1. Travis WD, Brambilla E, Noguchi M, et al. International Association for the Study of Lung Cancer/American Thoracic Society/European Respiratory Society international multidisciplinary classification of lung adenocarcinoma. *J Thorac Oncol.* 2011;6:244-285.
2. Dunnill MS, Gatter KC. Cellular heterogeneity in lung cancer. *Histopathology.* 1986;10:461-475.

Women's preferences regarding options for management of atypical, borderline or low-grade cervical cytological abnormalities: a review of the evidence

Sadique MZ, Legood R (London School of Hygiene and Tropical Medicine, UK)

Cytopathology 23:161-166, 2012

Objectives.—To review the evidence on women's preferences for and valuation of alternative management pathways following identification of low-grade cytological abnormalities as part of routine cervical cancer screening. The aim was to identify empirical studies evaluating women's preferences regarding alternative management pathways and to compare the impact of alternative elicitation methods on results.

Methods.—A systematic review of the literature was conducted using the online bibliographic information service PubMed database. Empirical studies were identified that elicited general preferences, utilities or valuations based on willingness to pay (WTP) with respect to management of low-grade cytology results. Data were extracted on the methodology used and the empirical results.

Results.—Where quality of life data were elicited directly from patients that were undergoing management of low-grade abnormalities utilizing direct elicitation techniques such as WTP, general preference questionnaires and the Euroqol, the studies tended towards a preference in favour of HPV testing (and colposcopy referral if HPV positive) rather than repeat cytology. In contrast, where studies included the general population and presented hypothetical scenarios of treatment pathways, and explicitly tried to incorporate assessment of process utility, the evidence indicated a slight tendency to favour repeat cytology.

Conclusion.—Consideration of patient preferences in the management of low-grade cytology is important for designing screening protocols. The reviewed studies indicate that potentially different conclusions may be drawn depending on the elicitation methodology and selection of participants in the research.

▶ Sadique and Legood evaluate the role of patient centeredness in empirical studies in determining the most appropriate management strategy in the care of women who have atypical, borderline, or low-grade Pap test results. Not surprisingly, the method of elicitation of the response and patient population affects the choice of the most appropriate management strategy. These data reflect both the biases of the investigators who have contributed to the field and the individuals who have participated in the studies. These data serve as a reminder to pathologists that patient preferences regarding the follow-up of laboratory test results are challenging to measure and that non—patient-centered systems may make assumptions in even how to determine best strategies. For further reading, see reference list.[1,2]

S. Raab, MD

References

1. Whynes DK, Woolley C, Philips Z. Management of low-grade cervical abnormalities detected at screening: which method do women prefer? *Cytopathology.* 2008; 19:355-362.
2. Melnikow J, Kuppermann M, Birch S, Chan BK, Nuovo J. Management of the low-grade abnormal Pap smear: What are women's preferences? *J Fam Pract.* 2002;51:849-855.

Factors contributing to false-negative and potential false-negative cytology reports in SurePath™ liquid-based cervical cytology

Gupta N, John D, Dudding N, et al (Royal Hallamshire Hosp, Sheffield, UK)

Cytopathology 24:39-43, 2013

Objectives.—The characteristics of false-negative conventional cervical cytology smears have been well documented, but there is limited literature available for liquid-based cytology (LBC), especially SurePath™ samples. We aimed to assess the characteristics of false-negative SurePath LBC samples.

Methods.—Over a period of 5 years, an audit of false-negative reports in SurePath cervical cytology was undertaken. In a workload of 183,112 samples, 481 (0.3%) false negatives were identified using two routes: those detected by routine laboratory internal quality control (rapid prescreening) ($n = 463$) and those reported as normal (true false negatives) with concurrent high-grade cervical histology ($n = 18$). Ninety-five false-negative cases with a subsequent biopsy reported as at least cervical intraepithelial neoplasia grade 2 (CIN2+) were reviewed for a number of different cytomorphological features.

Results.—Of 95 samples with subsequent CIN2+, 30.5% predominately contained microbiopsies/hyperchromatic crowded cell groups (HCGs), 27.3% sparse dyskarytotic cells, 4.2% pale cell dyskaryosis, 6.3% small dyskaryotic cells; 3.2% were misinterpreted cells, 8.4% contained other distracting cells, 7.4% were low contrast, 5.3% were unexplained and 7.4% were true negatives. The mean number of microbiopsies/HCGs in that category was 4.6. The mean number of abnormal cells in the sparse dyskaryotic cell category was 13.8.

Conclusions.—Microbiopsies/HCGs were the commonest reason for false negatives. They were usually present in sufficient numbers to be detected but interpretation could be problematic. Dispersed single abnormal cells were usually not identified because of their scarcity or the presence of distracters (Table 1).

► In this fascinating article, Gupta et al performed a root cause analysis of cervical intraepithelial neoplasia grade 2 false-negative SurePath Pap tests. The authors found (amazingly to my mind) that 88 of 95 cases had diagnostic cells that fit into a number of categories, as described in Table 1. Because these cell groups may retrospectively be recognized, we may hypothesize that retrospective methods of detection may be translated into prospective methods of detection and prevention. The first point to recognize is that the underlying problem is interplay between sampling and cognitive failures. The sampling issues will need to be addressed by technological, preparation, and sampling skill investigation. The cognitive issues also have a number of deeply lying latent factors dealing with training, work structure (eg, solitary practitioners practicing in environments with little assistance), and safety systems (the use of checklists that limit bias

TABLE 1.—The number of Microbiopsies and Abnormal Cells in Each Category (Using the Predominant Category for Each Case) of False-Negative Cases ($n = 88{:}95$ Minus 7 True False Negative)

Count	Number of Cases: Misinterpreted Microbiopsies	Sparse Dyskaryosis	Pale Cell Dyskaryosis	Small Cell Dyskaryosis	Misinterpreted Cells	Distracters	Low Contrast	Unexplained
Number of microbiopsies								
0	0	11	0	3	1	1	2	1
0–5	3	11	3	3	0	4	3	1
6–10	13	4	1	0	0	3	2	1
11–15	5	0	0	0	1	0	0	1
16–20	2	0	0	0	0	0	0	0
21–25	2	0	0	0	1	0	0	0
26–30	2	0	0	0	0	0	0	0
>30	2	0	0	0	0	0	0	1
Total	29 (4)*	26 (3)*	4 (1)*	6 (1)*	3	8 (2)*	7	5
Number of abnormal cells								
0	5	0	0	0	0	3	1	1
0–5	1	4	0	0	0	1	0	0
6–10	3	4	2	3	1	1	1	0
11–15	9	10	1	0	0	2	4	0
16–20	5	3	0	2	1	0	1	0
21–25	2	2	0	1	0	0	0	1
26–30	1	2	1	0	1	0	0	0
>30	3	1	0	0	0	1	0	3
Total	29 (4)*	26 (3)*	4 (1)*	6 (1)*	3	8 (2)*	7	5

*(n) Number of true false-negative samples in each category.

and improved focus on specific criteria). The solution does not solely lie in simply recognizing root causes. For further reading, see reference list.[1,2]

S. Raab, MD

References

1. Evered A. What can cytologists learn from 25 years of investigations in visual search? *Br J Biomed Sci.* 2005;62:182-192.
2. Studeman KD, Ioffe OB, Puszkiewicz J, Sauvegeot J, Henry MR. Effect of cellularity on the sensitivity of detecting squamous lesions in liquid-based cervical cytology. *Acta Cytol.* 2003;47:605-610.

Large performance variation does not affect outcome in the Finnish cervical cancer screening programme

Lönnberg S, Nieminen P, Kotaniemi-Talonen L, et al (Finnish Cancer Registry, Helsinki, Finland; Helsinki Univ Central Hosp, Finland; et al)

Cytopathology 23:172-180, 2012

Objective.—Cytology screening for prevention of cervical cancer can reduce incidence and mortality by more than 80% in settings with good organization and rigorous quality control. Audit studies are essential for reaching and maintaining a high quality of screening. The aim of this study was to evaluate variation in performance indicators by screening laboratory and assess the impact on the effectiveness of screening as indicated by cervical intraepithelial neoplasia grade 3 and above (CIN3+) rates after a negative screen.

Methods.—Seven cytology screening laboratories operating during 1990–1999 with a total of 953 610 screening tests performed were included in the study. By linking screening and cancer register files, all cases of CIN3+ diagnosed in the screened population were identified. For 395 CIN3+ cases with a preceding negative screen and 787 controls, a re-evaluation of smears was undertaken to uncover false negative screening tests. Performance parameters and rates of CIN3+ after a negative screen were analysed for interlaboratory heterogeneity.

Results.—The rates of follow-up recommendations and referrals varied by up to 3.6- (2.8–10.2%) and 4.0-fold (0.03–0.12%), respectively. CIN1, CIN2 and CIN3+ screen detection rates differed by up to 8.5- (0.02–0.17%), 5.4- (0.05–0.25%) and 3.3-fold (0.05–0.18%). False negative rates determined by re-evaluation showed up to 2.1-fold differences (29–62%). Rates of CIN3+ after a negative screen (0.023–0.048%) and as a proportion of total CIN3+ (15–31%) in the screened population were low and did not vary significantly.

Conclusions.—There were large variations in the sensitivity–specificity trade-off between laboratories, reflected in all performance indicators as well as in the test validity estimates of the re-evaluation phase, but not in screening effectiveness. Even though performance variations do not always have an impact on the effectiveness of screening, they lead to variations in cost, treatment and psychological burden, and should be addressed.

▶ Lönnberg and coauthors report that gynecologic cytopathology laboratories showed significant differences in several quality assurance parameters, including false-negative rates determined by re-evaluation, but these differences did not affect cervical cancer prevention effectiveness. However, these differences affected other quality metrics such as patient centeredness and efficiency. Consequently, the authors argue that we do not know the most appropriate trade-off between sensitivity and specificity, but that these Finnish laboratories essentially provided safe service. A theory to be tested based on these results is that overdiagnosis, based on fear of litigation or other factors, may not lead to meaningful increased cervical cancer prevention. For further reading, see reference list.[1,2]

S. Raab, MD

References

1. Kotaniemi-Talonen L, Nieminen P, Hakama M, et al. Significant variation in performance does not reflect the effectiveness of the cervical cancer screening programme in Finland. *Eur J Cancer.* 2007;43:169-174.
2. Kotaniemi-Talonen L, Anttila A, Malila N, et al. Screening with a primary human papillomavirus test does not increase detection of cervical cancer and intraepithelial neoplasia 3. *Eur J Cancer.* 2008;44:565-571.

Assessment of Manual Workload Limits in Gynecologic Cytology: Reconciling Data From 3 Major Prospective Trials of Automated Screening Devices

Renshaw AA, Elsheikh TM (Baptist Hosp, Miami, FL; Cleveland Clinic, OH)
Am J Clin Pathol 139:428-433, 2013

Previous prospective studies have shown different results when comparing automated and manual screening of gynecologic cytology. The results of 3 large prospective studies were reviewed and relative sensitivity used as a gold standard. No significant differences could be shown in relative sensitivity between the ThinPrep Imaging System and the FocalPoint GS Imaging System ($P > .05$). When manual screening was restricted to less than 6 hours per day, 50 or fewer slides per day, and at least 6 minutes per slide (<10 slides/h), the relative sensitivity for automation was significantly lower for atypical squamous cells of undetermined significance and above (ASC+) (0.81; 95% confidence interval [CI], 0.79-0.83) than when manual screening was not restricted (1.07; 95% CI, 1.03-1.10). All 3 sites that screened 10 or more slides per hour manually had a relative sensitivity for automation that was significantly higher for high-grade squamous intraepithelial lesions and above (HSIL+) than for the remaining groups who screened less than 10 slides per hour (1.40 [95% CI, 1.22-1.60] vs 0.97 [95% CI, 0.95-1.00]). These results suggest that location finding of abnormalities (ASC+) may be more strongly associated with time spent screening per day, whereas classification/interpretation skills (HSIL+) may depend on time spent on an individual case. There is no evidence that automated screening devices are more sensitive than manual screening performed at lower well-defined workloads. More restricted workloads (≤41 slides/d, ≤4.5 h/d) for manual screening may perform significantly better than automated screening devices as measured by histologic cervical intraepithelial neoplasia 2 and above.

▶ As a field, we have much to learn about the cognitive processes of cytotechnologists and cytopathologists in their review of slides. Kahneman[1] wrote that cognitive processes may be divided into 2 types: fast thinking and slow thinking. Slow thinking is rationale deliberate thought, and, in pathology, this is demonstrated by trainees, who are learning criteria and pattern, and more experienced personnel, who may slow down in their thought processes and rationally deliberate on cases that appear slightly different and need more time. Fast thinking is pattern recognition and involves the quick leap from criteria and pattern to diagnosis. The errors that occur with these 2 forms of cognition differ, and it is important to determine the types of errors that are occurring in the cognitive processes of a cytopathologist and cytotechnologist to determine the methods to limit error. The article by Renshaw and Elsheikh indirectly studies this issue by examining accuracy in using automated devices. However, the challenge in understanding the real issue is based on understanding process rather than outcome. The authors did not find a difference in outcomes, but it is unclear if the underlying cognitive processes are different using different screening methods.

S. Raab, MD

Reference

1. Kahneman D. *Thinking, fast and slow.* Penguin Books Limited; London, United Kingdom; 2011.

11 Hematolymphoid

Anaplastic Large Cell Lymphoma: A Potential Pitfall in the Differential Diagnosis of Melanoma

Pulitzer M, Brady MS, Blochin E, et al (Memorial Sloan-Kettering Cancer Ctr, NY; et al)

Arch Pathol Lab Med 137:280-283, 2013

The diagnosis of metastatic melanoma can be complicated by absent characteristic cytology, melanin, or antigen expression in a suspect tumor, putting the pathologist at risk for incorrectly diagnosing recurrent melanoma while missing a second malignancy. We report a 69-year-old man with a history of acral melanoma, metastatic to inguinal nodes, presenting with an ipsilateral thigh nodule. Histology showed a proliferation of pleomorphic cells in the dermis and subcutis, suspicious for melanoma. S100, Melan-A, and HMB-45 immunohistochemistry were negative. However, microphthalmia-associated transcription factor and CD117 labeled the neoplasm, prompting consideration of a late metastatic melanoma with loss of antigen expression. Subsequent immunolabeling for CD4, CD43, and CD30 and clonal Tcell gene rearrangements enabled the correct diagnosis of cutaneous anaplastic large cell lymphoma. This case illustrates a pitfall in evaluating tumors in patients with known metastatic melanoma, and emphasizes the need for broad-spectrum immunohistochemistry in cases that are not clear-cut.

▶ Pulitzer and colleagues describe that large cell lymphoma may mimic a metastatic malignant melanoma to the skin, especially in patients who have a history of malignant melanoma. The histologic separation of these entities may be difficult in some cases, especially in patients who have amelanotic variants. Pulitzer recommends that the immunohistochemical study panel should be expanded to include markers such as CD4, CD34, and CD30. Presumably, other large, single-cell malignancies are in the differential diagnosis, and the authors do not describe if other markers would be beneficial in a strategic exclusion approach. For further reading, see reference list.[1,2]

S. Raab, MD

References

1. Brauns TC, Schultewolter T, Dissemond J, Maschke J, Goos M. C-Kit expression in primary cutaneous T-cell lymphomas. *J Cutan Pathol.* 2004;31:577-582.
2. Callaway MP, Briggs JC. The incidence of late recurrence (greater than 10 years): an analysis of 536 consecutive cases of cutaneous melanoma. *Br J Plast Surg.* 1989;42:46-49.

Comparison Between 1-Needle Technique Versus 2-Needle Technique for Bone Marrow Aspiration and Biopsy Procedures

Al-Ibraheemi A, Pham T, Chen L, et al (Univ of Texas Med School, Houston; Trinity Univ, San Antonio, TX)
Arch Pathol Lab Med 137:974-978, 2013

Context.—Bone marrow examination is essential for diagnosis and staging of hematologic disorders. Traditionally, the bone marrow biopsy and aspirate are obtained with 2 needles at 2 separate sites. This approach is associated with significant discomfort, procedural time, and occasionally, morbidity. Although previous observations had suggested that a single-needle technique at one site is a simpler and less-painful procedure, there had been concern that the 1-needle technique may yield a suboptimal biopsy for diagnosis.

Objective.—To conduct a systematic comparison of multiple parameters of bone marrow biopsy specimens obtained by the traditional 2-needle technique versus the 1-needle technique for bone marrow collection.

Design.—We retrospectively evaluated 20 biopsy specimens obtained by each of the 2 mentioned techniques by comparing the morphologic quality of the biopsy, biopsy length, and biopsy cellularity.

Results.—We found that the 1-needle technique yielded an adequate biopsy for diagnosis. The measured parameters of the samples obtained by the 1-needle versus 2-needle techniques were similar.

Conclusion.—This study suggests that the 1-needle technique may be preferred for bone marrow aspirate and biopsy.

▶ Al-Ibraheemi et al provide evidence that a one-needle technique for procuring bone marrow tissue yielded adequate material for diagnosis. The study involved only a limited number of samples, and it would be interesting to conjecture if there are specific patient characteristics that could be used to predict if the 2-needle technique would be useful in specific patient subsets. For further reading, see reference list.[1,2]

S. Raab, MD

References

1. Islam A. Bone marrow aspiration before bone marrow core biopsy using the same bone marrow biopsy needle: a good or bad practice? *J Clin Pathol.* 2007;60: 212-215.
2. Lee SH, Erber WN, Porwit A, Tomonaga M, Peterson LC, International Council for Standardization in Hematology. ICSH guidelines for the standardization of bone marrow specimens and reports. *Int J Lab Hematol.* 2008;30:349-364.

12 Techniques/Molecular

Deep ion sequencing of amplicon adapter ligated libraries: a novel tool in molecular diagnostics of formalin fixed and paraffin embedded tissues

Becker K, Vollbrecht C, Koitzsch U, et al (Univ of Cologne, Germany; Univ Hosp Cologne, Germany)

J Clin Pathol 66:803-806, 2013

Due to the advanced progress in personalised therapy concepts for non-small cell lung cancer (NSCLC), we applied the ion semiconductor sequencing (ISS) approach to molecular diagnosis of NSCLC, analysing a set of therapy relevant gene loci. DNA from macrodissected tumour samples of formalin fixed biopsies was used for PCR amplification of *EGFR* exons 18, 19, 21 and *KRAS* exon 1. A total of 128 PCR products were analysed by conventional termination sequencing as well as by ISS. Sensitivity of ISS was additionally determined using 100–10 000 copies of reference mutants. All somatic mutations detected by direct Sanger sequencing were also identified by ISS. No additional mutants were detected. Running samples with limited copies of mutated alleles revealed high sensitivity, detecting less than 10% (2500 copies) mutants in a human wild type background. In conclusion, multiplexed mutation analyses by ISS is an efficient technology that can easily be linked to existing PCR approaches in molecular pathology.

▶ Becker et al describe a novel approach to the molecular diagnosis of non–small cell lung cancer using ion semiconductor sequencing. One of their take-home messages is that the use of any pre-existing polymerase chain reaction (PCR) products of well-established PCR protocols is possible. For additional reading, see reference list.[1,2]

S. Raab, MD

References

1. Hadd AG, Houghton J, Choudhary A, et al. Targeted, high-depth, next-generation sequencing of cancer genes in formalin-fixed, paraffin-embedded and fine-needle aspiration tumor specimens. *J Mol Diagn*. 2013;15:234-247.
2. Quail MA, Smith M, Coupland P, et al. A tale of three next generation sequencing platforms: comparison of Ion Torrent, Pacific Biosciences and Illumina MiSeq sequencers. *BMC Genomics*. 2012;13:341.

Molecular genetic testing for lung adenocarcinomas: a practical approach to clinically relevant mutations and translocations

Dacic S (Univ of Pittsburgh Med Ctr, PA)

J Clin Pathol 66:870-874, 2013

There is a consensus that molecular testing of the lung carcinoma should be the standard of care in the clinical management of patients with lung carcinoma. Recent practice guidelines in oncology and pathology recommend that all advanced and metastatic non-small-cell lung carcinoma with adenocarcinoma histology undergo biomarker testing for epidermal growth factor receptor gene (*EGFR*) mutations and anaplastic lymphoma kinase gene (*ALK*) rearrangements. Other types of non-small-cell carcinoma may be considered for such testing if they occur in never-smokers. The landscape of targetable biomarkers in non-small-cell carcinoma is changing rapidly, and demand for clinical testing beyond *EGFR* mutations and *ALK* gene rearrangements is increasing. Many patients may test positive for other 'drivers'. As a result, they may be treated with approved biomarker-driven therapies or may be eligible to receive investigational agents in clinical trials. This creates challenges for treating physicians and pathologists such as obtaining sufficient tissue for molecular testing and standardisation of molecular testing in clinical laboratories. This review will focus on the most important lung carcinoma biomarkers predictive of response and will discuss proposed routine molecular testing in clinical practice.

▶ Dacic provides a good review of epidermal growth factor receptor and anaplastic lymphoma kinase testing in patients who have lung carcinoma with adenocarcinoma histology. As Dacic indicates, molecular testing of lung adenocarcinoma is emerging as the standard of care. For additional reading, see reference list.[1,2]

S. Raab, MD

References

1. Smouse JH, Cibas ES, Jänne PA, Joshi VA, Zou KH, Lindeman NI. EGFR mutations are detected comparably in cytologic and surgical pathology specimens of nonsmall cell lung cancer. *Cancer.* 2009;117:67-72.
2. Kalikaki A, Koutsopoulos A, Trypaki M, et al. Comparison of EGFR and K-RAS gene status between primary tumours and corresponding metastases in NSCLC. *Br J Cancer.* 2008;99:923-929.

Fluorescence confocal microscopy for pathologists

Ragazzi M, Piana S, Longo C, et al (IRCSS Santa Maria Nuova Hosp, Reggio Emilia, Italy; et al)

Mod Pathol 1-12, 2013

Confocal microscopy is a non-invasive method of optical imaging that may provide microscopic images of untreated tissue that correspond almost perfectly to hematoxylin- and eosin-stained slides. Nowadays, following two confocal imaging systems are available: (1) reflectance confocal microscopy, based on the natural differences in refractive indices of subcellular structures within the tissues; (2) fluorescence confocal microscopy, based on the use of fluorochromes, such as acridine orange, to increase the contrast epithelium-stroma. In clinical practice to date, confocal microscopy has been used with the goal of obviating the need for excision biopsies, thereby reducing the need for pathological examination. The aim of our study was to test fluorescence confocal microscopy on different types of surgical specimens, specifically breast, lymph node, thyroid, and colon. The confocal images were correlated to the corresponding histological sections in order to provide a morphologic parallel and to highlight current limitations and possible applications of this technology for surgical pathology practice. As a result, neoplastic tissues were easily distinguishable from normal structures and reactive processes such as fibrosis; the use of fluorescence enhanced contrast and image quality in confocal microscopy without compromising final histologic evaluation. Finally, the fluorescence confocal microscopy images of the adipose tissue were as accurate as those of conventional histology and were devoid of the frozen-section-related artefacts that can compromise intraoperative evaluation. Despite some limitations mainly related to black/white images, which require training in imaging interpretation, this study confirms that fluorescence confocal microscopy may represent an alternative to frozen sections in the assessment of margin status in selected settings or when the conservation of the specimen is crucial. This is the first study to employ fluorescent confocal microscopy on surgical specimens other than the skin and to evaluate the diagnostic capability of this technology from pathologists' viewpoint.

▶ Ragazzi et al reported on the potential use of confocal microscopy in surgical pathology. Ragazzi et al described that fluorescence confocal microscopy offered some advantages over frozen-section analysis: (1) shorter turnaround time, (2) preservation of tissue integrity for routine histologic examination, and (3) detection of adipose tissue, which often is difficult to detect in routine frozen sections. It is possible that confocal microscopy could be used to avoid frozen sections and evaluate surgical margins in some specimen types and to evaluate small tissue specimens. Of course, several barriers in the implementation of confocal microscopy would need to be overcome, including the education of pathologists. However, this technology could be beneficial in improving surgical pathology quality metrics such as timeliness and efficiency. For additional reading, see reference list.[1,2]

S. Raab, MD

References

1. Gareau DS, Jeon H, Nehal KS, Rajadhyaksha M. Rapid screening of cancer margins in tissue with multimodal confocal microscopy. *J Surg Res.* 2012;178:533-538.
2. Gareau DS, Li Y, Huang B, Eastman Z, Nehal KS, Rajadhyaksha M. Confocal mosaicing microscopy in Mohs skin excisions: feasibility of rapid surgical pathology. *J Biomed Opt.* 2008;13:054001.

Are we counting mitoses correctly?

Yigit N, Gunal A, Kucukodaci Z, et al (Gulhane Military Med Academy and School of Medicine, Ankara, Turkey)

Ann Diagn Pathol 17:536-539, 2013

The number of mitotic figures in a predefined area is essential in pathologic evaluation for most tumors. This information sometimes provides clues in differentiating neoplastic lesions from nonneoplastic ones and sometimes in defining and grading of the tumors as well as prognosticating expected lifetime of the patient. As a generally accepted concept, scanning a certain number of consecutive nonoverlapping areas that are rich in viable tumor cells is required. Invasion fronts or the periphery of the tumors is preferred for counting mitosis. The target area to be counted for mitotic activity for various tumors is standardized as the number of mitosis in an established number of high-power fields. However, suggested mitotic counts, which constitute the basis of these studies, were obtained via the old microscopes, which usually had narrower visual fields than the state-of-the-art microscopes. Because the visual fields of the present microscopes provide larger areas compared with the older ones, corrections in mitosis counting are needed to make them compatible with the criteria, which had been put forward in the original reference studies (Table 2).

▶ Yigit et al emphasize important points in the technique of mitotic figure counting. Older microscopes, which were used to first obtain mitotic counts for specific diseases, had narrower visual fields compared with current microscopes. Table 2 shows the mean number of high-power fields that pathologists should count for specific disease entities for specific purposes (eg, grading and diagnosis).

S. Raab, MD

TABLE 2.—Suggested Mitosis or Specific Cell Types Counting Criteria for Different Entities and Related Corrections When Using 20- or 22-mm Ocular Lenses

			The instruments that was used in the original studies (mm^2)				The mean number of HPF that should be scanned for the correction when used 20- or 22-mm ocular lenses	
Entity	Purpose	Accepted criteria in the original reference studies	Ocular lens diameter (mm)	Field area per HPF (mm^2)	Total number of HPF	Total scanned area in the original studies	20 mm	22 mm
Soft tissue tumors [8]	Mitosis scoring for FNCLCC grading	Score 1: 0-9 mitosis Score 2: 10-19 mitosis Score 3: ≥20 mitosis	18.8	0.173	10	1.73	8.8	7.3
GIST [4]	Determination of aggressive behavior	≤5 mitosis >5 mitosis	14	0.10	50	5	25	21
Meningioma [1]	Determination of aggressive behavior	Meningioma: <4 mitosis Atypical meningioma: 4-20 mitosis Anaplastic meningioma: ≥20 mitosis	18	0.16	10	1.6	8	6.7
Follicular lymphoma [5]	Grading	Grade 1: 0-5 centroblast/1 HPF Grade 2: 6-15 centroblast/1 HPF Grade 3: N15 centroblast/1 HPF	18	0.16	10 HPF/10	1.6/10	8 HPF/10	6.7 HPF/10
Invasive ductal carcinoma of the breast (NOS) [3]	Mitosis counting for histological scoring	Score 1: 0-7 mitosis Score 2: 8-14 mitosis Score 3: ≥15 mitosis	20	0.20	10	2	10	8.4
Melanoma [9]	Determination of prognostic factor	Good prognostic factor: <1/mm^2 Bad prognostic factor: ≥1/mm^2	–	–	–	1	5	4.2
Carcinoid tumor of the lung [12]	Classification	Typical carcinoid: ≤1 mitosis/mm^2 Atypical carcinoid: ≥2 mitosis/mm^2	20	0.20	10	2	10	8.4
Neuroendocrine tumors of the gastrointestinal system [2]	Grading	Grade 1: <2 mitosis Grade 2: 2-20 mitosis Grade 3: >20 mitosis	20	0.20	10	2	10	8.4
Eosinophilic esophagitis [6]	Diagnosis	15 eosinophil/1 HPF	20	0.196	5 HPF/5	0.98	5 HPF/5	4.1 HPF/5
Colorectal adenocarcinoma [7]	Intratumoral lymphocyte counting	≥3 lymphocyte/1 HPF	20	0.196	5 HPF/5	0.98	5 HPF/5	4.1 HPF/5

Editor's Note: Please refer to original journal article for full references.

False positivity in HER2 testing of breast cancer: novel paths for approaching an old dilemma

Nunes CB, Rocha RM, Buzelin MA, et al (Federal Univ of Minas Gerais, Belo Horizonte, Brazil; AC Camargo Hosp, São Paulo, Brazil)

J Clin Pathol 66:946-950, 2013

Aims.—Variability in determining HER2 status has been reported, especially, differences in sensitivity and specificity among commercially available antibodies, with false positive and false negative results. We compared the sensitivity and specificity of five anti-HER2 antibodies by immunohistochemistry (IHC), using the new dual colour brightfield in situ hybridisation (DDISH) as the gold standard, on invasive breast carcinomas (IBC) arrays.

Material and Methods.—Serial sections from tissue microarrays (TMA) containing 200 preselected primary IBC were submitted to DDISH (VENTANA INFORM HER2 Dual ISH assay), and immunohistochemistry, using Dako A0485 and HercepTest (polyclonal), Novocastra CB11 (mouse monoclonal), NeoMarkers SP3 and Ventana 4B5 (rabbit monoclonal).

Results.—From the initial 200 cases, 184 were assessed by DDISH and IHC. The concordance among the antibodies was considered very good (kappa statistics varied from 0.82 to 0.9). The overall concordance between IHC and DDISH ranged from 94.1% for CB11 to 96.6% for A0485. The antibodies A0485, HercepTest, SP3 and 4B5 were over 95% sensitive and specific. CB11 was the most specific antibody (97.1%). 60% (CB11) to 83.3% (SP3) of the 2+ cases showed no gene amplification by DDISH. False negative cases varied from 0.5% (A0485) to 3.8% (CB11) of the

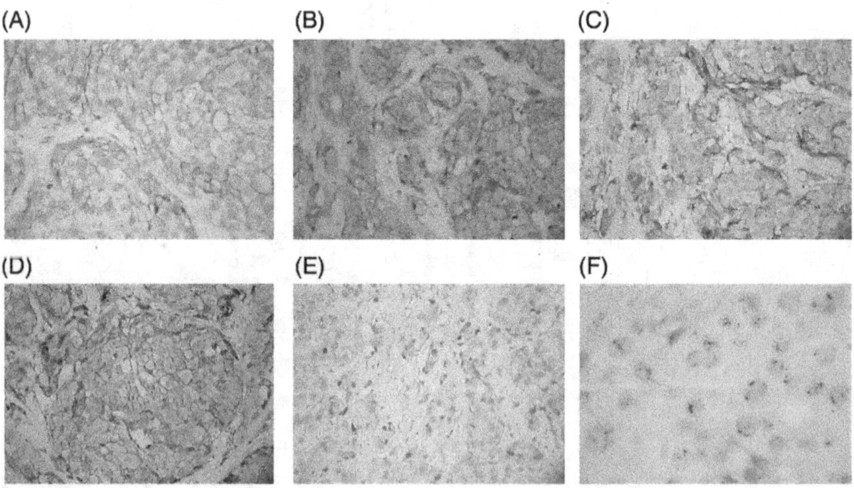

FIGURE 1.—HER2 protein expression and gene amplification in a discordant case. (A) 4B5 2+ immunostaining 400X; (B) HercepTest 3+ immunostaining; (C) A0485 2+ immunostaining 400X; (D) SP3 3+ immunostaining 400X; (E) CB11 1+ immunostaining 400X, (F) DDISH demonstrating HER2 amplification 1000X. (Reprinted from Nunes CB, Rocha RM, Buzelin MA, et al. False positivity in HER2 testing of breast cancer: novel paths for approaching an old dilemma. *J Clin Pathol.* 2013;66:946-950.)

TABLE 5.—Sensitivity and Specificity of Anti-HER2 Antibodies Compared with DDISH

Antibodies	Sensitivity	(95% CI)	Specificity	(95% CI)
A0485	98.4	(90.0 to 99.9)	95.3	(87.7 to 98.5)
HercepTest	95.4	(86.2 to 98.8)	95.2	(88.6 to 98.2)
CB11	89.0	(78.1 to 95.1)	97.1	(91.3 to 99.2)
SP3	97.0	(88.8 to 99.5)	95.2	(88.6 to 98.2)
4B5	96.9	(88.2 to 99.4)	94.8	(87.7 to 98.1)

cases, and false positive from 1.6% (CB11) to 2.7% (HercepTest, SP3 and 4B5) of the 184 cases.

Conclusions.—There was very good agreement among the five anti-HER2 antibodies. CB11 was the most specific antibody, but showed more false negative cases. A0485, SP3, 4B5 and HercepTest were highly sensitive and specific, but showed more false positive cases (Fig 1, Table 5).

► Accurately determining the HER2 status for women with breast cancer is challenging for pathologists. This study shows the 5 commercial antibodies in immunohistochemical analysis. These antibodies show slightly different levels of specificity and sensitivity (Table 5), and it is critically important for pathologists to know that these differences exist. Fig 1 shows an example of a discordant case. For further reading, please see reference list.[1,2]

S. Raab, MD

References

1. Hicks DG, Kulkarni S. HER2+ breast cancer: review of biologic relevance and optimal use of diagnostic tools. *Am J Clin Pathol.* 2008;129:263-273.
2. Schiavon BN, Jasani B, De Brot L, et al. Evaluation of reliability of FISH versus Brightfield Dual-probe In Situ Hybridization (BDISH) for frontline assessment of HER2 status in breast cancer samples in a community setting: influence of poor tissue preservation. *Am J Surg Pathol.* 2012;36:1489-1496.

Gene of the month: *KRAS*

Chetty R, Govender D (Oxford Univ Hosps Trust and Univ of Oxford Univ, UK; Groote Schuur Hosp, Cape Town, South Africa)
J Clin Pathol 66:548-550, 2013

This is a general overview of KRAS, its structure and role in pertinent cancers. Also its role in determining adjuvant therapy is discussed Table 1.

► The gene of the month series by the *Journal of Clinical Pathology* summarizes the role of genes in the field of oncology. In this example, *KRAS* is highlighted by Chetty and Govender. Table 1 shows the percentage of different cancers that have the *KRAS* mutation. Notably, patients who have metastatic colon cancer and *KRAS* mutations in codons 12 or 13 of exon1 do not benefit

TABLE 1.—*KRAS* Mutations in Various Cancer Types

Cancer Type	% KRAS Mutations
Gastrointestinal tract	61
Pancreas	57–90
Biliary tract	28
Lung	16
Endometrium	15
Ovary	14
Prostate	8
Uterine cervix	7
Liver	6
Thyroid	2

from anti–epidermal growth factor receptor therapy. For additional reading, see reference list.[1,2]

S. Raab, MD

References

1. Wang HL, Lopategui J, Amin MB, Patterson SD. KRAS mutation testing in human cancers: the pathologist's role in the era of personalized medicine. *Adv Anat Pathol.* 2010;17:23-32.
2. Hirsch FR, Varella-Garcia M, Bunn PA Jr, et al. Epidermal growth factor receptor in non-small-cell lung carcinomas: correlation between gene copy number and protein expression and impact on prognosis. *J Clin Oncol.* 2003;21:3798-3807.

PART II

LABORATORY MEDICINE

13 Laboratory Management and Outcomes

Transformation of Pathologists: Responding in a Volatile, Uncertain, Complex, and Ambiguous Environment

Hernandez JS, Allen TC (Mayo Clinic, Scottsdale, AZ; Univ of Texas Health Science Ctr Tyler)

Arch Pathol Lab Med 137:603-605, 2013

Background.—Pathologists are suffering a general discontent, frustration, disappointment, and even burnout. These negative attitudes develop in response to their current environment, which is characterized by volatility, uncertainty, complexity, and ambiguity (VUCA). What this means and how pathologists can turn things around were discussed.

VUCA Causes and Responses.—Pathologists experience volatility in the rapidly changing state of molecular/genetic/personalized/tailored medicine. Uncertainty can be related to political agitation over the current state of health care delivery and spending. Complexity can come from the constantly changing and increasing demands on pathology-resident education. Ambiguity arises when pathologists try to satisfy the different demands placed on them in private and academic spheres. In response to these influences, pathologists find that they can no longer offer straightforward answers to straightforward questions, but must deal with a new set of communication and practice behaviors.

Best Responses.—To counteract the influence of VUCA, pathologists need to prepare themselves to cope with the challenges in different and novel ways. To counteract volatility, pathologists must ask laboratory teams to translate their data into information that can be used, then practice communicating clearly and in ways that others can understand. Volatility can then become vision. Uncertainty can be managed by instituting challenges to the mental models that pathologists generally use. Red-teaming can help. This approach introduces a devil's advocate to offset the influence of "group-think." Flexibility in planning can also neutralize the effects of uncertainty. These moves turn uncertainty to understanding. Complexity can be addressed by developing collaborative leaders who see the big picture and lead peers to work collaboratively, thereby achieving more corporately than can be done individually. Aiming for permanent solutions must be supplanted by seeking to evaluate situations critically and applying resources creatively. Complexity can then be changed into clarity. Finally, ambiguity can create inefficiency and missed opportunities, leading to conflict and destruction of the framework of an organization. Instead pathologists should listen well, think divergently, and establish incremental dividends. As a result, they will become more agile and able to survive in a VUCA world.

Conclusions.—Pathologists need to change quickly and completely to adapt to the new challenges that face their profession. Future leaders in this area must develop capabilities for internal resilience and convey that to their followers. They need to do the right thing, be transparent about their efforts, and then be quiet about it. It will not be comfortable, but it will be an effective strategy for turning a difficult situation into one that is guided by vision and marked by understanding, clarity, and agility.

▶ In previous articles, the authors have noted the general discontent among pathologists with their changing work environment and reinforced that, even so, pathologists must remain ever professional. They did not, however, delve into the causes of the discontent, frustration, and malaise that are too often seen among pathologists nor how they might be handled. Why are so many pathologists frustrated and disappointed and sometimes burned out? Why do so many pathologists believe their contracts with society have been broken? What exactly is today's reality? What has happened, and what can be done about it? Today pathologists live in a VUCA world: VUCA—volatility, uncertainty, complexity, and ambiguity—is an acronym used to describe an environment of volatility: "the nature and dynamics of change, and the nature and speed of change forces and change catalysts"; uncertainty: "the lack of predictability, the prospects for surprise, and the sense of awareness and understanding of issues and events"; complexity: "the multiplex of force, the confounding of issues, and the chaos and confusion that surround an organization"; and ambiguity "the haziness of reality, the potential for misreads, and the mixed meanings of conditions; cause-and-effect confusion." Pathologists experience all 4 of these environments. This article expands on these concepts.

M. G. Bissell, MD, PhD, MPH

Federal Laboratory–Business Commercialization Partnerships

Walejko GK, Hughes ME, Howieson SV, et al (Science and Technology Policy Inst (STPI), Washington, DC)

Science 337:1297-1298, 2012

Background.—Federal laboratories offer resources such as multidisciplinary teams of scientists and engineers; large, complex facilities; and work on classified research that are not available in other settings. Such laboratories are being asked by government agencies to engage in and facilitate partnerships with businesses to produce commercial uses for their research.

Challenges face both the laboratories and the businesses with which they seek to form partnerships. Self-reported data were used to reveal the current status of transfer of federal laboratory technologies to market via numerous pathways.

Challenges and Changes.—Often businesses are unaware of the existence of federal laboratories or are unclear about their resources. Web sites often omit inventions available for licensing, provide sparse descriptions of ongoing research, and generally keep laboratories invisible. To increase the federal laboratories' online presence, the Department of Energy's (DOE's) Energy Efficiency and Renewable Energy (EERE) office has provided a portal for DOE laboratory patents related to research. The National Institutes of Health (NIH) also lists available licensing opportunities and offers an electronic catalog so companies can locate unpatented biologic materials. A public database for federally owned inventions has also been made available.

Companies may be hindered by slow negotiations to access research because of legal rules and regulations. E-mail and other streamlined agreements are being offered, along with the use of partnership intermediaries who can broker deals between businesses and laboratories. These services may be especially helpful to small businesses.

Researcher Issues.—Technology transfer is the responsibility of federal laboratory researchers, yet many do not include assessments of such efforts in performance reviews. Incentives to commercialize are lacking for federal researchers, with royalty payments capped at $150,000 per year. Providing sufficient incentives to researchers at government-owned and government-operated (GOGO) facilities while avoiding potential conflicts of interest can be a challenge.

Federal researchers may also be unaware about how to develop partnerships with industry and may lack business training. Now laboratories are trying to increase the business culture of their researchers through workshops and formal training.

Often laboratories develop early-stage technologies that require work to make them commercially feasible. To overcome this limitation, federal laboratories are exploring methods for developing early-stage technologies into products that can be commercially viable. The use of intermediaries who help to provide technology maturation funds is also being explored. In addition, unexpected research results may have commercial applications, and laboratories are being encouraged to discover and exploit these through entrepreneur-in-residence programs and technology scouts.

Conclusions.—Federal laboratories are being called upon to contribute to the economic development of the country either through partnerships or through other methods of technology transfer. Policy-makers should consider how economic development fits within the context of federally funded research and development.

▶ US federal laboratories, government owned and either government operated or contractor operated, spent $40.4 billion on research and development

(R&D) in 2009. This represents 30% of US federally funded R&D obligations. Federal laboratories offer unique resources, including multidisciplinary teams of scientists and engineers, large and complex facilities, and ability to work on classified research. Given these resources and increasing calls for greater returns on federally funded R&D investment, the US government has solicited the laboratories to engage and facilitate partnerships with businesses to produce commercial technologies. The authors discuss challenges to such partnerships and the strategies that federal laboratories have used in attempts to overcome them. Previous studies of such efforts are outdated and limited to particular laboratories. The current analysis relies on self-reported information; many efforts have not yet been rigorously evaluated. The focus is on the transfer of federal laboratory technologies to market through a variety of pathways, including joint research projects between industry and laboratories under cooperative R&D agreements and patents, licenses, and creation of start-ups. Federal laboratories transfer technology in other ways, including published research dissemination, researcher training, and standards development.

M. G. Bissell, MD, PhD, MPH

Laboratory Test Utilization Program: Structure and Impact in a Large Academic Medical Center

Warren JS (Univ of Michigan, Ann Arbor)

Am J Clin Pathol 139:289-297, 2013

In 2008, the University of Michigan Health System (UMHS) created a Laboratory Test Utilization Program that included the establishment of a Laboratory Formulary Committee under the imprimatur of the Faculty Group Practice, the Office of Clinical Affairs, the Department of Pathology, and UMHS hospital administration. A critical component of the program is UM-CareLink, an order entry system for inpatients and inpatient-like venues. UM-CareLink allows very basic decision support comment prompts. Through the application of peer-reviewed medical evidence, input by medical content experts, excellent cooperation by medical staff, and close oversight by Pathology of the Sendout Laboratory, this program has led to a robust process of test utilization oversight, excellent communication with clinical services, and significant UMHS activity-adjusted reductions in laboratory expense.

▶ Based on studies that have found no clear-cut correlation between numbers of laboratory tests ordered per patient and clinical outcomes and studies that have found significant geographic variations in test usage, also without differences in clinical outcomes, it is clear that excessive use and/or waste of laboratory resources contribute to the overall cost of health care. Currently, the direct cost of laboratory and pathology testing is believed to account for 4% ($60 billion per year) of health care costs. The rapid emergence of molecular diagnostics and whole-genome sequence-based testing portends an even greater relative contribution to overall health care costs. The economy-crippling upward trend in health care costs, coupled with an opportunity to more efficiently use laboratory testing resources, create an imperative to address the latter. Faculty members of the Department of Pathology at the University of Michigan (UM), in collaboration with departmental administrative and technical staff and with active participation by the UM Health System (UMHS) administration and clinical colleagues, have engaged for more than 15 years in a systematic and comprehensive approach to effectively rationalize laboratory resources. The overarching structure of this approach includes laboratory organization (transfer of laboratories to pathology, consolidation of laboratories within pathology, and maintenance of pathology-directed laboratory information technology and phlebotomy services), implementation of lean operations principles, pathology oversight of UMHS point-of-care testing (instrument selection, training oversight, and quality control), aggressive deployments of technological approaches (eg, automation), systematic make-buy analyses with resultant new test additions and old test discontinuations, aggressive multispecialty focus on the unit cost and utilization of blood products, aggressive price negotiations with commodity and laboratory services vendors, and laboratory test utilization management. The focus of this article is specifically the structure, operation, and impact of the UMHS Laboratory Test Utilization Program.

M. G. Bissell, MD, PhD, MPH

Should we customise critical value procedure according to patient origin and laboratory turnaround time?

Salinas M, López-Garrigós M, Gutiérrez M, et al (Hospital Universitario de San Juan, San Juan de Alicante, Spain; et al)

J Clin Pathol 66:269-272, 2013

Introduction.—Our routine laboratory critical value notification procedure is based on a short list of six fundamental critical values. The report system for our Stat laboratory is not based on this 'short list'; instead, critical values are always reported according to the patient clinical context and the previous laboratory results. The aim of our work is to show how a critical value notification procedure based on a rigid list of values and thresholds can result in completely different results depending on whether the tests are requested in a stat or a routine manner.

Material and Methods.—We reviewed the number of critical value notifications based on the short list for the routine laboratory. For the stat laboratory, we studied the number of real notifications based on the pathologist validation of the individualised situation of the patient and calculated the number of notifications that would have been reported if the routine short list would have been used instead.

Results.—The number of critical values that would have been reported if using the routine short list in stat laboratory was high when compared with the number of critical values that were really reported.

Conclusions.—Using a rigid list of laboratory values to notify critical values resulted in completely different results depending on whether the tests were requested in stat or routine. Reporting only really unexpected values through an individual custom-made reporting procedure may avoid the wasting of time and resources and raising false alarms among referring physicians and patients.

▶ Laboratory critical values are those values that identify life-threatening conditions requiring prompt medical intervention. The concept has evolved over the years, and currently accreditation agencies (the most widely accepted standard is ISO EN 15189:2007) define and require clinical laboratories to list critical limits, formulate notification procedures, and document critical results. Most laboratories attend to a variety of patients (eg, inpatients, primary care, emergency outpatients), and laboratory results that may be critical for some patients may be rather normal for others (eg, intensive care unit, dialysis, oncology). Furthermore, the improvement in technology and laboratory processes makes it possible to produce short laboratory response times; very often, it is possible for the requesting physician to check for results electronically immediately after they have been verified by the pathologist, when the patient may still be at hand. In this scenario, it is becoming increasingly difficult to establish a single critical value list to be used in the different situations that occur daily in a clinical laboratory. It seems more appropriate to adapt the test list and thresholds, as well as the notification procedure, to the type of patient, the laboratory response time, and to the requester, in the interest of efficiency. Instead of taking into account just the result value, it seems more sensible to also consider other information, such as the change in the current test result from previous results, the patient's characteristics, and the ordering provider. The aim of this study is to show how a critical value reporting system using a single list of values and thresholds can result in completely different results depending on whether the laboratory tests are requested in a stat or routine manner and to describe a flexible notification system, adapted to the requester and patient clinical situation, which may take into account the variability of the patient population and may help overcome this limitation.

M. G. Bissell, MD, PhD, MPH

Teaching Laboratory Medicine to Medical Students: Implementation and Evaluation

Molinaro RJ, Winkler AM, Kraft CS, et al (Emory Univ, Atlanta, GA)
Arch Pathol Lab Med 136:1423-1429, 2012

Context.—Laboratory medicine is an integral component of patient care. Approximately 60% to 70% of medical decisions are based on laboratory results. Physicians in specialties that order the tests are teaching medical students laboratory medicine and test use with minimal input from laboratory scientists who implement and maintain the quality control for those tests.

Objective.—To develop, implement, and evaluate a 1.5-day medical student clinical laboratory experience for fourth-year medical students in their last month of training.

Design.—The experience was devised and directed by laboratory scientists and included a panel discussion, laboratory tours, case studies that focused on the goals and objectives recently published by the Academy of Clinical Laboratory Physicians and Scientists, and medical-student presentations highlighting salient points of the experience. The same knowledge quiz was administered at the beginning and end of the experience and 84 students took both quizzes.

Results.—A score of 7 or more was obtained by 16 students (19%) on the initial quiz, whereas 34 (40%) obtained the same score on the final quiz; the improvement was found to be statistically significant ($P = .002$; $t = 3.215$), particularly in 3 out of the 10 questions administered.

Conclusions.—Although the assessment can only measure a small amount of knowledge recently acquired, the improvement observed by fourth-year medical students devoting a short period to learning laboratory medicine principles was encouraging. This medical student clinical laboratory experience format allowed teaching of a select group of laboratory medicine principles in 1.5 days to an entire medical school class.

▶ Very little formal education in laboratory medicine currently exists in most traditional medical school curricula. Pathology has traditionally been taught as an independent 6- to 12-month course with an emphasis on pathogenesis and how tissues are affected from the anatomic pathology perspective but with little emphasis on laboratory medicine. To compound the issue, many medical schools have modified their curricula, so the different topics are presented in a more integrated context. As a result, physicians in different specialties teach medical students the tests they use. This instruction occurs without input from the clinical laboratory professionals who have implemented the tests in the clinical laboratory and have the training to understand their utility, their limitations, and the regulatory components necessary for providing the service. In 2011, the authors implemented a CAPSTONE course at their institution in the final month of the students' fourth year, after the National Resident Matching Program. The primary goal of the CAPSTONE course was to ensure that students were ready for the next phase of their medical education by focusing on the Accreditation Council for Graduate Medical Education core competencies, including Systems-Based Practice. All fourth-year medical students were required to attend the CAPSTONE modules and were graded on a pass/fail basis determined by attendance and participation. The Department of Pathology and Laboratory Medicine sought, and was granted, a 1.5-day module to provide a laboratory medicine curriculum as a component of the Systems-Based Practice during CAPSTONE. The goals of the Medical Student Clinical Laboratory Experience (MSCLE) were to showcase hospital laboratories through tours and to illustrate the fundamentals of laboratory medicine that have been described by the Academy of Clinical Laboratory Physicians and Scientists performing case-based discussions. In this article, the authors describe the MSCLE that was devised and directed by laboratory scientists.

M. G. Bissell, MD, PhD, MPH

Utilization of Stat Test Priority in the Clinical Laboratory: A College of American Pathologists Q-Probes Study of 52 Institutions

Volmar KE, Wilkinson DS, Wagar EA, et al (Rex Pathology Associates, Raleigh, NC; Virginia Commonwealth Univ, Richmond; Univ of Texas MD Anderson Cancer Ctr, Houston; et al)

Arch Pathol Lab Med 137:220-227, 2013

Context.—Utilization of stat testing priority is a balance between safe, efficient patient management and resource expenditure.

Objective.—To determine the rate of stat testing, compare rates among institutions, and determine the distribution of turnaround time expectations for different turnaround time priorities.

Design.—During a 7-day period, participants prospectively determined the total number of chemistry, hematology, and coagulation billable tests from inpatients and emergency department patients. Among these, the total numbers of billable tests performed stat were identified. Laboratories also reported the levels of test priority they offered and turnaround expectations for each level of test priority.

Results.—Fifty institutions submitted data for the study, with 2 additional participants submitting partial results. Participants identified 639 589 chemistry, hematology, and coagulation billable tests, with 229 896 (35.9%) performed stat. The stat rate varied from 21.3% at the 10th percentile to 55.4% at the 90th percentile, with a median of 37.0% of participants' tests performed stat. Laboratories include a mean of 206 tests in chemistry, hematology, and coagulation test menus, with 67% of these tests offered stat. The fraction of the test menu offered stat varied from 29.0% at the 10th percentile to 97.8% at the 90th percentile, with a median of 73.3%of tests on the menu offered stat. The most common number of testing priorities offered by participating laboratories was 3 (44.2%).

Conclusions.—Among the 52 participating laboratories, the median stat testing rate was 37.0% and a median 73.3% of the test menu was offered stat.

► Laboratories generally offer at least 2 turnaround priority levels, routine and stat, *stat* from the Latin statim (immediately or without delay). Failure to meet stat expectations is a frequent source of dissatisfaction for both physician and nursing users of laboratory services and may lead to requests for near-patient testing, such as satellite stat laboratories or point-of-care testing. Under such circumstances, there is potential for duplication of equipment, duplication of personnel, and use of smaller analyzers with lower throughput. Thus, increased stat testing rates may increase costs relative to routine central laboratory testing. The overuse of stat testing may also create a situation in which the stat test request is no longer handled in a significantly different fashion from a routine test. Underutilization of stat testing may hinder safe and efficient patient management. The optimal use of stat testing must strike a balance between patient safety and laboratory resource expenditure. This Q-Probes study was designed to establish prevailing rates of stat testing and to determine what practice and demographic variables may influence those rates.

M. G. Bissell, MD, PhD, MPH

Rate of Occult Specimen Provenance Complications in Routine Clinical Practice

Pfeifer JD, Liu J (Washington Univ School of Medicine, St Louis, MO)

Am J Clin Pathol 139:93-100, 2013

Occult specimen provenance complications (SPCs), which occur when there is an absence of any direct or indirect indication that a specimen switch or contamination may have occurred, constitute a significant patient safety and medical-legal problem because they can lead to misdiagnosis. However, the rate at which occult SPCs occur is unknown because, by definition, this category of errors is not identified by standard laboratory practices. In this study, we evaluated a data set comprising almost 13,000 prostate biopsies that were prospectively tested for specimen provenance errors as part of routine clinical practice. The frequency of occult type 1 errors (a complete transposition between patients) and type 2 errors (contamination of the patient's tissue with 1 or more unrelated patients) was 0.26% and 0.67%, respectively; every urology practice setting and surgical pathology laboratory type with a representative sample size experienced at least 1 type 1 and 1 type 2 error during the study period. Overall, the mean frequency of SPCs across practice settings was 0.22% for type 1 errors and 1.69% for type 2 errors. The type 1 rate showed no correlation with a surgical pathology laboratory setting or urologic practice group setting; the type 2 rate correlated solely with a surgical pathology laboratory setting. The occult SPC rate in this limited data set provides an estimate of the scope of the problem of potential misdiagnosis as a result of occult specimen provenance errors in routine clinical practice.

▶ The rate at which occult specimen identification errors, also known as specimen provenance complications (SPCs), occur is unknown because, by definition, this category of errors is not identified by standard laboratory practices. Data from the REDUCE (Reduction by Dutasteride of Prostate Cancer Events) trial suggest that undetected SPCs occur at a rate of up to 0.5%, but because the REDUCE trial was a multicenter international trial, it is uncertain whether the documented error rate is representative of specimens processed exclusively in the United States. To obtain some measure of the rate of occult specimen identity errors in the US, the authors contacted a private laboratory that markets a system designed to detect occult SPCs in routine clinical practice (the know error® system). The laboratory agreed to provide them with unfettered access to their dataset from testing for occult SPCs in the setting of transrectal prostate biopsy performed to rule out adenocarcinoma of the prostate (a dataset comprising almost 13 000 biopsy specimens, which were prospectively tested for specimen provenance using STR analysis, in real time, as part of routine clinical practice).

The results of their analysis of this dataset not only provide an estimate of the rate of occult SPCs in the United States but also demonstrate that errors occur across the range of practice settings and diagnostic laboratories.

M. G. Bissell, MD, PhD, MPH

Determination of Turnaround Time in the Clinical Laboratory: "Accessioning-to-Result" Time Does Not Always Accurately Reflect Laboratory Performance

Stotler BA, Kratz A (Columbia Univ College of Physicians and Surgeons, NY; New York-Presbyterian Hosp)

Am J Clin Pathol 138:724-729, 2012

Laboratories often focus on computer-generated components of turnaround time (TAT) reports that capture time from sample accessioning to reporting of results, and use this indicator to determine performance. This study assesses limitations of "accessioning-to-results" times and details ways in which to evaluate laboratory-controlled TAT. Samples were sent via pneumatic tube and times from arrival to accessioning were determined. Staffing was increased and the delay between sample arrival and accessioning was measured again. Significant delays were seen between specimen arrival and accessioning, which were not captured with computer-generated TAT reports. When TAT was calculated to include these delays, the TAT goal was not achieved. Increasing the number of employees significantly decreased delays. Laboratories must ensure that TAT reports encompass all laboratory-controlled parts of the testing processes. Analysis of causes for discrepancies between computer reports and clinician perceptions, combined with targeted measurements and well-designed interventions, can decrease TAT and improve service.

▶ Clinical laboratories take pride in being extremely data driven. Many quality indicators are continuously monitored, analyzed, and used to allocate resources and improve service. These quality indicators include the turnaround times (TATs) necessary to report laboratory results to clinical staff. The total TAT for laboratory assays includes the entire interval from ordering of the test to the clinician's awareness of the result (ie, brain-to-brain). It consists of the intervals from order placement to specimen collection as well as the time necessary for transport to the laboratory, accessioning in the laboratory, centrifugation, aliquoting, additional preanalytic steps if necessary, transport times within and between laboratories, analysis time, the time after completion of analysis until result verification, and the time it takes for the clinical team to be informed of the result. Lack of full control over phlebotomy and specimen transport makes it difficult for the laboratory to address delays caused in the preanalytic stages that take place outside the laboratory. In addition, ordering and collection times are not always fully documented for all samples, and it is currently not possible to determine when clinicians become aware of most laboratory results. Thus, it is impossible for laboratories to use the total TAT as a quality assurance measure. "Accessioning" by the laboratory is defined as ordering the assay in the laboratory information system (LIS) or as scanning the bar-coded samples as received. "Result time" is defined as the release of finalized results into the hospital's electronic medical record. In contrast to ordering and collection times, the accessioning and result times are always well documented for all samples in the LIS; therefore, it is easy to obtain detailed reports on the accessioning-to-result component of the total TAT. Thus, most laboratories focus on the accessioning-to-result time in their TAT reports. Although this approach does not encompass the total TAT, it is generally accepted as the best representation of those elements of the TAT that the laboratory controls. The current report documents an important limitation of the accessioning-to-result verification time, describes a way to address this limitation, and shows how careful attention to feedback from clinical staff and proactive data collection can be used to improve clinical laboratory performance. Specifically, this study quantifies the interval between sample arrival in the laboratory to sample accessioning in the LIS and discusses how this delay, often not captured with standard TAT reports, affects laboratory service.

M. G. Bissell, MD, PhD, MPH

Managing demand for laboratory tests: a laboratory toolkit

Fryer AA, Smellie WSA (Univ Hosp of North Staffordshire NHS Trust, Hartshill, UK; Bishop Aukland General Hosp, UK)

J Clin Pathol 66:62-72, 2013

Healthcare budgets worldwide are facing increasing pressure to reduce costs and improve efficiency, while maintaining quality. Laboratory testing has not escaped this pressure, particularly since pathology investigations cost the National Health Service £2.5 billion per year. Indeed, the Carter Review, a UK Department of Health-commissioned review of pathology services in England, estimated that 20% of this could be saved by improving pathology services, despite an average annual increase of 8%–10% in workload. One area of increasing importance is managing the demands for pathology tests and reducing inappropriate requesting. The Carter Review estimated that 25% of pathology tests were unnecessary, representing a huge potential waste. Certainly, the large variability in levels of requesting between general practitioners suggests that inappropriate requesting is widespread. Unlocking the key to this variation and implementing measures to reduce inappropriate requesting would have major implications for patients and healthcare resources alike. This article reviews the approaches to demand management. Specifically, it aims to (a) define demand management and inappropriate requesting, (b) assess the drivers for demand management, (c) examine the various approaches used, illustrating the potential of electronic requesting and (d) provide a wider context. It will cover issues, such as educational approaches, information technology opportunities and challenges, vetting, duplicate request identification and management, the rôle of key performance indicators, profile composition and assessment of downstream impact of inappropriate

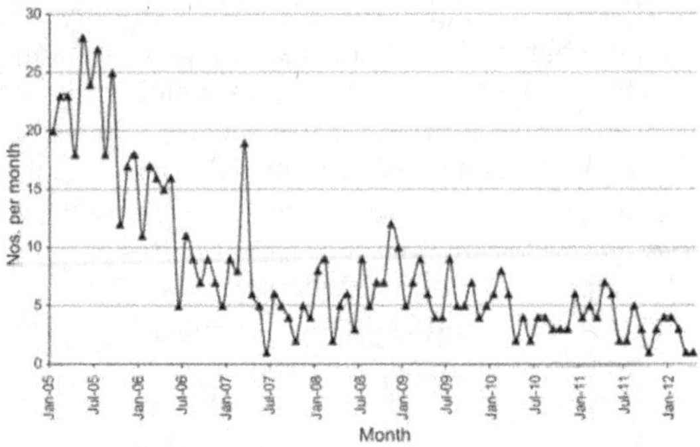

FIGURE 1.—Change in number of tests sent for urine toxicology screening (including drugs of abuse screens) per month following implementation of request vetting (two phases: October 2005 and June 2006). (Reprinted from Fryer AA, Smellie WSA. Managing demand for laboratory tests: a laboratory toolkit. *J Clin Pathol.* 2013;66:62-72, with permission from the BMJ Publishing Group Ltd.)

requesting. Currently, many laboratories are exploring demand management using a plethora of disparate approaches. Hence, this review seeks to provide a 'toolkit' with the view to allowing laboratories to develop a standardised demand management strategy (Fig 1).

▶ Like other sectors of the health economy, laboratory medicine is under increasing pressure to remove inefficiencies and reduce costs, while maintaining or improving standards. In the United Kingdom, this is reflected in a Department of Health drive to make £500 million in savings in laboratory medicine by a package of measures, including large-scale laboratory reorganization. Attention has focused on laboratory medicine as a potential source of savings, presumably because its costs are perceived as being easily identifiable and quantifiable, despite the fact that expenditure on this area accounts for only 3% to 4% of the UK national health budget. However, in an attempt to meet targets such as those outlined in the Carter Report, laboratories are increasingly looking at demand management as a means of reducing the cost of unnecessary pathology investigations. Estimates of inappropriate requesting vary greatly among studies, although the Carter Report gave an overall estimate of around 25%. This review examines the drivers for demand management, investigates how we define and detect an inappropriate request, and provides tools to limit such requests. It also discusses the wider impact of implementation of demand management approaches. It provides a series of specific recommendations with a view to helping the reader develop a wide-ranging demand management strategy (Fig 1).

M. G. Bissell, MD, PhD, MPH

Evaluating the Connections Between Primary Care Practice and Clinical Laboratory Testing: A Review of the Literature and Call for Laboratory Involvement in the Solutions

Smith ML, Raab SS, Fernald DH, et al (Mayo Clinic, Scottsdale, AZ; Univ of Colorado Denver, Aurora; Univ of Washington, Seattle; et al)
Arch Pathol Lab Med 137:120-125, 2013

Context.—Growing evidence has demonstrated a high frequency of quality gaps in laboratory medicine, with recent studies estimating that 15% to 54% of primary care medical errors reported by primary care physicians and staff are related to the testing process. However, there is lack of evidence-based performance metrics in the preanalytic and postanalytic phases of the testing pathway for primary care practices.

Objective.—To use results of the literature review to assist in the development of quality indicators that could improve preanalytic and postanalytic processes in primary care–based laboratory medicine.

Data Sources.—Literature in Ovid/MEDLINE from 2001 through 2011 was searched as a primary source of information. Ninety-five peer-reviewed and non–peer-reviewed publications were retrieved following title and abstract review and 10 articles were reviewed in their entirety by the authors. A systematic review of the literature was conducted regarding the connections between clinical laboratories and primary care offices and the resulting errors. Root causes of errors were categorized into 7 major themes: process failures, delays, communication gaps, errors in judgment and cognition, influence of minorities/language, practice culture, and lack of patient centeredness. Selected articles were evaluated for evidence quality using the Systematic Evidence Review and Evaluation

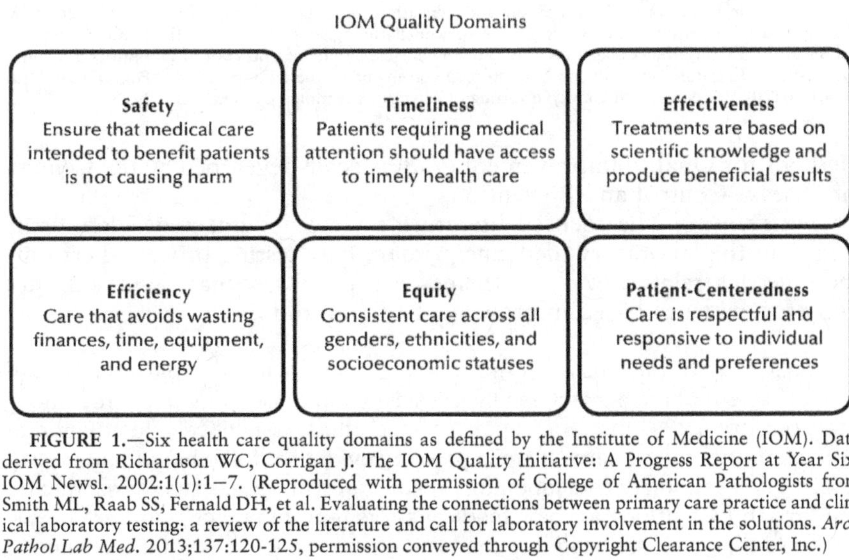

FIGURE 1.—Six health care quality domains as defined by the Institute of Medicine (IOM). Data derived from Richardson WC, Corrigan J. The IOM Quality Initiative: A Progress Report at Year Six. IOM Newsl. 2002:1(1):1–7. (Reproduced with permission of College of American Pathologists from Smith ML, Raab SS, Fernald DH, et al. Evaluating the connections between primary care practice and clinical laboratory testing: a review of the literature and call for laboratory involvement in the solutions. *Arch Pathol Lab Med.* 2013;137:120-125, permission conveyed through Copyright Clearance Center, Inc.)

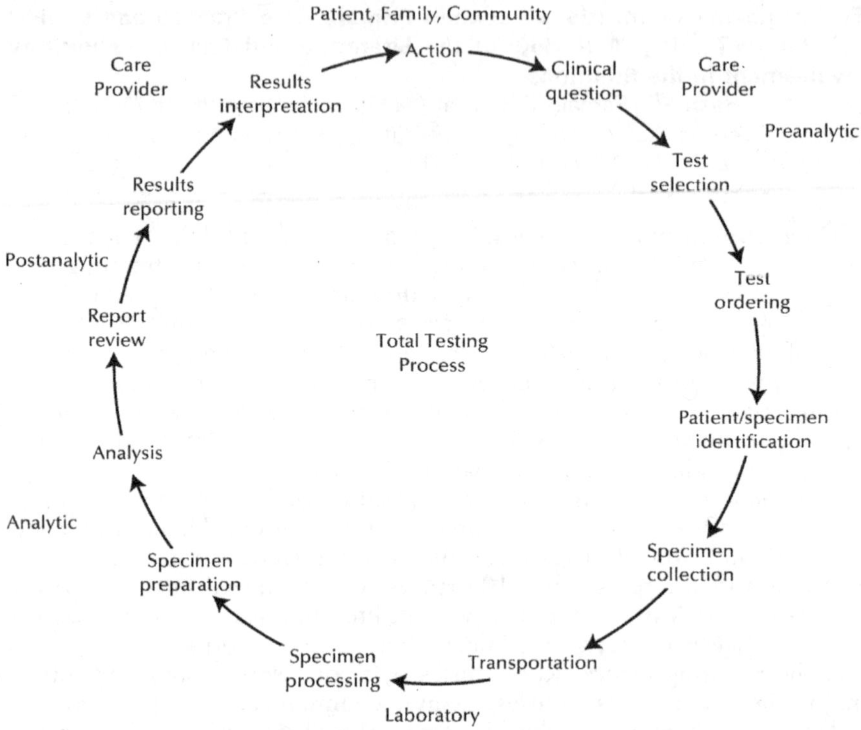

FIGURE 2.—The total testing process begins with a clinical question and the care provider and patient. Each larger step in the process comprises many smaller steps, and laboratory medicine is the sum total of all testing steps. Adapted with permission from Boone J. Presentation at the Institute on Critical Issues in Health Laboratory Practice: Managing for Better Health, September 23–26, 2007; Atlanta, GA: Centers for Disease Control and Prevention; and Barr JT, Silver S. The total testing process and its implications for laboratory administration and education. Clin Lab Manage Rev. 1994;8:526–542. (Reproduced with permission of College of American Pathologists from Smith ML, Raab SS, Fernald DH, et al. Evaluating the connections between primary care practice and clinical laboratory testing: a review of the literature and call for laboratory involvement in the solutions. *Arch Pathol Lab Med.* 2013;137:120-125, permission conveyed through Copyright Clearance Center, Inc.)

Methods for Quality Improvement grading scale developed by the Centers for Disease Control and Prevention.

Conclusions.—The focused literature review documented 7 key error themes in the laboratory medicine/primary care testing process. Performance metrics related to these themes are proposed that deserve future study for evidence-based improvement (Figs 1 and 2).

▶ Primary care physicians order many laboratory tests for their patients. Recent estimates are that the average family physician and general internist order laboratory testing in 29% and 38% of patient encounters, respectively. In addition to high laboratory test volume, there is growing evidence of the high frequency of quality gaps in primary care laboratory medicine, with recent studies estimating that 15% to 54% of primary care medical errors reported by primary care physicians and their staff are related to the testing process. Because of the volume of laboratory testing and the high frequency of medical errors that come from laboratory testing, there is a need for improved quality in the area.

The Institute of Medicine (IOM) provides a framework for understanding the quality of health care by defining it as the degree to which health services for individuals and populations increase the likelihood of desired health outcomes and are consistent with current professional knowledge. The IOM further classifies quality into 6 domains: safety, timeliness, effectiveness, efficiency, equity, and patient centeredness (Fig 1). In laboratory medicine, multiple studies have shown that the majority of errors or gaps in quality take place in the preanalytic and postanalytic phases of the total testing pathway (TTP). The TTP is a systems-based framework for the evaluation of the interactions, connections, and activities involved in the testing process (Fig 2). As Fig 2 shows, the process is circular and includes the preanalytic, analytic, and postanalytic phases of the testing cycle. Cognitive tasks are required at multiple steps, by both the primary care provider and the laboratory. When errors are categorized into general process categories, frequent preanalytic errors involve inadequate sample collection, inappropriate sample transportation, and incorrect test requests for patients. Frequent categories of postanalytic errors include delivery of duplicate reports and delays in receiving reports. Additionally, the connection between health care quality and communication is an issue of critical importance, especially in laboratory medicine. Poor communication among health care providers is the root cause of most medical errors, including sentinel events. Handoffs are especially critical processes in which communication failures place patients at risk. Much attention has been directed at quality initiatives within the analytic phases of testing in the laboratory with quality control programs, such as the College of American Pathologists' quality improvement programs and laboratory accreditation. Given the high frequency of these quality gaps in laboratory testing and the relative lack of laboratory quality initiatives aimed at improving the quality of testing in one of these phases, there is a critical need for the development of evidence-based performance metrics in the preanalytic and postanalytic phases of the TTP.

M. G. Bissell, MD, PhD, MPH

14 Clinical Chemistry

Design of Tumor Biomarker–Monitoring Trials: A Proposal by the European Group on Tumor Markers

Sölétormos G, Duffy MJ, Hayes DF, et al (Univ of Copenhagen, Hillerød, Denmark; Univ College Dublin, Ireland; Univ of Michigan Comprehensive Cancer Ctr, Ann Arbor; et al)

Clin Chem 59:52-59, 2013

A major application of tumor biomarkers is in serial monitoring of cancer patients, but there are no published guidelines on how to evaluate biomarkers for this purpose. The European Group on Tumor Markers has convened a multidisciplinary panel of scientists to develop guidance on the design of such monitoring trials. The panel proposes a 4-phase model for biomarker-monitoring trials analogous to that in use for the investigation of new drugs. In phase I, biomarker kinetics and correlation with tumor burden are assessed. Phase II evaluates the ability of the biomarker to identify, exclude, and/or predict a change in disease status. In phase III, the effectiveness of tumor biomarker–guided intervention is assessed by measuring patient outcome in randomized trials. Phase IV consists of an audit of the long-term effects after biomarker monitoring has been included into standard patient care. Systematic well-designed evaluations of biomarkers for monitoring may provide a stronger evidence base that might enable their earlier use in evaluating responses to cancer therapy.

▶ Although serologic tumor biomarkers are primarily used to monitor the response of cancer patients to therapy and to provide early indication of changes in tumor burden, no consensus yet exists about the optimal design and conduct of longitudinal trials involving serial monitoring of tumor biomarkers. The web site of the Enhancing the Quality and Transparency of Health Research (EQUATOR) initiative provides a comprehensive catalog of recommendations for promoting transparent and accurate reporting of medical research studies, as does an excellent complementary review. Few of the publications cited specifically refer to tumor markers, however, and those that do have generally focused on the diagnostic, prognostic, or predictive use of measurements made at a single time point, rather than by serial monitoring. To address this issue, the European Group on Tumor Markers has established a multidisciplinary international panel, the MONITOR Working Group, with the aim of developing recommendations to stimulate improvements in the design of trials that assess the use of serial tumor biomarker measurements. Many previously reported monitoring trials were fishing expeditions, rather than well-designed, hypothesis-driven investigations.

Consequently, it has often been difficult to conclude whether observed changes in the biomarker investigated influenced clinical decision making, for example, by prompting early requests for additional diagnostic tests (including imaging) or by a change in therapy. In this report, the MONITOR Working Group proposes an approach to the design of longitudinal tumor biomarker trials that is analogous to that used to evaluate new therapeutic drugs. Although this proposal is flexible and does not dictate a specific trial design or analytical strategies, it is likely to be most relevant to reasonably well-characterized serum biomarkers.

M. G. Bissell, MD, PhD, MPH

Unresolved Discrepancies between Cannabinoid Test Results for Infant Urine

Barakauskas VE, Davis R, Krasowski MD, et al (Univ of Utah School of Medicine, Salt Lake City; ARUP Laboratories Inc., Salt Lake City UT; Univ of Iowa Hosps and Clinics, Iowa City)

Clin Chem 58:1364-1367, 2012

Background.—False-positive drug screen results for tetrahydrocannabinol (THC) have been observed. This study investigated the rate of unconfirmed positive screen results in infant and noninfant urine samples and evaluated possible reasons for differences.

Methods.—The rate of unconfirmed positive THC screen results for urine samples was determined retrospectively in 2 independent data sets (n = 14 859, reference laboratory; n = 21 807, hospital laboratory) by comparing positive immunoassay-based drug screen results with the associated results of confirmation tests. We then assessed the rate of positive THC screens for samples with varying likelihoods of cannabinoid presence to evaluate the contribution of infant-specific urine constituents to positive results. Finally, a method to detect a THC metabolite (11-hydroxy-Δ^9-THC) that occurs in meconium was developed to determine its prevalence in infant urine.

Results.—Positive screen results failed to confirm more frequently in samples from infants (47%) than in non-infants (0.8%). The hospital laboratory observed a similar discrepancy with a different immunoassay. Infant samples with a high likelihood of containing cannabinoids despite negative confirmatory results had a similar rate of positive screening results (50%, n = 20), whereas all samples with a low likelihood of containing cannabinoids screened negative (n = 23). 11-Hydroxy-Δ^9-THC was not detected in any infant urine sample tested (n = 16).

Conclusions.—Conventional confirmatory methods for THC may be inappropriate for urine samples from infants. Our results suggest that one or more currently unrecognized THC-associated compounds are responsible for positive THC screen results for infant urine, as opposed to an infant-associated interference.

▶ Drug-of-abuse screening in neonates is used to determine whether an infant has been exposed to drugs or to confirm maternal drug use during pregnancy.

Among the possible testing algorithms, the Substance Abuse and Mental Health Services Administration recommends confirmation of positive results obtained in an immunoassay screen by an independent method, which typically involves chromatographic separation coupled with mass spectrometric detection. Two positive results obtained with different analytical methods and different aliquots of the same sample confirm the presence of a drug. Many of these principles are applied in clinical testing. Owing to the specialized instrumentation commonly used, confirmation is often performed by reference laboratories that may not be aware of the results of the initial screen. Tetrahydrocannabinol (THC) exposure is often assessed in urine by targeting the major urinary metabolite, 11-nor-delta9carboxy-THC (9-COOH-THC), although upward of 100 different metabolites are thought to occur. Although 9-COOH-THC is the most common target of confirmatory assays, immunoassay screens cross-react with other THC metabolites to varying degrees. At ARUP Laboratories, both immunoassay screening and a liquid chromatography-tandem mass spectrometry (LC-MS/MS) confirmatory method are available for urine THC testing. The screening assay (Syva Emit II Plus; Siemens Healthcare Diagnostics) has a cutoff of 20 μg/L 9-COOH-THC, but it shows greater than 45% cross-reactivity with hydroxy metabolites of THC. In contrast, the LC-MS/MS confirmatory assay measures only 9-COOH-THC after alkaline hydrolysis of the glucuronide adducts (5-μg/L cutoff). Anecdotal evidence has surfaced over the last year that urine samples from infants that show positive results in a urine THC drug screen often do not confirm positive findings when referred for quantitative testing by LC-MS/MS. In response to these observations, the authors undertook this study.

M. G. Bissell, MD, PhD, MPH

Quantifying the Accuracy of a Diagnostic Test or Marker

Linnet K, Bossuyt PMM, Moons KGM, et al (Univ of Copenhagen, Denmark; Univ of Amsterdam, the Netherlands; UMC Utrecht, the Netherlands)
Clin Chem 58:1292-1301, 2012

Background.—In recent years, increasing focus has been directed to the methodology for evaluating (new) tests or biomarkers. A key step in the evaluation of a diagnostic test is the investigation into its accuracy.

Content.—We reviewed the literature on how to assess the accuracy of diagnostic tests. Accuracy refers to the amount of agreement between the results of the test under evaluation (index test) and the results of a reference standard or test. The generally recommended approach is to use a prospective cohort design in patients who are suspected of having the disease of interest, in which each individual undergoes the index and same reference standard tests. This approach presents several challenges, including the problems that can arise with the verification of the index test results by the preferred reference standard test, the choice of cutoff value in case of a continuous index test result, and the determination of how to translate accuracy results to recommendations for clinical use. This first in a series of 4 reports presents an overview of the designs of single-test accuracy studies and the concepts of specificity, sensitivity, posterior probabilities (i.e., predictive values) for the presence of target disease, ROC curves, and likelihood ratios, all illustrated with empirical data from a study on the diagnosis of suspected deep venous thrombosis. Limitations of the concept of the diagnostic accuracy for a single test are also highlighted.

Conclusions.—The prospective cohort design in patients suspected of having the disease of interest is the optimal approach to estimate the accuracy of a diagnostic test. However, the accuracy of a diagnostic index test is not constant but varies across different clinical contexts, disease spectrums, and even patient subgroups.

▶ Diagnostic tests, like any other medical intervention, require proper evaluation before their introduction and recommendation for use in clinical practice. The major categories of test evaluation studies are analytical validity, clinical validity, and clinical utility. The focus here is on studies that examine the clinical validity and clinical utility of a test. Considering the basic principles and the state of the art in the evaluation of the clinical accuracy of diagnostic biomarkers and other medical tests, in such accuracy studies the results of one or more tests under evaluation (ie, index tests) are compared with the results of the prevailing clinical reference standard or method. This reference standard or method is the test or strategy that is clinically used to determine the presence or absence of the disease of interest (ie, target disease). Such accuracy studies provide information about the degree of agreement in results from the index tests and the presence or absence of disease, that is, the reference standard results. Additionally, these studies provide information about the frequency of types of errors (ie, false-positive and false-negative test results) by the index test compared with the reference standard. Although an index test may provide a more accurate, more timely, or less invasive identification of the target disease compared with the reference standard, this does not automatically translate to improved therapeutic management, let alone to improved patient health or cost effectiveness of care in general. Consequently, increasing attention is being paid to studies that examine the utility of a test in terms of these latter aspects or outcomes. These so-called clinical utility studies are directed at documenting the degree to which the actual use of a test leads to improved therapeutic management and, consequently, improved patient outcomes or, more generally, cost effectiveness of provided care.

M. G. Bissell, MD, PhD, MPH

Alternative Calibration Strategies for the Clinical Laboratory: Application to Nortriptyline Therapeutic Drug Monitoring

Olson MT, Breaud A, Harlan R, et al (Johns Hopkins Hosp, Baltimore, MD; et al)

Clin Chem 59:920-927, 2013

Background.—The addition of a calibration curve with every run is both time-consuming and expensive for clinical mass spectrometry assays.

We present alternative calibration strategies that eliminate the need for a calibration curve except as required by laboratory regulations.

Methods.—We measured serum nortriptyline concentrations prospectively in 68 patients on 16 days over a 2-month period using a method employing calibration schemes that relied on the measurement of the response ratio (RR) corrected by the response factor (RF), i.e., a measurement of the RR for an equimolar mixture of the analyte and internal standard. Measurements were taken with contemporaneous RF (cRF) measurements as well as sporadic RF (sRF) measurements. The measurements with these alternative calibration schemes were compared against the clinical results obtained by interpolation on a calibration curve, and those differences were evaluated for analytical and clinical significance.

Results.—The differences between the values measured by cRF and sRF calibration and interpolation on a calibration curve were not significant ($P = 0.088$ and $P = 0.091$, respectively). Both the cRF and sRF-based calibration results demonstrated a low mean bias against the calibration curve interpolations of 3.69% (95% CI, −15.8% to 23.2%) and 3.11% (95% CI, −16.4% to 22.6%), respectively. When these results were classified as subtherapeutic, therapeutic, or supratherapeutic, there was categorical agreement in 95.6% of the cRF calibration results and 94.1% of the sRF results.

Conclusions.—cRF and sRF calibration in a clinically validated liquid chromatography–tandem mass spectrometry assay yields results that are analytically and clinically commensurate to those produced by interpolation with a calibration curve.

▶ The growing use of liquid chromatography–tandem mass spectrometry (LC-MS/MS) in the clinical laboratory brings with it the ability to perform a broad range of quantitative assays with a single instrument. After the initial expenditure involved in purchasing an instrument, one expensive feature of clinical MS as it is usually practiced in the United States is the generation of a calibration curve for calculating results each time the assay is run, in contrast to the biannual calibration required by the Clinical Laboratory Improvement Amendments. Contemporaneous calibration curve measurement for MS assays originated when the instruments were less stable than the ones currently in use in the clinical laboratory. Earlier instruments required more correction for day-to-day variability. Alternatives to repetitive calibration curve measurement have been shown in one study. These strategies rely on the analyte-to-stable isotope response ratio corrected for the response factor (RF)—the ratio of an equimolar analyte and stable isotope ratio solution. Two variations of this approach are contemporaneous RF (cRF)-based calibration, in which the RF is measured for each assay batch, and sporadic RF (sRF)-based calibration, in which the RF is used over multiple days unless there is quality control failure or major instrumental change. cRF- and sRF-based calibrations have been called *one-point* and *no-point calibration*, respectively, and no-point calibration has also been called *internal calibration*. However, because all standard MS assays rely on internal calibration, the use of this term is too broad. In addition, the terms *one-point* and *no-point calibration* do not fully describe processes used in the calibration scheme. As such, the terms *cRF-* and *sRF-based calibration* are used here and recommended to avoid future ambiguities. The usefulness of these approaches has been shown in pharmacokinetics investigations and basic science research. These laboratories generally analyze large batches of samples over a short period, whereas clinical laboratories analyze small numbers of patient samples as they are received. Thus, the impetus to decrease the calibration overhead is even more important in the clinical laboratory than it is in these other environments. Here, the authors describe the prospective use of these alternative calibration approaches for measuring the serum concentration of the tricyclic antidepressant nortriptyline in a clinical laboratory environment.

M. G. Bissell, MD, PhD, MPH

Evaluation of the health effects of occupational exposure of analytic laboratory workers processing illicit drug investigation files

Bentur Y, Bentur L, Rotenberg M, et al (Technion-Israel Inst of Technology, Haifa; Sheba Med Ctr, Tel Hashomer, Israel; et al)
Clin Toxicol 51:237-242, 2013

Introduction.—The Analytic Laboratory of Israel Police processes illicit drug files. In recent years, workers of this laboratory have complained of health problems. Limited information exists on the effect of occupational exposure to illicit drugs; biomonitoring was never done.

Objective.—To assess health effects and systemic absorption of illicit drugs in workers of the Analytic Laboratory occupationally exposed to illicit drugs.

Methods.—A prospective cohort study using health and occupational questionnaires, clinical assessments, and monitoring of urinary excretion of illicit drugs was conducted. The study included three blocks of one week each. At each week workers were assessed at the beginning (baseline), and the assessments were repeated at the end of the three working days. Urine specimens were analyzed for illicit drugs in an independent laboratory. Demographic, clinical, occupational, and laboratory data were subjected to descriptive analysis, and paired Student's *t*-test, chi-square analysis, and repeated measures model.

Results.—Twenty-seven workers (age, 39.2 ± 8.3 years; 77.8% females) were included, yielding 122 paired samples. The following parameters were reduced at the end of shift compared with baseline: diastolic blood pressure (71.2 ± 11.2 and 77.2 ± 13.6 mmHg, respectively, $p < 0.0001$), FEV1 (98.3 ± 14.6% and 100.7 ± 12.7%, respectively, $p < 0.0001$), FVC (101.4 ± 13.7% and 103.7 ± 14.0%, respectively, $p = 0.003$), and FEF25-75 (85.7 ± 18.0% and 89.6 ± 18.7%, respectively, $p = 0.01$). Main health complaints included headache, fatigue, and dry eyes. No illicit drug was detected in the urine specimens.

Conclusion.—It is suggested that the health concerns of the laboratory workers were not related to the absorption of illicit drugs; environmental conditions (e.g. inadequate ventilation and respirable dust) can contribute to these concerns.

▶ According to the 2009 survey of the Israel Anti-Drug Authority, the estimated number of illegal drug users in Israel is about 321 000, of whom 60 000 are youth of school age (excluding inhalant users). The main illicit drugs reported include marijuana, hashish, heroin, cocaine, and synthetic drugs (eg, amphetamines). Drug dealers in Israel continuously market new derivatives, especially of stimulants, for example, cathinone and amphetamine derivatives. The Analytic Laboratory, Laboratory of Identification and Forensic Science of Israel Police, is largely involved in the identification of illicit drugs. This enables police to locate and prosecute illegal drug manufacturers and dealers. The Analytic Laboratory opens about 18 000 drug investigation files annually, which are processed by about 25 workers. During recent years, the number of drug investigation files (especially for cathinone, amphetamine, and methamphetamine derivatives) reaching the Analytic Laboratory has been increasing, and currently they constitute about 10% of all investigation files. These files deal with about 500 000 capsules, tens of kilograms of powders, and 50 000 to 100 000 tablets per year. In 2003, a female worker suffered from cough, dyspnea, severe headache, dizziness, palpitations, and near-syncope shortly after opening a large bag with substance and inhaling the powder; it was later identified as cathinone. Since then, some of the workers of the Analytic Laboratory have complained of sporadic headaches, dizziness, nausea, cough, sneezing, and eye and skin irritation. A limited number of publications on occupational exposure to drugs of abuse can be found in the medical literature. The results of these studies were based on the questionnaires and were limited by response and recall biases or by description of voluntary calls to a poison center. No biomonitoring of illicit drugs was done for the workers included in these studies. None assessed analytic laboratory workers occupationally exposed to illicit drugs. The objective of this study was to assess the health effects and systemic absorption of illicit drugs in workers of the Analytic Laboratory of Israel Police who are occupationally exposed to these drugs.

M. G. Bissell, MD, PhD, MPH

Short- and Long-term Individual Variation in Cardiac Troponin in Patients with Stable Coronary Artery Disease

Nordenskjöld AM, Ahlström H, Eggers KM, et al (Örebro Univ Hosp, Sweden; Uppsala Univ, Sweden; et al)
Clin Chem 59:401-409, 2013

Background.—A rise or fall of cardiac troponin is a prerequisite for the diagnosis of acute myocardial infarction. Defining significant changes requires knowledge of both biological and analytical variation. The short-term biological variation of cardiac troponin in healthy individuals is 3%–48%. However, healthy individuals may not be representative for patients in whom cardiac troponin measurement is often of clinical importance.

Therefore, we studied the individual variation of cardiac troponin in patients with symptoms of stable coronary artery disease.

Methods.—Twenty-four patients scheduled for elective coronary angiography were included. Blood samples were drawn once at enrollment and serially at six 4-h intervals on the day before coronary angiography. Cardiac troponin was measured with hs-cTn assays from Abbott Laboratories (premarket cTnI assay) and Roche Diagnostics (Elecsys® cTnT assay with two different lots).

Results.—The short-term individual variation in cardiac troponin I (cTnI) was 14%, the reference change value (RCV) 49%, and RCV-log-normal (rise/fall) 54%/−35%. The corresponding values for cTnT were 7%, 23%, and 26%/−21%. The long-term variation for cTnI was 24%, RCV 69%, and RCV-log-normal (rise/ fall) 97%/−49%. The corresponding values for cTnT were 11%, 32%, and 37%/−27%.

Conclusions.—The short-term individual variation of cardiac troponin in patients with symptoms of stable coronary artery disease is similar to the biological variation previously demonstrated in healthy individuals. Our results suggest that a change in cardiac troponin concentrations of >50% can be used in attempting to diagnose acute myocardial injury. To detect significant long-term changes in cardiac troponin concentrations, larger changes will be required.

▶ Measurement of cardiac troponin is a prerequisite for the diagnosis or exclusion of acute myocardial infarction (AMI) and, thus, essential in the evaluation of patients with chest pain. Guidelines advocate the use of a cardiac troponin cutoff concentration at the 99th percentile of a healthy control group, together with a rising and/or falling pattern. The identification of dynamic changes is critical, because increased but relatively stable concentrations of cardiac troponin can be observed in chronic diseases, such as severe renal insufficiency and congestive heart failure. The ability to separate dynamic changes associated with acute myocardial injury from fluctuations caused by analytical imprecision and/or biological variation requires not only data in patients with AMI but also comparative data in healthy individuals and, where possible, those with cardiovascular disease (Fig 1 in the original article). Patients with stable coronary artery disease, chest pain, and no AMI are among those who eventually are seen in emergency departments with chest pain necessitating evaluation for myocardial injury. The authors hypothesized that the individual variation in cardiac troponin concentrations might be higher in patients with coronary artery disease compared with healthy individuals. Therefore, the individual variation of cardiac troponin in these patients might be more appropriate for calculating the degree of rise or fall needed to separate changes caused by acute myocardial damage from spontaneous changes seen in patients without acute myocardial injury. Accordingly, the aim of this study was to evaluate the short- and long-term individual variation of cTnI and cTnT, with 2 different troponin assays, in patients with verified or highly suspected but putatively stable coronary artery disease.

M. G. Bissell, MD, PhD, MPH

Unleashing the Power of Proteomics to Develop Blood-Based Cancer Markers

Taguchi A, Hanash SM (Fred Hutchinson Cancer Res Ctr, Seattle, WA)
Clin Chem 59:119-126, 2013

Background.—There is an urgent need for blood-based molecular tests to assist in the detection and diagnosis of cancers at an early stage, when curative interventions are still possible, and to predict and monitor response to treatment and disease recurrence. The rich content of proteins in blood that are impacted by tumor development and host factors provides an ideal opportunity to develop noninvasive diagnostics for cancer.

Content.—Mass spectrometry instrumentation has advanced sufficiently to allow the discovery of protein alterations directly in plasma across no less than 7 orders of magnitude of protein abundance. Moreover, the use of proteomics to harness the immune response in the form of seropositivity to tumor antigens has the potential to complement circulating protein biomarker panels for cancer detection. The depth of analysis currently possible in a discovery setting allows the detection of potential markers at concentrations of less than 1 μg/L. Such low concentrations may exceed the limits of detection of ELISAs and thus require the development of clinical assays with exquisite analytical sensitivity. Clearly the availability for discovery and validation of biospecimens that are highly relevant to the intended clinical application and have been collected, processed, and stored with the use of standard operating procedures is of crucial importance to the successful application of proteomics to the development of blood-based tests for cancer.

Summary.—The realization of the potential of proteomics to yield blood biomarkers will benefit from a collaborative approach and a substantial investment in resources.

▶ For disease investigation, the profiling of blood constituents, notably serum and plasma, using protein characterization technologies holds long-standing interest because of the easy accessibility of this circulating fluid and its rich content of proteins that inform scientists about the health status of an individual (Fig 1 in the original article). The available methodologies to analyze proteins have evolved dramatically over the last few decades. The initial method consisted of 1-dimensional protein separations, which was followed by the use of 2-dimensional polyacrylamide gel electrophoresis coupled with Edman sequencing. The advent of mass spectrometry, coupled with the sequencing of human and other genomes, has had a dramatic impact on the field of proteomics. The capabilities of current proteomics technologies in terms of coverage of the proteome and depth of analysis that can be achieved in a quantitative manner are truly astounding compared with just a decade ago. Recent advances include substantial increases in speed, analytical sensitivity, and dynamic range, and the availability of multiple fragmentation techniques. Equally important is orthogonal sample fractionation before mass spectrometry. Yet, there remains a perception that proteomics technologies are inadequate to address the protein complexities inherent in cells, tissues, and biological fluids. Here, the authors outline strategies for the application of proteomics to the development of blood-based cancer markers.

M. G. Bissell, MD, PhD, MPH

Serum human epididymis protein 4 vs carbohydrate antigen 125 for ovarian cancer diagnosis: a systematic review

Ferrarow S, Braga F, Lanzoni M, et al (Universitá degli Studi, Milano, Italy)

J Clin Pathol 66:273-281, 2013

Background.—Human epididymis protein 4 (HE4) measurements in serum have been proposed for improving the specificity of laboratory identification of ovarian cancer (OC).

Objective.—To critically revise the available literature on the comparison between the diagnostic accuracy of HE4 and carbohydrate antigen 125 (CA-125) to confirm the additional clinical value of HE4.

Methods.—A literature search was undertaken on electronic databases and references from retrieved articles; articles were analysed according to predefined criteria. Meta-analyses for HE4 and CA-125 biomarkers with OR, diagnostic sensitivity, specificity, positive (LR+) and negative (LR−) likelihood ratios as effect sizes were performed.

Results.—16 articles were originally included in metaanalyses, but two for HE4 and one for CA-125 were eliminated as outliers. Furthermore, for HE4 a publication bias was detected. ORs for both HE4 (37.2, 95% CI 19.0 to 72.7, adjusted for publication bias) and CA-125 (15.4, 95% CI 10.4 to 22.8) were significant, although in a heterogeneous set of studies ($p < 0.0001$). By combining sensitivity and specificity, the overall LR+ and LR− were 13.0 (95% CI 8.2 to 20.7) and 0.23 (95% CI 0.19 to 0.28) for HE4 and 4.2 (95% CI 3.1 to 5.6) and 0.27 (95% CI 0.23 to 0.31) for CA-125, respectively.

Conclusions.—HE4 measurement seems to be superior to CA-125 in terms of diagnostic performance for identification of OC in women with suspected gynaecological disease. Due to the high prevalence of OC in post-menopausal women and the need for data focused on early tumour stages, more studies tailored on these specific subsets are needed.

▶ Carbohydrate antigen 125 (CA-125) is the established biomarker for detecting ovarian cancer (OC) recurrence and monitoring therapeutic response. In addition, recent guidelines recommend its measurement in the primary care setting in women with suggestive symptoms or those at high risk for OC, in combination with pelvic ultrasound scan, even though some investigators have discouraged this application because of the low sensitivity of the test, which is even worse in early-stage tumors (approximately 50%). Overall, CA-125 effectiveness in the identification of the malignancy is threatened by its low diagnostic specificity. In fact, this glycoprotein is widely distributed on the surface of cells of mesothelial origin in various benign and malignant conditions other than OC. Among a wide spectrum of biomarkers recently proposed to aid in the diagnosis of women with suspected OC, human epididymis protein 4 (HE4) is undoubtedly the most promising. Its measurement was, from the beginning, proposed to improve the diagnostic specificity of CA-125, just maintaining a similar sensitivity. HE4 has homology with some secreted serine protease inhibitors and was reported to be amplified in some CA-125–deficient OCs, whereas its expression is lower in normal ovarian tissue, ovarian benign disease, and low malignant potential tumors. After preliminary studies confirming genomic and immunohistochemical findings on HE4, a large body of literature has been recently produced. Despite the low number of initially available studies, recent guidelines resorting to a meta-analytic approach have suggested HE4 be used as an aid in OC diagnosis. In addition, a systematic review (SR) has been recently published reporting better diagnostic performance in terms of sensitivity, specificity, and likelihood ratios for HE4 than for CA-125. However, the type of included studies, the applied selection criteria, and the statistical approach used to synthesize the evidence could be criticized. Exploiting the more recent increase of studies on the comparison of HE4 and CA-125 diagnostic performances for OC, the authors designed an SR to critically revise available literature, overcoming the above-reported threats of Yu's SR. In particular, they sought to provide a synthesis of the available evidence on the diagnostic accuracy of the tests by considering only those studies evaluating both markers on the same case series. Methodologically, a stepwise selection of the studies and a further application of proper summary receiving operating curves analysis were used to strengthen the evidence.

M. G. Bissell, MD, PhD, MPH

Toxicological analysis of blood and urine samples from female victims of alleged sexual assault

Jones AW, Holmgren A, Ahlner J (Natl Board of Forensic Medicine, Linköping, Sweden)

Clin Toxicol 50:555-561, 2012

Background.—The toxicological analysis of blood and urine samples from victims of alleged sexual assault represents a crucial part of the forensic evidence when this crime is investigated.

Material and Methods.—We searched a national forensic toxicology database (TOXBASE) to find cases registered as sexual assault, rape, including date-rape that the police had requested the analysis of ethanol and other drugs. Between 2008 and 2010, N = 1460 such cases met this criteria. After immunological screening of urine or blood samples, all positive results were verified by more specific analytical methods, such as gas chromatography-mass spectrometry (GC-MS) for illicit drugs. A large number of prescription drugs and their metabolites were determined by capillary GC with nitrogen-phosphorous (N-P) detector. GC with flame ionization detector (FID) was used to analyze ethanol and gamma-hydroxybutyrate (GHB) in blood at limits of quantitation (LOQ) of 0.1 g/L and 8 mg/L, respectively.

Results.—The average age (± standard deviation) of all victims was 24 ± 10.3 years and 72% were between 15 and 29 years. Ethanol and other drugs were not detected in 31% of cases (N = 459). Blood-ethanol was positive in N = 658 cases at mean, median and highest concentrations of 1.23 g/L, 1.22 g/L and 4.3 g/L, respectively. Ethanol plus drugs were present in N = 188 cases (13%) and one or more other drugs alone in N = 210 cases (14%). Cannabis (marijuana) and amphetamines were the major illicit drugs, whereas diazepam, alprazolam, zopiclone as well as newer antidepressants were the major prescription drugs identified.

Conclusions.—The mean age of victims of sexual assault in Sweden, the proportion of drug positive to drug negative cases, the predominance of ethanol positive cases as well as the types of other drugs showed a remarkably good agreement in two studies spanning a period of 8 years.

▶ Drug-facilitated sexual assault (DFSA) conjures up the image of a perpetrator adding a chemical substance to a person's food or drink to render the person incapacitated for the purpose of committing an illicit sexual act. Drug-facilitated crimes attract a lot of attention from the news media, government agencies, as well as reports in scientific journals. When investigating DFSA, it is obviously important to determine whether drugs had been taken voluntarily, which is often the case with the legal drug ethanol. Moreover, it is important to establish whether the victims were taking any prescription or recreational drugs at the time the offense was committed. In most of the previous investigations of DFSA, the principal toxicologic finding has been a positive blood alcohol concentration (BAC). The presence of fast-acting hypnotic or knock-out drugs, as exemplified by chloral hydrate, γ-hydroxybutyrate, z-hypnotics (zaleplon, zolpidem, zopiclone), and flunitrazepam is seldom verified. However, because many of these drugs have short elimination half-lives, the concentration in blood or urine might have decreased below the analytical limits of quantitation by the time specimens were collected from the victims. Ethanol is a legal drug, and depending on the amount ingested, the speed of drinking, the person's age, and previous experience with alcohol, ethanol-induced effects might range from mild euphoria to unconsciousness. Ethanol influences people in different ways from no discernible effects to excitement, loss of inhibitions, and dangerous behavior, including engaging in unplanned sexual activities. There is often a fine line between consensual sex and sexual assault, especially when both parties are under the influence of alcohol. Excessive binge drinking resulting in high BAC (> 2.0 g/L) often leads to gross intoxication and incapacitation in novice drinkers.

This article reports the toxicologic results from analysis of blood and urine samples from female victims of alleged sexual assault or rape that came to the attention of the police in Sweden between 2008 and 2010. The victims of this crime are representative of the whole country, and the toxicologic results were compared and contrasted with an earlier investigation covering the years 2003 to 2007.

M. G. Bissell, MD, PhD, MPH

Serum testosterone, dihydrotestosterone and estradiol concentrations in older men self-reporting very good health: the healthy man study

Sartorius G, Spasevska S, Idan A, et al (Concord Hosp, Clayton, Victoria, Australia; et al)

Clin Endocrinol 77:755-763, 2012

Objective.—To determine serum concentrations, intra-individual variability and impact of age-related co-morbidities on serum testosterone (T), dihydrotestosterone (DHT), estradiol (E_2) and estrone (E_1) in older men.

Design.—Observational, repeated measures study.

Participants.—Men ($n = 325$) with 40 years and older self-reporting very good or excellent health.

Measurements.—Standardized history, physical examination and collection of nine blood samples at fixed time intervals were measured over 3 months (three at 20 min intervals on days 1 (fasting) and 2 (non-fasting), one at days 7, 30 and 90). Serum T, DHT, E_2 and E_1 ($n = 2900$, > 99% of scheduled samples) measured by liquid chromatography-tandem mass spectrometry (LC-MS) were analysed by linear mixed model analysis with fasting, age and obesity as covariables.

Results.—Mean serum T did not vary with age ($P = 0{\cdot}76$) but obesity ($-0{\cdot}35$ nm per body mass index (BMI) unit, $P < 0{\cdot}0001$) and ex-smoker status ($-1{\cdot}6$ nm, $P < 0{\cdot}001$) had significant effects. Serum DHT was increased with age ($+0{\cdot}011$ nm per year, $P = 0{\cdot}001$) but decreased with obesity ($-0{\cdot}05$ nm per BMI unit, $P < 0{\cdot}0001$). Serum E_2 did not vary with age ($P = 0{\cdot}31$) or obesity ($P = 0{\cdot}12$). Overnight fasting increased (by 9–16%, all $P < 0{\cdot}001$) and reduced variability in morning serum T, DHT, E_2 and E_1. Non-fasting serum T and DHT were stable over time (day, week, month or 3 months; $P > 0{\cdot}28$).

Conclusions.—Serum T, DHT and E_2 displayed no decrease associated with age among men over 40 years of age who self-report very good or excellent health although obesity and ex-smoking status were associated with decreased serum androgens (T and DHT) but not E_2. These findings support the interpretation that the age-related decline in blood T accompanying non-specific symptoms in older men may be due to accumulating age-related co-morbidities rather than a symptomatic androgen deficiency state.

▶ The decline in blood testosterone (T) during male aging is well known from numerous observational studies since the advent of T immunoassay in the early 1970s. Such studies are typically cross-sectional and obtain only a single blood sample for T measurement. More recent longitudinal studies involving serial blood sampling have appeared, although many are still relying on single blood samples per time point, which frequently are inconsistent. Although causality cannot be ascribed from observational studies, the coincidence of declining blood T concentrations with nonspecific symptoms that are consistent with, but not diagnostic of, androgen deficiency (AD) has led to the andropause hypothesis, which postulates that these symptoms may be caused by age-related AD. Using the analogy of unequivocal hormone deficiency states, such as pathologically based AD in young men and menopause in women, this proposes that symptomatic age-related AD may contribute a reversible component to deterioration in somatic and reproductive health of older men. Definitive testing of this hypothesis requires a placebo-controlled, randomized clinical trial that remains a prospect for the future. The alternative view is that the decline in blood T levels in older men is a consequence of the accumulation of comorbidities of aging, which can depress blood T levels unrelated to the coincidental, nonspecific symptoms of chronic disease that resemble those of AD. This alternative hypothesis, whereby blood T is effectively a nonspecific barometer of (ill)-health, cannot be proven directly but would be a plausible interpretation if the andropause hypothesis is refuted. In the interim, while the andropause hypothesis remains untested, consensus clinical guidelines and analysis of large-scale observational studies tentatively define age-related AD (andropause, late-onset hypogonadism) providing tacit support for unproven T treatment of older men, according to criteria that combine nonspecific symptoms and blood T thresholds into a putative diagnosis of age-related AD. This study aimed to measure age-specific serum concentrations of the major sex steroids (T, DHT, and E2) among healthy older men as well as estimate the within-individual variability and the impact of common age-related comorbidities (obesity, smoking).

M. G. Bissell, MD, PhD, MPH

Albuminuria Prevalence in First Morning Void Compared with Previous Random Urine from Adults in the National Health and Nutrition Examination Survey, 2009–2010

Saydah SH, Pavkov ME, Zhang C, et al (CDC, Atlanta, GA; et al)
Clin Chem 59:675-683, 2013

Background.—Albuminuria, defined as urine albumin/creatinine ratio (ACR) ≥30 mg/g, is a diagnostic component of chronic kidney disease (CKD). National estimates of ACR and CKD prevalence have been based on single random urine samples. Although 2 urine samples or a first morning void are known to produce different estimates of ACR, the impact of differing urine sampling schemes on nationally estimated rates of CKD is unknown.

Methods.—In 2009–2010, the National Health and Nutrition Examination Survey (NHANES) participants provided 2 untimed urine samples for sequential ACR measurement: an initial random urine collected in the NHANES mobile examination center and a subsequent first morning void collected at home. Rates of albuminuria were calculated in the overall population and broken down by demographics, diagnosed diabetes and hypertension status, and estimated glomerular filtration rate (eGFR).

Results.—Overall, 43.5% of adults with increased ACR (≥30 mg/g) in a random urine also had increased ACR in a first morning urine. This percentage was higher among individuals ≥50 years old (48.9%), males (53.3%), participants with diagnosed diabetes (56.3%) and hypertension (51.5%), and eGFR <60 mL/min/1.72m^2 (56.9%). The use of confirmed increased ACR (defined as the presence of ACR ≥30 mg/g in both samples taken within 10 days) to define CKD resulted in a lower overall prevalence (11.6%) than first morning urine (12.7%) or random spot urine only (15.2%).

Conclusions.—ACR measured on random urine samples appears to overestimate the prevalence of albuminuria compared to first morning urine collections.

▶ More than 10% of US adults meet the diagnostic criteria for chronic kidney disease (CKD), defined as reduced kidney function or the presence of kidney damage for at least 3 months regardless of kidney function. Kidney damage is ascertained by increased urinary markers, such as albuminuria, or by abnormal urinary sediment, abnormal imaging studies, or kidney biopsy. Albuminuria, defined by a urinary albumin-to-creatinine ratio (ACR) 230 mg/g, is often considered an early marker of glomerular kidney diseases and is associated with an increased risk of death independent of the level of kidney function. In the United States, previous studies have estimated the population prevalence of increased ACR as 7.8% on the basis of a single random urine sample. Owing to the high within-individual variation of ACR, clinical recommendations for diagnosing CKD when glomerular filtration rate is within reference intervals require that at least 2 urinary samples collected within 3 to 6 months contain 230 mg albumin per gram of creatinine in the absence of clinical or laboratory evidence of urinary tract infection. Although a 24-hour urine collection is considered the gold standard for detecting increased albumin excretion, this method is laborious and prone to collection error and, therefore, impractical for surveillance. ACR measured in a spot morning urine collection correlates well with the timed excretion rate in cross-sectional studies and is a strong predictor of kidney disease progression in longitudinal studies. ACR measurements in random, untimed urine samples generally show a higher within-person biological CV than is found for first or second morning samples. However, comparisons between studies are difficult because of lack of standardized methodology. In the US, persistence of albuminuria, on the basis of a repeat examination at the National Health and Nutrition Examination Survey (NHANES) Mobile Examination Center, was previously estimated at approximately 63% in a subsample of adult participants from 1988 to 1994. It is not known if changes in the demographics and disease characteristics of the US population since the early 1990s have influenced this estimate. In NHANES 2009-2010, 2 urine samples were collected for ACR determination in participants 6 years of age and older, including initial random spot urine at the Mobile Examination Center and a subsequent first morning void at home. This report presents distributions of random and first morning urine measures, measures of agreement between the 2 urine collections, and highlights related to methodologic issues and differences in national prevalence estimates for CKD (Fig 1 in the original article).

M. G. Bissell, MD, PhD, MPH

15 Clinical Microbiology

CHROMagar Yersinia, a New Chromogenic Agar for Screening of Potentially Pathogenic *Yersinia enterocolitica* Isolates in Stools

Renaud N, Lecci L, Courcol RJ, et al (Lille Univ Med Ctr, France)

J Clin Microbiol 51:1184-1187, 2013

CHROMagar Yersinia (CAY) is a new chromogenic medium for the presumptive detection of virulent *Yersinia enterocolitica* in stools. Based on a comparative analysis of 1,494 consecutive stools from hospitalized patients, CAY was found to be just as sensitive as the reference medium (cefsulodin-irgasan-novobiocin agar) but was significantly more specific and had a very low falsepositive rate. CAY reduces the workload (and thus costs) for stool analysis and can therefore be recommended for routine laboratory use.

▶ In temperate and cold areas of the world, *Yersinia enterocolitica* is the third most common human bacterial enteropathogen. Although it mainly causes sporadic cases of gastroenteritis, outbreaks have been reported. The species is subdivided into 6 biovars (IA, IB, 2, 3, 4, and 5) and can also be separated into serogroups on the basis of the somatic (O) antigens, some of which are common to 2 or more biovars. However, the pathogenicity of the various serogroups of *Y enterocolitica* is heterogeneous. When considering the 30 O serogroups, most of the strains isolated from humans with diarrhea come from serogroups O:3; O:5,27; O:8; and O:9. Biovar IA strains are generally considered to be nonpathogenic because they lack (in contrast to biovars I band 2 to 5) the p YV plasmid that is essential for bacterial virulence isolation of *Y enterocolitica* from stools, which is fastidious because it is frequently outgrown by other Enterobacteriaceae. Partially selective media containing antimicrobial cocktails have been proposed to facilitate *Y enterocolitica* recovery from fecal specimens, and the semiselective cefsulodin-irgasan-novobiocin (CIN) agar developed more than 30 years ago is still the medium most widely used by medical microbiologists for this purpose. A *Y enterocolitica* chromogenic medium (YeCM) has been used for quality control in the food industry. In fact, YeCM was shown to be just as sensitive as CIN and was well suited for rapid detection of virulent *Y enterocolitica* in the tonsils of slaughtered pigs, the main animal reservoir of strains that are pathogenic in humans. However, YeCM has not been evaluated in a clinical microbiology setting in humans. CHROMagar Yersinia (CAY) is a new, selective, chromogenic medium for the presumptive identification of pathogenic *Y enterocolitica* colonies. The latter are colored mauve after 48 hours of incubation at 28°C (the species' optimal growth temperature), whereas nonpathogenic strains of the species and occasional isolates of other *Enterobacteriaceae* grow as metallic blue colonies after as little as 24 hours of incubation at the same temperature. In this study, the authors evaluated the performance of CAY relative to the CIN reference medium for the routine detection of pathogenic *Y enterocolitica* in stools from patients with diarrhea.

M. G. Bissell, MD, PhD, MPH

Assessment of Real-Time PCR Assay for Detection of *Rickettsia* spp. and *Rickettsia rickettsii* in Banked Clinical Samples

Kato CY, Chung IH, Robinson LK, et al (Ctrs for Disease Control and Prevention, Atlanta, GA)

J Clin Microbiol 51:314-317, 2013

Two novel real-time PCR assays were developed for the detection of *Rickettsia* spp. One assay detects all tested *Rickettsia* spp.; the other is specific for *Rickettsia rickettsii*. Evaluation using DNA from human blood and tissue samples showed both assays to be more sensitive than nested PCR assays currently in use at the CDC.

▶ *Rickettsia rickettsii*, the causative agent of Rocky Mountain spotted fever (RMSF), is a tick-borne bacterial agent that is a member of the spotted fever group rickettsiae. Symptoms of this disease may include, but are not limited to, high fever, headache, and rash, with the potential for a fatal outcome. National case fatality rates are less than 1% but can approach 7% in some regions to which it is highly endemic; a fatal outcome may be averted with timely administration of doxycycline. In the United States, serologic tests are most often used to diagnose RMSF with seroconversion (4-fold titer increase from acute to convalescent phase) by immunofluorescence assay, the gold standard. However, serologic test results are frequently negative during the acute phase of illness, and currently available molecular tests are not reliable for use in management when applied to acute-phase blood samples, which may have very few organisms. Clinical management of suspected RMSF cases based on test results is not recommended, partly because of diagnostic assay limitations, and physicians must treat suspected cases empirically. Although empirical treatment of suspected cases will always be recommended, the development of more sensitive molecular tests that could be applied to patient specimens during the acute phase of illness will enhance the identification of nonfatal cases, improve the timeliness of public health actions after identification of a case, and aid national surveillance efforts by better defining the spectrum and burden of tick-borne rickettsial infections.

M. G. Bissell, MD, PhD, MPH

Detection of Hepatitis C Virus Transmission by Use of DNA Mass Spectrometry

Ganova-Raeva LM, Dimitrova ZE, Campo DS, et al (Ctrs for Disease Control and Prevention, Atlanta, GA; et al)

J Infect Dis 207:999-1006, 2013

The molecular detection of transmission of rapidly mutating pathogens such as hepatitis C virus (HCV) is commonly achieved by assessing the genetic relatedness of strains among infected patients. We describe the development of a novel mass spectrometry (MS)—based approach to identify HCV transmission. MS was used to detect products of base-specific cleavage of RNA molecules obtained from HCV polymerase chain reaction fragments. The MS-peak profiles were found to reflect variation in the HCV genomic sequence and the intrahost composition of the HCV population. Serum specimens originating from 60 case patients from 14 epidemiologically confirmed outbreaks and 25 unrelated controls were tested. Neighbor-joining trees constructed using MS-peak profile-based Hamming distances showed 100% accuracy, and linkage networks constructed using a threshold established from the Hamming distances between epidemiologically unrelated cases showed 100% sensitivity and 99.93% specificity in transmission detection. This MS-based approach is rapid, robust, reproducible, cost-effective, and applicable to investigating transmissions of other pathogens.

► Hepatitis C virus (HCV) is a human pathogen belonging to the Flaviviridae family. Accurate identification of HCV strains involved in transmission can be achieved by matching the genetic compositions of viral populations sampled from infected hosts. Because HVR1 is one of the most variable regions of the HCV genome, analysis of intrahost HVR1 variants is frequently used for identification of and tracking HCV transmissions. Such analysis involves (1) separation of individual HVR1 variants either by genetic cloning of polymerase chain reaction (PCR) amplicons or by PCR cloning, using endpoint limiting dilution of complementary DNA and (2) sequencing of these variants. Next-generation sequencing technologies couple the separation of genetic variants with sequencing, thus simplifying significantly the assessment of viral heterogeneity. However, the high rate of sequencing errors generated per DNA read and the problematic representation of intrahost viral heterogeneity are potential hindrances to adopting next-generation sequencing approaches to the detection of transmissions. DNA mass spectrometry (MS) provides a different platform for genetic analysis of viral strains. It has successfully been adopted for resequencing, microbial typing, and single nucleotide polymorphism discovery. Here, the authors describe the development of an MS approach for identification of genetic equivalence among HCV strains involved in outbreaks. It does not entail separation and sequencing of viral variants; rather, it uses patterns of MS peaks generated from the entire intrahost viral population. They found the MS approach to be as accurate as previously established molecular technologies in the detection of HCV transmission but significantly more cost effective and less time consuming.

M. G. Bissell, MD, PhD, MPH

Using the rate of bacterial clearance determined by real-time polymerase chain reaction as a timely surrogate marker to evaluate the appropriateness of antibiotic usage in critical patients with *Acinetobacter baumannii* bacteremia

Chuang Y-C, Chang S-C, Wang W-K (Natl Taiwan Univ, Taipei; Univ of Hawaii, Honolulu)

Crit Care Med 40:2273-2280, 2012

Objective.—Bacteremia caused by *Acinetobacter baumannii* is becoming more frequent among critically ill patients, and has been associated with high mortality and prolonged hospital stay. Multidrug resistance and delay in blood culture have been shown to be significant barriers to appropriate antibiotic treatment. Quantitative polymerase chain reaction assays were recently used to monitor bacterial loads; we hypothesized that the rate of bacterial clearance determined by quantitative polymerase chain reaction can be used as a timely surrogate marker to evaluate the appropriateness of antibiotic usage.

Design.—Prospective observational study.

Setting.—University hospital and research laboratory.

Patients.—Patients with culture-proven *A. baumannii* bacteremia in the intensive care units were prospectively enrolled from April 2008 to February 2009.

Interventions.—Plasmid Oxa-51/pCRII-TOPO, which contained a 431-bp fragment of the *A. baumannii*-specific *Oxa-51* gene in a pCRII-TOPO vector, was used as the standard. Sequential bacterial DNA loads in the blood were measured by a quantitative polymerase chain reaction assay.

Measurements and Main Results.—We enrolled 51 patients with *A. baumannii* bacteremia, and examined 318 sequential whole blood samples. The initial mean bacterial load was 2.15 log copies/mL, and the rate of bacterial clearance was 0.088 log copies/mL/day. Multivariate linear regression using the generalized estimation equation approach revealed that the use of immunosuppressants was an independent predictor for slower bacterial clearance (coefficient, 1.116; $p < .001$), and appropriate antibiotic usage was an independent predictor for more rapid bacterial clearance (coefficient, −0.995; $p < .001$). Patients with a slower rate of bacterial clearance experienced higher in-hospital mortality (odds ratio, 2.323; $p = .04$).

Conclusions.—Immunosuppression and appropriate antibiotic usage were independent factors affecting the rate of clearance of *A. baumannii* bacteremia in critical patients. These findings highlight the importance of appropriate antibiotic usage and development of effective antibiotics against *A. baumannii* in an era of emerging antibiotic resistance. The rate of bacterial clearance could serve as a timely surrogate marker for evaluating the appropriateness of antibiotics.

▶ *Acinetobacter baumannii* is a nonfermenting gram-negative Aerobic coccobacillus, and is the most virulent species in the *Acinetobacter calcoaceticus-A baumannii* complex. Health care—associated infections caused by *A baumannii* are increasing among patients in intensive care units. These infections are associated with high mortality and a prolonged length of hospital stay. In addition to pneumonia, bacteremia is the most common presentation of *A baumannii* infection and is associated with high mortality. The emergence of antimicrobial resistance of *A baumannii* has limited the available therapeutic options. Timely and appropriate antibiotic usage is critical for the treatment of patients with sepsis; however, barriers to this practice include the decreased sensitivity and delays in the processing time from positive growth to determination of susceptibility profiles by traditional blood cultures. Moreover, risk factors for multidrug-resistant *A baumannii* infections may also impact survival, making the evaluation of treatment response to antibiotics very difficult. The authors hypothesized that the appropriate use of antibiotics leads to a higher rate of bacterial clearance and better outcomes, and that the rate of bacterial clearance can be used to evaluate the appropriateness of antimicrobial therapy in a timely manner. In this prospective, observational study of patients with *A baumannii* bacteremia, they followed up sequential bacterial DNA loads in the blood using a quantitative real-time polymerase chain reaction assay and investigated the relationship of clearance of bacteremia to antibiotic use and other factors.

M. G. Bissell, MD, PhD, MPH

Cytomegalovirus DNA in Semen and Blood Is Associated With Higher Levels of Proviral HIV DNA

Gianella S, Anderson CM, Vargas MV, et al (Univ of California-San Diego, La Jolla)

J Infect Dis 207:898-902, 2013

Over three-fourths of human immunodeficiency virus (HIV)—infected men who have sex with men (MSM) have at least one herpesvirus detected in their semen, and cytomegalovirus (CMV) is the most prevalent. The presence of CMV is associated with higher T-cell immune activation and with HIV disease progression in treated and untreated individuals. In this study of 113 antiretroviral (ART)—naive HIV-infected MSM, we found that CMV replication in blood and semen was associated with higher levels of HIV DNA in peripheral blood mononuclear cells. These observations suggest that interventions aimed to reduce CMV replication and, thus, systemic immune activation could decrease the size of the latent HIV reservoir.

▶ Over three-fourths of human immunodeficiency virus (HIV)—infected men who have sex with men have at least one actively replicating herpesvirus detected in their semen, and cytomegalovirus (CMV) is the most prevalent. Although the interactions between herpesviruses and HIV are relevant to HIV transmission, the role of herpesviruses in HIV pathogenesis may be equally important. Presence of CMV is associated with HIV disease progression and higher T-cell immune activation. Such immune activation can blunt $CD4^+$ T-cell recovery during antiretroviral therapy and lead to premature mortality. Moreover, immune activation in response to CMV may be responsible for accelerated immunosenescence in HIV-infected and HIV-uninfected individuals. Because activated T cells undergo extensive cell division and differentiation, the authors hypothesized that bystander proliferation of HIV-infected $CD4^+$ T cells could be an important factor in determining the size of the HIV proviral reservoir. The latent HIV reservoir is established during primary HIV infection, but the mechanisms that maintain this reservoir are unclear. It is, therefore, particularly important to understand which factors contribute to increase the immune activation and which mechanisms drive and modulate the establishment of the viral reservoir during the earliest phase of HIV infection. Here, the authors investigated the relationships between CMV replication in semen and paired peripheral blood mononuclear cells (PBMCs) and estimated the duration of infection, the HIV DNA level in PBMCs, the HIV RNA load in blood plasma, and $CD4^+$ T-cell numbers.

M. G. Bissell, MD, PhD, MPH

Is It Time to Replace the Tuberculin Skin Test With a Blood Test?

LoBue PA, Castro KG (Ctrs for Disease Control and Prevention, Atlanta, GA)

JAMA 308:241-242, 2012

Background.—The eradication of tuberculosis (TB) before the 22nd century will require substantial improvements in the diagnosis and treatment of latent tuberculosis infection (LTBI) to prevent its progression. Medication regimens with shorter durations, specifically, 12 weekly doses rather than 9 months of doses, have the potential to increase the rates of treatment completion. A replacement for the tuberculin skin test (TST) has been sought as well, with the most likely candidate being interferon-γ-release assays (IGRAs). TST measures the induration after inoculation. IGRAs detect ex vivo interferon-γ production by peripheral blood mononuclear cells exposed to peptides that are designed to simulate *Mycobacterium tuberculosis* antigens. A comparison of the current status of TST and IGRAs was undertaken.

Strengths.—IGRAs require a single visit rather than the two visits needed for TST–one to be inoculated and one to read the results 48 to 72 hours later. IGRAs also use an objective measure rather than relying on human interpretation of induration. IGRAs use peptides that simulate specific *M tuberculosi* antigens rather than the purified protein derivative used in TSTs. Purified protein derivative contains several *M tuberculosis* antigens that cross-react with bacilli Calmette-Guérin (BCG) and many nontuberculous mycobacteria. The peptides are seldom found in nontuberculous mycobacteria and never in BCG. Finally, IGRAs have been tested in many populations, although some of these sample sizes were small.

Limitations.—TST performs poorly in predicting which patients will eventually develop TB disease, with only 5% to 10% of those with positive TST results progressing. It has been difficult to test IGRA ability in this area because of ethical concerns and limited sample size. Another limitation is the cost of IGRAs, which can be three times the cost of TST. Cost-effectiveness studies have yielded inconsistent results for the two diagnostic approaches. Finally, there have been unexpected reports of unusually high rates of initially positive IGRA results and high IGRA conversion rates among health care workers who are frequently tested in relatively low-risk-for-TB situations. This may reflect an inadequate or suboptimal cutoff for a positive result in all populations. TST has three cutoffs for a positive test based on pretest TB risk, with conversion to a positive result requiring a change of at least 10 mm in induration.

Conclusions.—Current evidence indicates that IGRAs are at least as reliable as TSTs for predicting future incident TB and may be slightly better. However, they are more costly than TSTs and do not improve the diagnostic result more than incrementally. The Centers for Disease Control and Prevention has recommended that IGRAs be used in place of TST in all situations where TST is currently used and may be preferred for individuals who have been BCG vaccinated or belong to groups with an historically low rate of return for TST readings, such as homeless persons. TST is preferred but IGRA is an acceptable alternative in situations involving young children. Programs and institutions should assess the availability, cost, and benefits of each method for their target populations.

▶ Effective diagnosis and treatment of latent tuberculosis infection (LTBI) to prevent progression to tuberculosis (TB) disease is one of the priority strategies for control, prevention, and eventual elimination of TB in the United States. Recent mathematical TB transmission modeling has shown that substantial improvements in addressing LTBI will be needed to eliminate TB before the 22nd century. Effective management of LTBI has been hampered by limitations of both treatment regimens and diagnostic tools. The advent of medication regimens with much shorter durations (eg, 12 weekly doses of isoniazid and rifapentine) than the current standard of 9 months of isoniazid is likely to lead to higher rates of treatment completion. Efforts have also been directed at finding a replacement for the tuberculin skin test (TST), which, despite its many limitations, has been the mainstay of LTBI diagnosis. Beginning in the 1990s, interferon-γ-release assays (IGRAs) were developed to diagnose LTBI. Currently, 2 US Food and Drug Administration–approved IGRAs are commercially available, QuantiFERON TB Gold In-Tube (Cellestis/Qiagen) and T-SPOT.TB (Oxford Immunotec). These blood tests detect ex vivo interferon-γ production by peripheral blood mononuclear cells exposed to peptides designed to simulate *Mycobacterium tuberculosis* antigens. IGRAs offer several practical and theoretical advantages over TST. IGRAs require only 1 patient visit as opposed to 2 for TST (one visit for placement and one visit for reading 48 to 72 hours later). IGRAs use an objective measurement of interferon-γ production as opposed to human measurement of induration for TST. Also, IGRAs use peptides simulating specific *M tuberculosis* antigens (early secretory antigenic target 6 [ESAT-6], culture filtrate protein 10 [CFP-10], TB7.7), whereas TST uses purified protein derivative. Purified protein derivative contains numerous *M tuberculosis* antigens that cross-react with bacille Calmette-Guérin (BCG) and many nontuberculous mycobacteria. ESAT-6, CFP-10, and TB7.7 are found in very few nontuberculous mycobacteria and are not found in BCG.

M. G. Bissell, MD, PhD, MPH

Respiratory Viral Coinfections Identified by a 10-Plex Real-Time Reverse-Transcription Polymerase Chain Reaction Assay in Patients Hospitalized With Severe Acute Respiratory Illness—South Africa, 2009–2010

Pretorius MA, Madhi SA, Cohen C, et al (Univ of the Witwatersrand, Johannesburg, South Africa; et al)

J Infect Dis 206:S159-S165, 2012

Background.—Data about respiratory coinfections with 2009 pandemic influenza A virus subtype H1N1 during the 2009–2010 influenza pandemic in Africa are limited. We used an existing surveillance program for severe acute respiratory illness to evaluate a new multiplex real-time polymerase chain reaction assay and investigate the role of influenza virus and other respiratory viruses in pneumonia hospitalizations during and after the influenza pandemic in South Africa.

Methods.—The multiplex assay was developed to detect 10 respiratory viruses, including influenza A and B viruses, parainfluenza virus types 1–3, respiratory syncytial virus (RSV), enterovirus, human metapneumovirus (hMPV), adenovirus (AdV), and rhinovirus (RV), followed by influenza virus subtyping. Nasopharyngeal and oropharyngeal specimens were collected from patients hospitalized with pneumonia at 6 hospitals during 2009–2010.

Results.—Validation against external quality controls confirmed the high sensitivity (91%) and specificity (100%) and user-friendliness, compared with other PCR technologies. Of 8173 patients, 40% had single-virus infections, 17% had coinfections, and 43% remained negative. The most common viruses were RV (25%), RSV (14%), AdV (13%), and influenza A virus (5%). Influenza virus, RSV, PIV type 3, and hMPV showed seasonal patterns.

Conclusion.—The data provide a better understanding of the viral etiology of hospitalized cases of pneumonia and demonstrate the usefulness of this multiplex assay in respiratory disease surveillance in South Africa.

▶ Pneumonia is a major cause of morbidity and mortality among children worldwide and causes 18% of all deaths among children less than 5 years of age. Viral infections have been shown to play a major role in acute respiratory infections in the developed world, but apart from a few articles on specific viruses, such as influenza virus and respiratory syncytial virus (RSV) in selected regions, data remain limited from sub-Saharan Africa. In April 2009, pandemic influenza

A virus subtype H1N1 (A[H1N1]pdm09) emerged as a new pathogen. South Africa reported 12 640 cases and 93 deaths during the first wave, from June through October 2009, the most of any country in Africa. Respiratory viruses traditionally associated with acute respiratory tract infection include influenza A and B viruses, RSV, parainfluenza virus (PIV) types 1-3, adenovirus, enterovirus, human metapneumovirus (hMPV), and rhinovirus. Although a few studies have determined the frequency of respiratory viruses in patients with acute lower respiratory tract illness in Africa, these studies have mainly been limited to single sites and to a limited number of viruses, and little has been reported on viral coinfections. Few data are available about the contribution of other respiratory viruses to respiratory tract infections during the recent influenza pandemic or their role in A(H1N1)pdm09 infections in Africa, and limited data are available from elsewhere. Comparative studies have found that real-time reverse transcription polymerase chain reaction (rRT-PCR) assays are substantially more sensitive than conventional methods, such as viral culture and immunofluorescence assays, for detecting respiratory viruses. Furthermore, compared with conventional PCR and other real-time methods, multiplex rRT-PCR has a significant advantage, as it permits simultaneous amplification of several viruses in a single reaction. This facilitates cost-effective diagnosis, enabling the detection of multiple viruses in a single clinical specimen. As part of a severe acute respiratory illness (SARI) surveillance program that commenced in February 2009 in South Africa, the authors developed a 2-step multiplex rRT-PCR assay that could detect 10 different viruses (influenza A and B viruses, RSV, enterovirus, hMPV, adenovirus, rhinovirus, and PIV types 1–3) to investigate the role of the most common respiratory viruses as etiologic agents in patients hospitalized with SARI in South Africa.

M. G. Bissell, MD, PhD, MPH

A Cohort Effect of the Sexual Revolution May Be Masking an Increase in Human Papillomavirus Detection at Menopause in the United States

Gravitt PE, Rositch AF, Silver MI, et al (Johns Hopkins Bloomberg School of Public Health, Baltimore, MD; et al)

J Infect Dis 207:272-280, 2013

Background.—Cohort effects, new sex partnerships, and human papillomavirus (HPV) reactivation have been posited as explanations for the bimodal age-specific HPV prevalence observed in some populations; no studies have systematically evaluated the reasons for the lack of a second peak in the United States.

Methods.—A cohort of 843 women aged 35–60 years were enrolled into a 2-year, semiannual follow-up study. Age-specific HPV prevalence was estimated in strata defined by a lower risk of prior infection (<5 self-reported lifetime sex partners) and a higher risk of prior infection (≥5 lifetime sex partners). The interaction between age and lifetime sex partners was tested using likelihood ratio statistics. Population attributable risk (PAR) was estimated using Levin's formula.

Results.—The age-specific prevalence of 14 high-risk HPV genotypes (HR-HPV) declined with age among women with <5 lifetime sex partners but not among women with ≥5 lifetime sex partners ($P = .01$ for interaction). The PAR for HR-HPV due to ≥5 lifetime sex partners was higher among older women (87.2%), compared with younger women (28.0%). In contrast, the PAR associated with a new sex partner was 28% among women aged 35–49 years and 7.7% among women aged 50–60 years.

Conclusions.—A lower cumulative probability of HPV infection among women with a sexual debut before the sexual revolution may be masking an age-related increase in HPV reactivation in the United States.

▶ Pooled and meta-analyses of age-specific human papillomavirus (HPV) prevalence have demonstrated considerable variability across geographic regions. A recent study updated the age-specific prevalence from a global analysis of 1 million women with normal cervical cytology findings. In all regions, the HPV prevalence was highest among younger women around the age of sexual debut. A second peak in HPV prevalence around the age of menopause was marked in Central and South America and Western Africa but absent in North America, Eastern and Southeast Asia, Eastern Europe, Northern Europe, and Western Europe. An attenuated menopausal peak prevalence was observed in South Asia, Southern Europe, and Southern Africa. Explanations for this variability include differences in relative prevalence of new partnerships at older ages, risk of HPV reactivation at older ages, and cohort effects. The lack of a second increase in HPV prevalence at menopause in the United States suggests that older US women are not having a significant increase in new sex partnerships at menopause and are not at risk of HPV reactivation, assuming no influence of a cohort effect. To investigate whether these assertions were valid, the authors compared differences in recent and lifetime sexual behaviors, by age group, to investigate the presence of a cohort effect in an older screening population in Baltimore, Maryland, and its impact on HPV prevalence estimates.

M. G. Bissell, MD, PhD, MPH

Diagnostic Accuracy of Histopathologic and Cytopathologic Examination of *Aspergillus* Species

Shah AA, Hazen KC (Univ of Virginia Health System, Charlottesville)
Am J Clin Pathol 139:55-61, 2013

To assess the diagnostic accuracy of histopathologic and cytopathologic examination (HCE) of *Aspergillus* species (spp), we performed an 11-year retrospective review to correlate surgical/cytology cases with a diagnosis of *Aspergillus* spp with their concurrent fungal culture results. Diagnostic accuracy was defined as the percentage of cases with culture-proven *Aspergillus* spp divided by the number of cases diagnosed as *Aspergillus* spp on HCE that had growth on fungal culture. Ninety surgical/cytology cases with concurrent fungal culture were reviewed, 58 of which grew a fungal organism. Of these 58 cases, 45 grew an Aspergillus spp, whereas 13 grew an organism other than *Aspergillus* spp, including both common (*Scedosporium, Fusarium*, and *Paecilomyces* spp) and uncommon mimickers (*Trichosporon loubieri*), resulting in a diagnostic accuracy of 78%. The low diagnostic accuracy indicates that several fungal organisms can morphologically mimic *Aspergillus* spp and can only be distinguished by fungal culture and DNA sequencing.

▶ *Aspergillus* species (spp) exist as septate molds and are a common cause of opportunistic mycoses in the immunocompromised host. *Aspergillus* spp can cause a range of clinical infections in the skin, eyes, ears, lung, and other organs. Histopathologic and cytopathologic examination (HCE), one of the major tools used in the diagnosis of these infections, is considered one of the criteria for diagnosing invasive fungal infections, as proposed by the European Organisation for Research and Treatment of Cancer/Invasive Fungal Infections Cooperative Group and the National Institute of Allergy and Infectious Diseases Mycoses Study Group Consensus Group. Early and accurate diagnosis of any fungal infection is critical. However, identification in histopathologic and cytopathologic specimens of *Aspergillus* spp can be challenging because a number of other fungal species are morphologically similar, such as *Scedosporium* spp, *Penicillium* spp, and *Fusarium* spp. Distinguishing these organisms from *Aspergillus* spp is essential in guiding treatment and patient outcomes. To date, few studies have assessed the accuracy of HCE in the diagnosis of aspergillosis. To assess the accuracy of the histopathologic and cytopathologic diagnosis of *Aspergillus* spp, the authors performed an 11-year retrospective review of all cytology and surgical pathology cases that had a diagnosis indicating the presence of *Aspergillus* spp and their concurrent fungal culture results.

M. G. Bissell, MD, PhD, MPH

Comparison of 2 Blood Culture Media Shows Significant Differences in Bacterial Recovery for Patients on Antimicrobial Therapy

Zadroga R, Williams DN, Gottschall R, et al (Univ of Minnesota, Minneapolis; Hennepin County Med Ctr, Minneapolis, MN; et al)
Clin Infect Dis 56:790-797, 2013

Background.—Antimicrobial removal devices in blood culture media are designed to remove antibiotics from the blood culture solution, thereby facilitating bacterial growth. How well these devices function clinically has not been established.

Methods.—All blood drawn for culture from adult inpatients and emergency department visitors in a level I trauma center was placed in paired BACTEC Plus and BacT/Alert FAN culture media and studied simultaneously, consecutively, and prospectively between 1 February and 30 September 2011. All cultures were processed per standard laboratory protocols.

Results.—Of 9395 total cultures collected, 1219 (13%) were positive, 831 were included, and 524 (33%) contained pathogens. BACTEC had a 4.5-hour faster detection time ($P < .0001$), and isolated exclusively 182 of

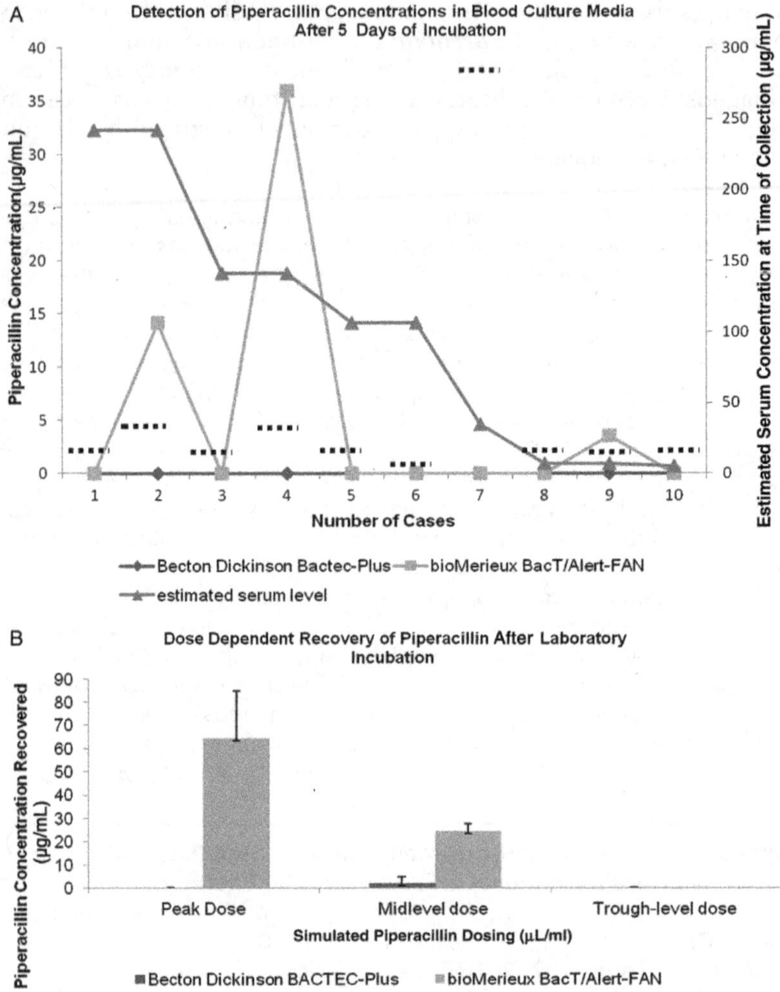

FIGURE 2.—*A*, Ten clinical samples containing aliquots of blood culture (BC) media with patients' blood were tested by high-performance liquid chromatography (HPLC). Microorganisms were preferentially recovered from BACTEC media for all cases except case 7. Triangles represent detection of piperacillin concentrations from BACTEC media (Becton Dickinson) after 5 days of incubation in the laboratory. Squares represent detection of piperacillin concentrations from BacT/Alert (bioMérieux) media after 5 days of incubation in the laboratory. Triangles represent estimated patient piperacillin concentrations present at the time of BC collection. Dashed lines represent the piperacillin minimum inhibitory concentration of the microorganism isolated in the case. Lower limit of piperacillin detection was 2.0 μg/mL. *Patient 4 received a 4.5-g dose of piperacillin and had received a total of 7 doses prior to BC collection. The time differential between piperacillin administration and collection of BC was on average 1 hour 40 minutes. *B*, Simulated peak, mid-, and trough-level doses of piperacillin were administered in vitro in triplicate into BACTEC and BacT/Alert aerobic BC bottles and incubated for 5 days in the laboratory prior to HPLC testing. Error bars indicate standard deviation between triplicate testing. Lower limit of piperacillin detection was 2.0 μg/mL. (Reprinted from Zadroga R, Williams DN, Gottschall R, et al. Comparison of 2 blood culture media shows significant differences in bacterial recovery for patients on antimicrobial therapy. *Clin Infect Dis.* 2013;56:790-797, by permission of the Infectious Diseases Society of America.)

524 (35%; $P < .001$) pathogens, 136 of 345 (39%) of the gram-positive cocci ($P < .001$), 48 of 175 (27%; $P = .02$) of the gram-negative rods, 101 of 195 (52%) of *Staphylococcus aureus* ($P < .001$), and 59 of 120 (49%; $P = .004$) septic events. If active antibiotics had been dosed 0–4 or 4–48 hours prior to culture collection, the odds of that culture growing in BACTEC were 4.8- and 5.2-fold greater, respectively, than of growing in BacT/Alert ($P < .0001$). Both were equivalent in the recovery of yeast and when no antimicrobials were dosed.

Conclusions.—BACTEC media has faster time to detection and increased bacterial recovery over the BacT/Alert media in the following categories: overall growth, pathogens, septic events, gram-positive cocci, gram-negative rods, *Staphylococcus aureus*, and cultures where antimicrobials were dosed up to 48 hours before culture collection (Fig 2).

▶ Bloodstream infections are a leading cause of morbidity and mortality in the United States and impact length of hospital stay and associated health care costs. Between 2000 and 2008, the number of hospital admissions for septicemia more than doubled. In 2011, the Agency for Healthcare Research and Quality identified hospital mortality rates for septicemia at levels 8 times higher than mortality derived from other hospital stays, and in 2009 septicemia was deemed the most expensive reason for hospitalization. In response to the increasing incidence and mortality from septicemia, numerous studies have attempted to qualify the laboratory's role in the diagnosis and identification of bloodstream pathogens and in guiding appropriate therapeutic interventions. Over the decades, significant advances have been made in laboratory blood culture systems, including the additions of enriched growth media, advances in automated agitation systems, and development of software that allows faster detection of bacterial growth via improved algorithms designed to track growth curves. Despite these technological advances, obtaining blood cultures (BCs) before initiating anti-infective therapy and ensuring appropriate fill volumes of 20 to 40 mL of blood per venipuncture within a single BC order remain key factors in the detection of adult bacteremia. Initiation of prompt and appropriate antimicrobial therapy in patients at risk for sepsis is a clinical goal. However, there has been concern that initiation of antimicrobial therapy before culture collection can delay pathogen recovery or, in some cases, artificially sterilize BCs. To address this, BC manufacturers have incorporated blood-broth ratios or proprietary antimicrobial removal systems into BC media to minimize the impact of antimicrobials present in the media. This study was a prospective, simultaneous, head-to-head comparison of aerobic BACTEC and BacT/Alert BC media in a clinical setting focusing on the impact of prior antimicrobial exposure on bacterial recovery, time to detection, and identification of septic events (Fig 2).

M. G. Bissell, MD, PhD, MPH

Real-time polymerase chain reaction testing for *Clostridium difficile* reduces isolation time and improves patient management in a small community hospital

Catanzaro M, Cirone J (Pocono Med Ctr, East Stroudsburg, PA)
Am J Infect Control 40:663-666, 2012

Background.—The impact of a switch from a toxin A/B enzyme immunoassay (EIA) to a polymerase chain reaction (PCR) method for detection of toxigenic *Clostridium difficile* was assessed for *C difficile* infection (CDI) rates, patient isolation-days, and CDI-related treatment.

Methods.—A 6-month retrospective study was done on symptomatic patients tested by the toxin A/B EIA and PCR assays. Data on the number of *C difficile* tests ordered, patient isolation-days, and treatment with metronidazole or vancomycin were collected. CDI rates were reported as cases per 10,000 patient-days, and differences between both groups were compared by χ^2 and Z-test analysis.

Results.—The CDI incidence was 11.2 and 12.7/10,000 patient-days in the EIA and PCR test periods, respectively ($P = .36$). Health care-associated CDI decreased from 4.4 per 10,000 patient-days during EIA testing to 0.9 per 10,000 patient-days during PCR testing ($P = .02$). A significant decrease in patient isolation-days ($P < .00001$), tests ordered ($P = .002$), and metronidazole treatment for patients with a negative C difficile test ($P = .02$) was observed with PCR testing.

Conclusion.—PCR testing is a viable option for small community hospitals, providing accurate and timely results for patient management and infection control. This can potentially lead to improved outcomes, increased patient satisfaction, and significant hospital cost savings.

▶ *Clostridium difficile* is an intestinal anaerobic bacterium found in 1% to 3% of healthy adults and is the leading cause of antibiotic-associated diarrhea in health care facilities. A recent survey of US hospitals by the Association for Professionals in Infection Control and Epidemiology estimated that the incidence of *C difficile* infections (CDI) is 13 per 1000 inpatients and that approximately 109 000 patients die annually from CDI, which is higher than previously estimated. In addition to increasing a patient's length of hospital stay, the cost of managing CDI is a nonreimbursable expense to many health care facilities. The recent guidelines by the Society for Healthcare Epidemiology of America and the Infectious Diseases Society of America address current practices for diagnosis and management of CDI patients, but many research gaps still exist. In the past 5 years, the authors' institution observed an increase in CDI cases among patients admitted to the facility, as well as during their hospitalization. In February 2008, environmental cleaning routines were changed, and isolation signs directing health care workers and visitors on hand hygiene were installed. When CDI rates spiked again in December 2008, despite educational and disinfection efforts, a new policy was initiated in which symptomatic patients were presumptively placed in isolation until toxigenic *C difficile* was ruled out by toxin A/B enzyme immunoassay (EIA), the test method used since 2002.

However, after several incidents of hospital-onset CDI in roommates of toxin A/B EIA-negative patients, the requirement for removing a patient from isolation was changed from 1 to 3 negative toxin A/B EIA stools. Although this appeared to control CDI transmission for some time, concerns were raised that patients remained in isolation longer than necessary, contributing to excess workload for care providers, increased costs for additional personal protective equipment, and repeat patient testing. Furthermore, this approach did not necessarily change the physicians' practice of treating symptomatic patients, regardless of the test results, and patient satisfaction was poor because of prolonged isolation. Polymerase chain reaction (PCR) assays have demonstrated higher sensitivity (93%-100%) than toxin A/B EIA (50%-73%) or cell culture cytotoxicity (58%-76%) methods for detection of toxigenic *C difficile* in symptomatic patients. The objective of this study was to assess the impact of switching from toxin A/B EIA to a rapid PCR-based method for toxigenic *C difficile* detection on overall CDI rates; health care-onset, health care facility—associated CDI; antibiotic therapy; and isolation days associated with assessment and management of CDI.

M. G. Bissell, MD, PhD, MPH

16 Hematology and Immunology

The Differential Diagnosis and Bone Marrow Evaluation of New-Onset Pancytopenia

Weinzierl EP, Arber DA (Stanford Univ, CA)

Am J Clin Pathol 139:9-29, 2013

New-onset pancytopenia can be caused by a wide variety of etiologies, leading to a diagnostic dilemma. These etiologies range from congenital bone marrow failure to marrow space-occupying lesions, infection, and peripheral destruction, to name a few. Bone marrow examination, in addition to a detailed clinical history, is often required for an accurate diagnosis. The purpose of this review is to provide a brief overview of many of the causes of new-onset pancytopenia in adults and children, with emphasis on bone marrow findings and recommendations of additional testing and clinical evaluation when needed, with the overall aim of aiding the pathologist's role as a consultant to the patient's treating physician.

▶ Pancytopenia is a common indication for bone marrow examination and can have numerous causes. Cytotoxic therapies, including myeloablative radiation therapy and chemotherapy, are common, but predictable, causes of pancytopenia in patients being treated systemically for neoplasia. New-onset pancytopenia outside this setting, in both children and adults, can prove to be a diagnostic dilemma, and causes include congenital and acquired bone marrow failure syndromes, marrow space-occupying lesions, peripheral destruction of hematopoietic cells, autoimmune disorders, infection, and ineffective marrow production. Often, the workup of new-onset pancytopenia is extensive and should include a detailed clinical, medication, recreational drug, and environmental exposure history. Although bone marrow examination often reveals an underlying condition causing pancytopenia, it is not always conclusive. Understanding the various disorders that may cause pancytopenia can aid in the recommendation of additional testing and clinical evaluation when the marrow studies are not specific for a single etiology. Here, the authors provide a systematic overview of many of the causes of new-onset pancytopenia.

M. G. Bissell, MD, PhD, MPH

Comparison of Automated Differential Blood Cell Counts From Abbott Sapphire, Siemens Advia 120, Beckman Coulter DxH 800, and Sysmex XE-2100 in Normal and Pathologic Samples

Meintker L, Ringwald J, Rauh M, et al (Hämatologie & Internistische Onkologie, Erlangen, Germany; Universitätsklinikum, Erlangen, Germany)
Am J Clin Pathol 139:641-650, 2013

Reliable automated blood cell characterization and quantification remain challenging in pathologic samples, whereas slide reviews due to unnecessary flagging should be avoided. We compared 4 modern hematology analyzers—Abbott Sapphire, Siemens Advia 120, Sysmex XE-2100, and Beckman Coulter DxH 800—regarding complete blood cell count (CBC), leukocyte differential count, and flagging efficacy in a total of 202 samples from hematology patients and normal controls. Manual differential count was used as reference. The analyzers exhibited very good correlation for CBC parameters. Neutrophils and eosinophils also showed very good correlations, whereas lymphocytes and monocytes correlated fairly. The Advia 120 displayed notably lower measurements for both parameters, which is attributable to classification of some events as large unstained cells. Basophil counts were unreliable with all analyzers. Flagging for blasts and immature granulocytes showed moderate sensitivity and specificity. Operators must not rely on blast flagging alone to detect leukemic samples with any analyzer.

▶ Modern hematology analyzers combine multiple techniques, such as absorption spectrometry, impedance, conductivity measurement, and flow cytometry, for cell counting and differentiation. Together with improved analytical algorithms and pattern recognition, automated cell differentiation is a rapid and cost-efficient method for complete blood cell count (CBC) and leukocyte differential count (LDC). Previous reports indicate that CBC and LDC among analyzers generally have good but not perfect agreement. Nonetheless, in various situations, accurate automated measurement is difficult or not possible (eg, immature cells, platelet clumps), and microscopy is triggered by the respective flags in the laboratory results. Therefore, the objective of modem hematology laboratories is to optimize the number of samples for which further, putative expensive action (eg, microscopic smear review) is needed while minimizing the number of false-negative results. The authors compared 4 modern analyzers, all top of the range from the respective manufacturers, regarding accordance of CBC and LDC among analyzers compared with microscopic smear review and flagging efficiency in normal and pathologic samples.

M. G. Bissell, MD, PhD, MPH

Comparison of a powered bone marrow biopsy device with a manual system: results of a prospective randomised controlled trial

Bucher CM, Lehmann T, Tichelli A, et al (Univ Hosp Basel, Switzerland)

J Clin Pathol 66:24-28, 2013

The diagnostic and clinical usefulness of a powered bone marrow biopsy device (OnControl()) versus a standard manual device (TRAP Hospital System) was studied. Primary endpoints were biopsy quality and patient pain during the procedure. Fifty patients underwent a total of 60 procedures by three expert operators in a randomised stratified fashion. Baseline demographic and clinical parameters were similar in both groups. The usage of conscious sedation, dosage of lidocaine/pethidin was similar between groups. Biopsy quality was rated 'sufficient for diagnosis' in 24/30 in the control group and 25/30 in the powered group ($p = 0.74$). Biopsy cylinder length, procedure time (from skin contact of the biopsy needle to placement of the biopsy cylinder in the formalin container) and patient reported pain during the procedure (T1), 15 min after the procedure (T2) and 3–5 days after the procedure (T3) there were comparable between groups. In the small subgroup of patients that did not receive conscious sedation (n = 15; manual 6, powered 9) significantly lower median pain scores were observed with the powered system (median pain score 3 vs 7; $p = 0.015$). Patients were satisfied with either device whether sedation was used (sedation: median 9 for both groups, range 3–10 (manual) and 0–10 (powered)) no sedation (median 8 (manual) vs 9 (powered)). In summary bone marrow biopsies taken with the manual or powered device produce similar technical and clinical results. If no conscious sedation is used, pain during the procedure appears to be lower with the powered system. The use of a powered system seems to be justified in selected patients.

▶ Recent studies have indicated that a powered bone marrow biopsy device (On Control, Vidacare) is superior to manual devices to obtain marrow aspirates and bone marrow biopsies. An uncontrolled, 3-center study using a first-generation device reported fast insertion into the bone marrow cavity and short aspiration times paired with low insertional and aspirational pain scores in 55 patients. Follow up-studies using a second-generation device allow for the extraction of a biopsy core cylinder after aspiration. A randomized study found that the new device produces significantly larger biopsies, shortens procedure time, and reduces intermediate-term pain. Two reports found significantly less insertional pain, significantly shortened procedure time, longer marrow biopsies, and better operator satisfaction. However, crush artifacts were more abundant with the powered system. Data from the authors' department, a large retrospective study, and repeated surveys have indicated that the manual procedure is very safe and that the diagnostic yield is generally high. However, in a fraction of patients, diagnostic yield is insufficient and could potentially be improved by larger biopsy specimens. The impact of the larger cylinders obtained with the powered device on their diagnostic value has not been addressed. The primary goal of this study was to determine the clinical relevance of differences in quality of cylinders obtained either with a standard manual device or a powered device. Further, the authors wanted to address the hypothesis that the powered system is less painful during and after the intervention, potentially leading to improved patient satisfaction.

M. G. Bissell, MD, PhD, MPH

Design and Feasibility of a Novel, Rapid, and Simple Fluorescence 26-Plex RT-PCR Assay for Simultaneous Detection of 24 Fusion Transcripts in Adult Acute Myeloid Leukemia

Laforêt M-P, Turlure P, Lippert E, et al (Univ of Limoges, France; CHU Bordeaux, Pessac, France; et al)

J Mol Diagn 15:186-195, 2013

Identification of chromosomal abnormalities is mandatory for classification of acute myeloid leukemia (AML), and the abnormalities have to be determined quickly, to allow patient enrollment in multicenter protocols and/or for selecting therapeutic strategies. Rapid AML molecular diagnosis is often difficult to achieve, however, because it is based on numerous different RT-PCR protocols. We developed a new RT-PCR method, one that does not require a nested step, to simultaneously detect all AML fusion transcripts from six major recurrent translocations found in adults: t(15;17)(q22;q12), inv(16)(p13.1q22) [t(16;16)(p13.1;q22)], t(8;21)(q22;q22), t(6;9)(p23;q34), t(9;22)(q34;q11), and t(10;11)(p13;q14). Specific primers for RT-PCR detection of the 24 fusion transcripts, along with two transcripts for controls, were designed for this 26-plex RT-PCR. Each PCR product had a different size and was separated by capillary electrophoresis. We also designed a multiplex positive control with 24 chimeric RNAs, corresponding to all chimeric RNAs tested. Compared with classical molecular biology protocols and cytogenetic analyses used as reference standards, results of the 26-plex RT-PCR method were concordant in all 204 (100%) cases of adult AML tested. Results were obtained in less than 24 hours. Because of the multiplex positive control, interpretation of the peaks was very easy, without any ambiguity. The tumor cell detection threshold was 1.5%.

► Precise molecular diagnosis of adult acute myeloid leukemia (AML) can be a challenging task for laboratories, because a detailed molecular characterization very often has to be given in less than 8 days to allow patient stratification and enrollment in multicenter therapeutic protocols. Currently, many molecular laboratories combine conventional cytogenetics with fluorescence in situ hybridization (FISH), and single reverse transcriptase polymerase chain reaction (RT-PCR); however, FISH is expensive and time consuming, and RT-PCR involves numerous different protocols. At the scale of one hospital center, these resources may be required for very few patients per year. The consensus molecular biology method for such diagnosis is presented in a Concerted Action BIOMED-I report, which describes up to 12 different single RT-PCRs with their corresponding nested PCRs. Attempts have been made to simplify or to accelerate procedures for molecular diagnosis of adult AML. Some studies have been based on electronic hybridization and fluorescence detection or biochips. Several multiplex RT-PCR systems have been described for detection of some of these fusion transcripts, but often using analysis of the amplified fragments by agarose gel electrophoresis stained with ethidium bromide; however, these orientation multiplex RT-PCRs had to be followed by different nested PCRs, specific for the suspected fusion transcripts, and had to be confirmed by sequencing. To date, none of the published techniques detect the 6 key translocations together in a simple multiplex RT-PCR and using capillary electrophoresis. Here, the authors describe a rapid and reproducible method to simultaneously detect 24 fusion transcripts using a 26-plex RT-PCR method. Each PCR product had a different size, and all PCR products could be separated by capillary electrophoresis. They also developed a multiplex positive control that includes all tested fusion transcripts; it is produced by in vitro transcription, controls all steps in the procedure after RNA purification, and provides a marker for the position of each PCR product after capillary electrophoresis.

M. G. Bissell, MD, PhD, MPH

IL-1 Family Members IL-18 and IL-33 Upregulate the Inflammatory Potential of Differentiated Human Th1 and Th2 Cultures

Blom L, Poulsen LK (Copenhagen Univ Hosp at Gentofte, Hellerup, Denmark)

J Immunol 189:4331-4337, 2012

The IL-1 family members IL-1β, IL-18, and IL-33 are potent cytokines in relationship to amplifying the CD4⁺ T cell cytokine production. To evaluate their impact on in vitro-differentiated human Th1 and Th2 cultures, such cultures were established from naive T cells, purified from healthy blood donors, and reactivated in the presence of IL-1β, IL-18, or IL-33. Interestingly, we observe modifying responses in Th1 and Th2 cultures induced by IL-18 or IL-33 but not by IL-1β, both contributing to amplify production of IL-5, IL-13, and IFN-γ. IL-18 or IL-33 stimulation of Th1 cultures resulted in increased IFN-γ and IL-13 production concurrent with reduced IL-10 gene transcription and secretion even though Th1 cultures, in contrast to IL-18Rα, had low ST2L expression. Furthermore, adding IL-18 to Th1 cultures promoted *Tbet* mRNA expression and production. Th2 cultures stimulated with IL-18 or IL-33 had an increased IL-5 secretion. Interestingly, E4BP4 gene expression and the percentage of E4BP4⁺ cells of the recently shown IL-10 transcriptional regulator E4BP4 correlated with IL-10 gene expression and protein secretion in Th1 cultures. Taken together, we report that the IL-1 family "alarmins" IL-18 and IL-33 in addition to amplifying both Th1- and Th2-associated cytokines block production of the regulatory cytokine IL-10 in Th1 cultures.

▶ CD4⁺ T cells are important in orchestrating appropriate responses to eliminate pathogens. CD4⁺ T cells start to proliferate and produce a diverse combination of cytokines depending on the type of pathogen, antigen-presenting cell, and the microenvironment cytokine milieu. Failure to dampen protective CD4$^+$ T-cell response after pathogen clearance can result in severe tissue inflammation and release of highly inflammatory cytokines, such as interleukin (IL)-18 and IL-33. The IL-1 family members IL-18 and IL-33 are highly inflammatory cytokines constitutively expressed in mucosal or barrier cell types, acting as regulators of innate and acquired immune responses by amplifying both Th1 and Th2 responses with or without T-cell receptor activation. The capacity of IL-18 and IL-33 to amplify the effector Th1 and Th2 cytokine production of IL-5, IL-9, IL-13, IFN-γ, and tumor necrosis factor-α suggests that they are endogenous activators of inflammatory responses, with implications for both autoimmune and allergic disorders. Recently, authors have established an in vitro system to examine tissue factors to modulate the cytokine production by differentiated CD4$^+$ T-cell subsets. In the present study, the authors used this system to demonstrate that IL-1 family member IL-18 or IL-33 stimulation, in addition to increasing both Th1 and Th2 proinflammatory cytokine production, represses IL-10 gene transcription and secretion in differentiated Th1l cultures. IL-33 or IL-18 stimulations of Th2 cultures promote additional IL-5 secretion. Furthermore, they found that *E4BP4*-positive gene expression and the percentage of E4BP4-positive cells correlate with IL-18-mediated and IL-33-mediated down-regulation of IL-10 gene transcription and secretion in differentiated Th1 cultures.

M. G. Bissell, MD, PhD, MPH

Chronic Activation of the Kinase IKKβ Impairs T Cell Function and Survival

Krishna S, Xie D, Gorentla B, et al (Duke Univ Med Ctr, Durham, NC; et al)
J Immunol 189:1209-1219, 2012

Activation of the transcription factor NF-κB is critical for cytokine production and T cell survival after TCR engagement. The effects of persistent NF-κB activity on T cell function and survival are poorly understood. In this study, using a murine model that expresses a constitutively active form of inhibitor of NF-κB kinase β (caIKKβ) in a T cell-specific manner, we demonstrate that chronic inhibitor of NF-κB kinase β signaling promotes T cell apoptosis, attenuates responsiveness to TCR-mediated stimulation in vitro, and impairs T cell responses to bacterial infection in vivo. caIKKβ T cells showed increased Fas ligand expression and caspase-8 activation, and blocking Fas/Fas ligand interactions enhanced cell survival. T cell unresponsiveness was associated with defects in TCR proximal signaling and elevated levels of B lymphocyte-induced maturation protein 1, a transcriptional repressor that promotes T cell exhaustion. caIKKβ T cells also showed a defect in IL-2 production, and addition of exogenous IL-2 enhanced their survival and proliferation. Conditional deletion of B lymphocyte-induced maturation protein 1 partially rescued the sensitivity of caIKKβ T cells to TCR triggering. Furthermore, adoptively transferred caIKKβ T cells showed diminished expansion and increased contraction in response to infection with *Listeria monocytogenes* expressing a cognate Ag. Despite their functional defects, caIKKβ T cells readily produced proinflammatory cytokines, and mice developed autoimmunity. In contrast to NF-κB's critical role in T cell activation and survival, our study demonstrates that persistent IKK-NF-κB signaling is sufficient to impair both T cell function and survival.

▶ Nuclear factor-kappa-B (NF-κB) is a ubiquitously expressed transcription factor that plays an important role in the survival and function of various immune cells. Emerging evidence suggests that chronic viral pathogens, such as human immunodeficiency virus-1 and human T-cell leukemia virus-1, often trigger NF-κB signaling in infected cells. An improved understanding of the effects of persistent NF-κB signaling on peripheral T-cell function may, therefore, reveal mechanisms that can be targeted to promote desirable outcomes during chronic disease. To study the functional and mechanistic consequences of T-cell specific inhibitor of NF-κB (IKK)—NF-κB hyperactivation, the authors expressed a conditional constitutively active allele of the inhibitor of NF-κB kinase β (caIKKβ) in the presence of Cre recombinase driven by the CD4 promoter (IKK mice). They report that uncontrolled IKKβ activation promotes T-cell apoptosis and attenuates responsiveness to T-cell receptor stimulation, in part, by increasing the expression of Fas ligand and B-lymphocyte—induced maturation protein 1, respectively. Diminished interleukin-2 production also contributed to defects in survival and proliferation. In vivo, IKK T cells mounted a compromised Ag-specific T-cell response to bacterial infection. Interestingly, only certain T-cell functions were selectively impaired by chronic IKKβ signaling: IKK T cells readily produced proinflammatory cytokines, and mice developed multiorgan inflammation. Their findings suggest that persistent IKKβ activity in T cells adversely affects function and survival, compromises Ag-specific responses, and promotes autoimmunity.

M. G. Bissell, MD, PhD, MPH

Pro-Apoptotic Protein Noxa Regulates Memory T Cell Population Size and Protects against Lethal Immunopathology

Wensveen FM, Klarenbeek PL, van Gisbergen KPJM, et al (Univ of Amsterdam, The Netherlands; et al)

J Immunol 190:1180-1191, 2013

Memory T cells form a highly specific defense layer against reinfection with previously encountered pathogens. In addition, memory T cells provide protection against pathogens that are similar, but not identical to the original infectious agent. This is because each T cell response harbors multiple clones with slightly different affinities, thereby creating T cell memory with a certain degree of diversity. Currently, the mechanisms that control size, diversity, and cross-reactivity of the memory T cell pool are incompletely defined. Previously, we established a role for apoptosis, mediated by the BH3-only protein Noxa, in controlling diversity of the effector

T cell population. This function might positively or negatively impact T cell memory in terms of function, pool size, and cross-reactivity during recall responses. Therefore, we investigated the role of Noxa in T cell memory during acute and chronic infections. Upon influenza infection, Noxa$^{-/-}$ mice generate a memory compartment of increased size and clonal diversity. Reinfection resulted in an increased recall response, whereas cross-reactive responses were impaired. Chronic infection of Noxa$^{-/-}$ mice with mouse CMV resulted in enhanced memory cell inflation, but no obvious pathology. In contrast, in a model of continuous, high-level T cell activation, reduced apoptosis of activated T cells rapidly led to severe organ pathology and premature death in Noxa-deficient mice. These results establish Noxa as an important regulator of the number of memory cells formed during infection. Chronic immune activation in the absence of Noxa leads to excessive accumulation of primed cells, which may result in severe pathology.

▶ A prominent candidate that potentially regulates immunologic memory cell formation is the proapoptotic protein Noxa (encoded by *Pmaip1*). During priming in the lymph node, T-cell activation, survival, and effector pool size are strictly limited by the availability of antigen (Ag), costimulatory molecules, nutrients, and cytokines. Even in the presence of all these factors, outgrowth of some activated T cells is favored over others, based on T-cell receptor (TCR) affinity. Previously, it has been shown that expansion and persistence of low-affinity effector cells is inhibited via competition-based apoptosis that mediates clonal dominance of high-affinity clones via the termination of low-affinity T cells. TCR affinity influences stability of the prosurvival molecule Mcl-1 via an interleukin-2R—mediated signaling loop. T cells lacking Noxa, the antagonist of Mcl-2, have a competitive advantage during priming, resulting in the survival and recruitment of increased numbers of low-affinity clones into the effector cell pool. This results in decreased numbers of high-affinity cells and reduced Ag responsiveness of the effector T-cell pool as a whole. Currently, it is unknown whether Noxa mediates similar effects during the formation of memory T cells.

In this study, the authors investigated how the absence of Noxa affects the formation, maintenance, and recall capabilities of memory T cells. The authors found that Noxa ablation results in enhanced diversity of the memory cell compartment and increased absolute memory cell numbers upon influenza infection. As a result of increased memory cell numbers, Noxa$^{-/-}$ mice form enlarged recall responses and have increased memory inflation during chronic mouse cytomegalovirus infection. In a transgenic model of persistent T-cell activation, effector T-cell accumulation ultimately led to severe organ pathology and premature death in mice deficient for Noxa. Their data show that control of memory precursor cell numbers via Noxa-mediated apoptosis is essential to prevent excessive immune responses upon reinfection.

M. G. Bissell, MD, PhD, MPH

Fine-Tuning of Regulatory T Cell Function: The Role of Calcium Signals and Naive Regulatory T Cells for Regulatory T Cell Deficiency in Multiple Sclerosis

Schwarz A, Schumacher M, Pfaff D, et al (Univ Hosp Heidelberg, Germany; et al)

J Immunol 190:4965-4970, 2013

The suppressor function of regulatory T cells (Tregs) is impaired in multiple sclerosis (MS), but the mechanisms underlying this deficiency are not fully understood. As Tregs counteract the sustained elevation of intracellular calcium, which is indispensable for full activation of conventional T cells (Tcons), we hypothesized that interference with this pathway might prompt MS-related Treg dysfunction. Using single-cell live imaging, we observed that Tregs rapidly reduce Ca^{2+} influx and downstream signals in Tcons upon cell contact, yet differ in their potency to efficiently suppress several target cells at the same time. Strikingly, individual Tregs harboring a $CD4^+$ $CD25^+$ $FOXP3^+$ $CD45RA^+$ naive phenotype suppressed significantly more adjacent Tcons than did $CD4^+$ $CD25^+$ $FOXP3^+$ $CD45RA^-$ memory Tregs. Some constituents even completely failed to dampen Tcon Ca^{2+} influx and were contained exclusively in the memory subset. In accordance with their more powerful suppressive performance, the Ca^{2+} signature was considerably enhanced in naive Tregs in response to TCR triggering, compared with the memory counterparts. MS Tregs displayed a significantly diminished suppression of mean Ca^{2+} influx in the sum of individual Tcons recorded. This reduced inhibitory activity was closely linked to decreased numbers of individual Tcons becoming suppressed by adjacent Tregs and, in turn, correlated with a marked reduction of naive subtypes and concomitant expansion of nonsuppressive memory phenotypes. We conclude that the superior achievement of naive Tregs is pivotal in maintaining Treg efficiency. As a consequence, MS Tregs become defective because they lack naive subtypes and are disproportionately enriched in memory cells that have lost their inherent downregulatory activity.

▶ $CD4^+$ $CD25^+$ $FOXP3^+$ regulatory T cells (Tregs) are key players in maintaining immunologic self-tolerance, and a functional Treg deficiency is associated with various autoimmune diseases, including multiple sclerosis (MS). The ability of Tregs derived from patients with MS to downregulate both proliferation and cytokine secretion of activated conventional T cells (Tcons) in vitro is impaired, and this dysfunctional state is linked to a possibly thymic-dependent imbalance between naive and more short-lived memory cells that make up the peripheral Treg population. In addition, other abnormalities in Tregs that constitute functionally heterogeneous subsets are likely to contribute to the Treg defect in MS. Thus, recent findings show that less-suppressive Tregs capable of producing interferon gamma (IFN-γ) are significantly increased in the peripheral blood of patients with MS and that certain subtypes of patient-derived memory Tregs exhibit a downscaled suppressive performance in response to distinct T cell—activating stimuli. Notably, the defective Treg state is ameliorated under disease-modifying treatment, indicating that pharmacologic modulation of Tregs might prove to be a promising strategy for restoring immunologic homeostasis in MS. In this article, the authors hypothesized that a difference in the ability to downregulate $Ca2^+$ influx in effector T cells might affect the suppressive performance of total Tregs and might be involved in the Treg defect that can be detected in patients with MS. They established an in-house, single-cell live imaging assay by which they could directly monitor $Ca2^+$ signatures in a multitude of individual cells exhibiting either a $CD4^+$ $CD25^+$ $FOXP3^+$ Treg or a $CD4^+$ $CD25^-$ FOXP3 Tcon phenotype and closely monitor the contact-dependent impact of a single Treg on $Ca2^+$ signaling in one or more adjacent Tcons. Because they have shown previously that homeostatic changes in the Treg compartment affect total Treg function, Tregs were further separated according to surface expression of CD45RA in naive and memory Treg subtypes. The authors used this experimental approach to screen for differences in the mode of suppression between cells isolated from peripheral blood of healthy donors vs those obtained from MS patients. The recorded $Ca2^+$ signaling components were correlated with the subordinate nuclear translocation of NFAT that propagates the $Ca2^+$ signal to the nucleus to initiate gene transcription, as, for example, for IFN-γ or interleukin-2. These readouts were complemented by assessing proliferative responses and cytokine release of TCR-triggered Tcons.

M. G. Bissell, MD, PhD, MPH

Complement in Immune and Inflammatory Disorders: Therapeutic Interventions

Ricklin D, Lambris JD (Univ of Pennsylvania, Philadelphia)

J Immunol 190:3839-3847, 2013

With the awareness that immune-inflammatory cross-talk is at the heart of many disorders, the desire for novel immunomodulatory strategies in the therapy of such diseases has grown dramatically. As a prime initiator and important modulator of immunological and inflammatory processes, the complement system has emerged as an attractive target for early and upstream intervention in inflammatory diseases and has moved into the spotlight of drug discovery. Although prevalent conditions such as age-related macular degeneration have attracted the most attention, the diverse array of complement-mediated pathologies, with distinct underlying mechanisms, demands a multifaceted arsenal of therapeutic strategies. Fortunately, efforts in recent years have not only introduced the first complement inhibitors to the clinic but also filled the pipelines with promising candidates. With a focus on immunomodulatory strategies, in this review we discuss complement-directed therapeutic concepts and highlight promising candidate molecules (Fig 1).

▶ Many concepts of modern drug discovery have deep roots in immunology research, with Paul Ehrlich's notions of the "magic bullet" and his "side-chain theory" being among the most prominent examples. The connection between these 2 disciplines has even intensified in recent years in view of biological

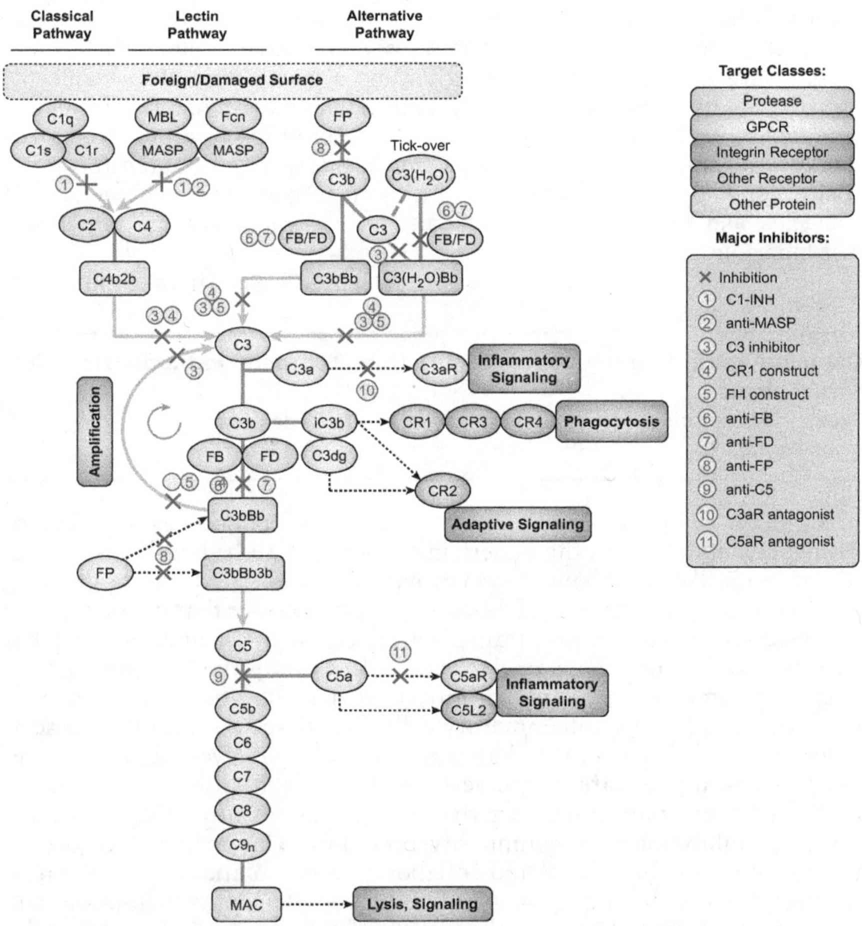

FIGURE 1.—Simplified scheme of the complement cascade with currently exploited targets of complement-directed therapeutic intervention. Only the AP C5 convertase (C3bBb3b) is shown for reasons of simplicity; however C5 convertases (C4b2b3b) can also be formed with contribution from the CP/LP. The enzymatic fragment of C2 is referred to as C2b (or 2b as part of the CP/LP convertases); the same fragment is designated as C2a in some publications. AP, Alternative pathway; C3(H2O), hydrolyzed C3; C1-INH, C1 inhibitor; C5L2, C5a receptor-like 2; CP, classical pathway; CR, complement receptor; FB, factor B; Fcn, ficolins; FD, factor D; FH, factor H; FP, factor P (properdin); GPCR, G protein–coupled receptor; LP, lectin pathway; MAC, membrane attack complex; MASP, mannose-binding lectin–associated protease; MBL, mannose-binding lectin. (Reprinted from Ricklin D, Lambris JD. Complement in immune and inflammatory disorders: therapeutic interventions. *J Immunol.* 2013;190:3839-3847, © 2013, The American Association of Immunologists, Inc.)

drugs such as monoclonal antibodies. Therapeutic immune modulation is increasingly recognized as a promising strategy for tackling inflammatory diseases; yet, it is in need of more selective modulators that help restore the immune balance and resolve inflammation. Fueled by the discovery of new functional roles, immune cross-talk mechanisms, and a growing number of disease associations, complement has emerged as focal point of interest in immunomodulatory and anti-inflammatory strategies. The variety of intervention points and high number of extracellular targets within the complement cascade (Fig 1), the availability of potent natural inhibitor templates, and a spike in structure/function insight have all contributed to rapid advances in the field of complement-related drug discovery. Although only 2 drugs with connection to complement are currently available in the clinic, ongoing research efforts have produced a plethora of innovative and diverse drug candidates that show great promise in many clinical conditions. In this review, we provide an overview of current therapeutic strategies and highlight drug candidates that are in preclinical or clinical development.

M. G. Bissell, MD, PhD, MPH

Complement in Immune and Inflammatory Disorders: Pathophysiological Mechanisms

Ricklin D, Lambris JD (Univ of Pennsylvania, Philadelphia)
J Immunol 190:3831-3838, 2013

Although acute or chronic inflammation is a common component of many clinical disorders, the underlying processes can be highly distinct. In recent years, the complement system has been associated with a growing number of immunological and inflammatory conditions that include degenerative diseases, cancer, and transplant rejection. It becomes evident that excessive activation or insufficient control of complement activation on host cells can cause an immune imbalance that may fuel a vicious cycle between complement, inflammatory cells, and tissue damage that exacerbates clinical complications. Although the exact involvement of complement needs to be carefully investigated for each disease, therapeutic modulation of complement activity emerges as an attractive target for upstream inhibition of inflammatory processes. This review provides an update about the functional and collaborative capabilities of complement, highlights major disease areas with known complement contribution, and indicates the potential for complement as a focal point in immunomodulatory strategies for treating inflammatory diseases (Fig 1).

▶ Inflammation is a recognized hallmark of disease, yet the knowledge about underlying mechanisms that shape the inflammatory response and its resolution has been largely extended in recent years. Given the classic perception of complement as a defense system against microbial intruders, it may appear surprising that this ancient pillar of innate immunity was identified as a contributor in various inflammatory pathologies. Yet it has become evident that complement not only acts as a sensor of pathogens but also recognizes diseased and damaged host cells, and it closely collaborates with other immune and defense systems to eliminate potential danger. This interplay serves as a vital triage system that tailors the immune response according to the threat level. However, insufficient, excessive, or poorly controlled complement activation can tip the balance between health and disease and lead to self-attack of host cells. In the worst case, a vicious

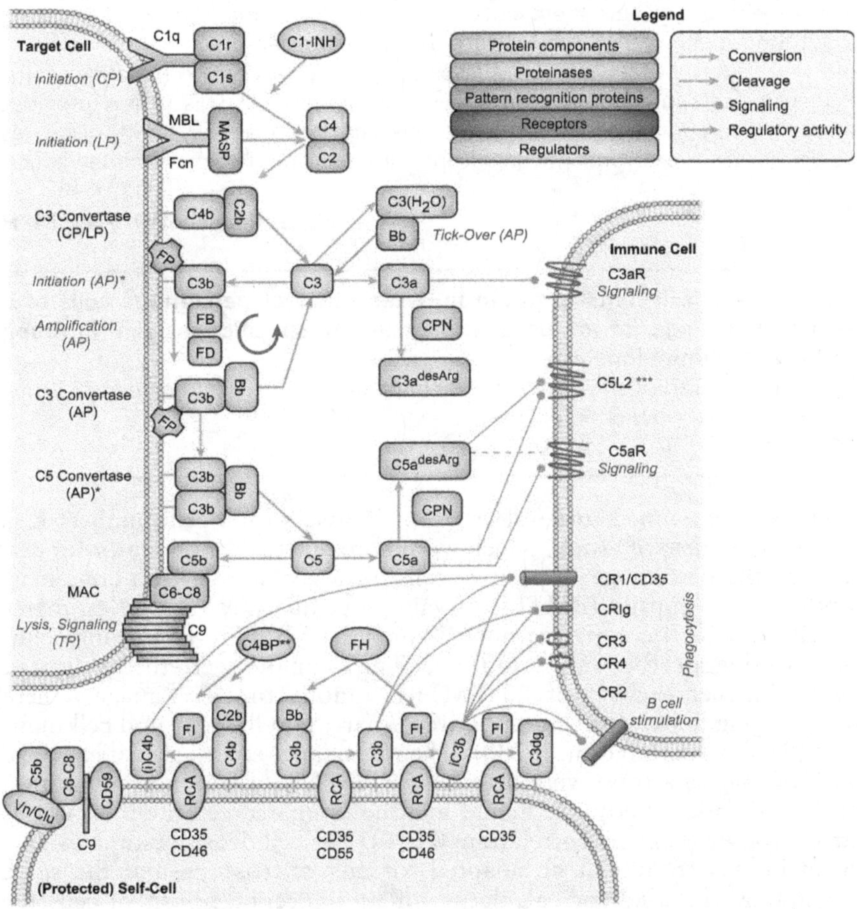

FIGURE 1.—Simplified scheme of the complement activation network. *Only part of the functional spectrum of factor P (FP) is visualized: FP may act as pattern-recognition molecule and recruit C3b from plasma to the target surface (alternative pathway [AP] initiation); additionally, it stabilizes both the AP C3 and C5 convertases. Only the AP C5 convertase (C3bBb3b) is shown; a CP/LP C5 convertase (C4b2b3b) is also formed. The enzymatic fragment of C2 is referred to as C2b in this review; the same fragment is sometimes designated as C2a in literature. **The regulation of the CP/LP C3 convertase is depicted a one-step process but follows a two-step mechanism similar to C3b, including decay acceleration (C4BP, CD35) and factor I (FI)—mediated degradation to iC4b (C4BP, CD35, CD46). ***The function of C5a receptor-like 2 (C5L2) is not fully described and may be content-specific; C5a and C5a-desArg bind equally well to C5L2, whereas their binding and signaling profiles on C5aR are distinct. The binding of C3adesArg to C5L2 remains controversial. C1-INH, C1 inhibitor; Clu, clusterin; CPN, carboxypeptidase-N; CR, complement receptor; FB, factor B; Fcn, ficolins; FD, factor D; FH, factor H; MAC, membrane attack complex; RCA, regulator of complement activation; Vn, vitronectin. (Reprinted from Ricklin D, Lambris JD. Complement in immune and inflammatory disorders: pathophysiological mechanisms. *J Immunol.* 2013;190:3831-3838, © 2013, The American Association of Immunologists, Inc.)

cycle between tissue damage, complement activation, and immune attack perpetually recreates inflammatory stimulators rather than resolving them. In view of this upstream position in inflammatory homeostasis, there is growing interest in understanding the role of complement in pathologic processes and in exploiting complement targets for therapeutic modulation. Fortunately, our knowledge about the functions of complement in health and disease has much improved, and new discoveries have found a fascinating cross-talk network that ties complement closely into the immune-inflammatory network. This review provides an update on complement and its dialogue with associated systems, discusses major disease areas, and indicates opportunities for therapeutic intervention (Fig 1).

M. G. Bissell, MD, PhD, MPH

Estimation of cell density to aid in assessment of percentage cells of a particular lineage or of cells expressing a specific antigen in bone marrow trephine biopsies

Al-Shieban S, Tadrous PJ, Naresh KN (Imperial College Healthcare NHS Trust, London, UK; Northwick Park Hosp, London, UK)
J Clin Pathol 66:155-159, 2013

The authors aimed to develop a tool to assess total cell numbers in a microscope's field of vision, which would provide the denominator for calculating the percentage of positive cells for a given antigen in bone marrow trephine biopsies (BMTBs) of varying cellularities. Precise estimates of cell densities were made from 179 images of BMTBs of varying cellularities using a cell-counting software. The estimates were then validated on an independent set of 20 BMTBs. Among the 179 images, there was a strong linear association between marrow cellularity and cell numbers (Pearson correlation: 0.788). Then standardised cell densities (cells/mm^2 of bone marrow) were deduced for BMTBs of varying cellularities. In the validation study, the actual and the estimated cell numbers correlated strongly (Pearson correlation: 0.990). The cell density estimates provided in this study can be adapted for any microscope and the same method can be used for calculation of the percentage-positive cells for any antigen (Table 1).

▶ The percentages of cells expressing an antigen (by immunohistochemistry) in bone marrow trephine biopsies (BMTBs) are an estimate and not an actual count. Although the precise counting of cells expressing a particular antigen (on immunostained slides) is relatively easy, counting all cells in the microscope's field of vision is difficult, and the lack of a denominator for the cells counted positive for an antigen hampers the documentation of a precise percentage. The number of cells in a microscope's field of vision with respect to BMTBs is highly variable and is dependent on the bone marrow cellularity. Other than cellularity, factors such as cell size, edema, and fibrosis can also influence the number of cells per field of vision. The authors have developed a tool that will aid in expressing the cells positive for a particular antigen as a percentage of all bone marrow cells. To achieve this, they have produced a quick reference table (Table 1) documenting the predicted cell densities of all bone marrow cells (in samples with

TABLE 1.—Cell Density in Bone Marrow Trephine Specimens of Differing Cellularities

Percentage Bone Marrow Cellularity	Number of Patients (n = 102)	Number of Images (n = 179)	Cell Count Within the Image (area = 0.03521 mm^2)	Cell Density Expressed as Cells per 1 mm^2 Bone Marrow	Estimated Cell Count in One 40× Objective Field (area = 0.336 mm^2)	Estimated Cell Count in One 60× Objective Field (area = 0.1465 mm^2)
15	2	5	7	199	67	29
20	2	7	38	1079	363	158
25	3	4	77	2187	735	320
30	4	4	113	3209	1078	470
35	5	5	152	4317	1451	632
40	10	10	188	5339	1794	782
45	6	18	225	6390	2147	936
50	14	22	263	7469	2510	1094
55	2	2	299	8492	2853	1244
60	8	12	335	9514	3197	1394
65	4	8	370	10 508	3531	1539
70	7	7	411	11 673	3922	1710
75	2	6	447	12 695	4266	1860
80	7	11	483	13 718	4609	2010
85	4	4	520	14 769	4962	2164
90	7	12	558	15 848	5325	2322
95	7	14	590	16 757	5630	2455
100	8	28	633	17 978	6041	2634

varying cellularities) and a table estimating cells with a 40× or a 60× field of vision that can be drafted for any microscope. These numbers can be used as the denominators for reporting percentages of cells expressing a particular antigen in BMTBs.

M. G. Bissell, MD, PhD, MPH

17 Transfusion Medicine and Coagulation

Analysis of prolonged storage on coagulation Factor (F)V, FVII, and FVIII in thawed plasma: is it time to extend the expiration date beyond 5 days?

Tholpady A, Monson J, Radovancevic R, et al (Univ of Texas Med School at Houston)

Transfusion 53:645-650, 2013

Background.—According to AABB standards, fresh-frozen plasma (FFP) should be thawed at 30 to 37°C and expire after 24 hours. An increase in the aggressive management of trauma patients with thawed plasma has heightened the risk of plasma waste. One way to reduce plasma waste is to extend its shelf life, given that the full range of therapeutic efficacy is maintained. We evaluated the effect of prolonged storage at 1 to 6°C on the activity of Factor (F)V, FVII, and FVIII in plasma thawed at 37 or 45°C.

Study Design and Methods.—Group O plasma from healthy donors (n=20) was divided into 10 pairs and frozen and stored at not more than −18°C. One sample from each pair was thawed at 37 or 45°C, and all were stored at 1 to 6°C. Samples were analyzed for FV, FVII, and FVIII activity on Days 0, 5, 10, 15, and 20.

Results.—Plasma thawing time was 17% less at 45°C than at 37°C. No differences were observed between thawing groups in coagulation activity of FV, FVII, and FVIII during the 20-day storage period ($p>0.12$). In both groups, the activity of FV and FVIII decreased over time but remained within a normal range at 10 days.

Conclusion.—Although levels of plasma clotting factors are reduced in storage, therapeutic levels of FV and FVIII are maintained in thawed plasma stored for up to 10 days at 1 to 6°C. Thawing of FFP at 45°C decreases thawing time but does not affect the activity of FV, FVII, and FVIII.

▶ Fresh-frozen plasma (FFP) has a 24-hour shelf life after thawing and requires careful attention to avoid waste and control clinical laboratory budgets. There is also a thawing delay of 30 to 35 minutes; thus, many facilities maintain a liquid inventory of plasma to meet urgent needs of trauma patients and massive bleeding situations. Although plasma inventories currently meet clinical need, the use of male-only plasma donors will decrease the amount of available plasma. This decrease in plasma inventory and the limited AB plasma are why it is advantageous to explore options on how to reduce plasma waste. Many laboratories, like the University of Texas, use thawed plasma that is stored at 1° to 6° for 5 days because studies have found that adequate clotting factor activity was retained. This policy has reduced the amount of waste, but they still waste over 500 units amounting to an annual loss of close to $35 000. Several studies have published data showing that beyond the 5-day expiration date, the clotting factors remain adequate. The authors in this study examined the clotting factor activity in plasma that was thawed and stored for up to 20 days. They also analyzed whether they could cut the thawing time of each unit by thawing the plasma at a temperature of 45°C. Pooled pairs of plasma for each sample were used to decrease the effect of one donor having exceptional or abnormal values, and only group O donors were used to minimize blood group–related variance. Their study found that there was an acute decline in factor activity through day 5 that plateaued through day 20. The residual clotting factor activity for FV and FVIII were within the laboratory's normal range through day 10. This indicates that extending the shelf life of thawed plasma to 10 days may reduce plasma waste and allow for more flexibility in inventory management. The thawing time was only decreased by 5 minutes but showed no difference in residual clotting factor activity between the groups. This did not seem like a large enough change in order to change practices if laboratories maintain a liquid inventory for urgent uses. Several publications in recent years have also demonstrated stable levels of coagulation factors past 5-day storage period. Limiting the storage time to 5 days may be overly conservative, and additional studies may give more support to change current standards if plasma inventory becomes insufficient for clinical demand. One specific variable that should be investigated is the risk of bacterial contamination with extending the length of storage time. Additionally, the concern that transfusing older blood products negatively affects patient outcome would need to be addressed.

H. Signorelli, DO

Human T-lymphotropic virus laboratory testing of maternal blood at time of cord blood donations and clinical implications

Glasser L, Cyrus S, Machan JT, et al (CBR Systems, Inc., Tucson, AZ; Creative Testing Solutions, Phoenix, AZ; Rhode Island Hosp and Lifespan, Providence)
Transfusion 53:1302-1308, 2013

Background.—In the United States, blood products are tested for infectious diseases including human T-lymphotropic virus (HTLV)-I/II. Positive results of maternal blood samples at the time of cord blood (CB) donation must be reported to mother and physician. Tests for HTLV have a high false-positive rate. This is problematic because there is no prenatal testing of the mother.

Study Design and Methods.—This study involves 119,769 maternal blood samples at time of CB donation and evaluates positive results for HTLV in screening tests, supplemental immunoassays, and nucleic acid tests (NATs). Infectious disease markers (IDMs) and maternal health histories of HTLV-positive and -negative mothers were compared.

Results.—Of 119,769 mothers donating CB, 545 tested positive with the screening test, 33 were positive with the supplemental tests, and two were positive with NAT. When indeterminate results were excluded from the supplemental test only six were positive. Eight of 34 mothers with positive or indeterminate supplemental test results had received intravenous immunoglobulin. There were no significant differences between HTLV-positive and -negative mothers with regard to the incidence of other IDMs.

Conclusions.—Testing maternal blood for HTLV is problematic for CB banks, obstetricians, and mothers because of the high false-positive rate. CB banks need rapid turnaround time and supplemental testing. If results on the latter are positive the obstetrician should be notified, educated, do follow-up testing, and counseling. Indeterminate results on supplemental tests are most likely false positives. We recommend that mothers with positive or indeterminate supplemental test results have follow-up NAT.

▶ Human T-cell lymphotropic virus (HTLV) was the first human retrovirus to be identified and was the first virus shown to be a cause of human malignancy. In 1989, the Centers for Disease Control and Prevention recommended the screening of all blood products for HTLV. Unlike screening routine blood donors, infectious disease testing for HTLV in mothers at the time of cord blood (CB) donation is unique because of implications with regard to breastfeeding. This study examines a large number of maternal blood samples collected at the time of CB donation. It evaluates HTLV positivity with the US Food and Drug Administration (FDA)-licensed chemiluminescent assay or enzyme immunoassay in maternal blood samples and compares methodologically different assays to determine the true prevalence of HTLV. It also assesses the relationship between mothers testing positive with the FDA-licensed screening test and other infectious disease markers, examines health history questionnaires, and discusses the clinical implications of a positive test result.

M. G. Bissell, MD, PhD, MPH

Laboratory evaluation of rapid test kits to detect hepatitis C antibody for use in predonation screening in emergency settings

O'Connell RJ, Gates RG, Bautista CT, et al (Walter Reed Army Inst of Res, Silver Spring, MD; US Military HIV Res Program, Fort Gordon, GA; US Army Blood Program, Falls Church, VA; et al)

Transfusion 53:505-517, 2013

Background.—Emergency whole blood transfusion is a lifesaving procedure employed on modern battlefields. Rapid device tests (RDTs) are frequently used to mitigate transfusion-transmitted infection risks.

Study Design and Methods.—A limited evaluation of the RDT formerly used on battlefields was performed using 50 donor plasma samples and commercially available panels. Five hepatitis C virus (HCV) RDTs with sufficient stated sensitivity and thermostability were assessed using 335 HCV-positive and 339 HCV-negative donor plasma samples, 54 seroconversion panel plasma samples, and 84 HCV-positive and 84 HCV-negative spiked whole blood under normal, hot, and cold storage conditions and normal and hot test conditions, plus an ease-of-use survey.

Results.—BioRapid HCV test sensitivity on donor plasma was 84% (95% confidence interval [CI], 70.9%-92.8%). Using all positive plasma samples, OraQuick HCV sensitivity exceeded all comparators (99.4%, 95% CI, 98.0%-99.9%, $p < 0.05$). Specificity was consistently high, led by OraQuick HCV at 99.7% (95% CI, 98.6%-100%), statistically superior only to Axiom HCV ($p < 0.05$). Using seroconversion panels, only OraQuick HCV showed equivalent or earlier HCV detection compared to the gold standard. Using spiked whole blood, specificity was consistently high, and sensitivity ranged significantly from 34.5% (95% CI, 25.0%-45.1%) for CORE HCV to 98.8% (95% CI, 94.3%-99.9%) for OraQuick HCV. All comparator RDTs were significantly less sensitive than OraQuick HCV at one or more stress condition.

Conclusion.—This HCV RDT comparison identified significant sensitivity differences, particularly using whole blood under extreme storage and testing conditions. These data support OraQuick HCV superiority and illustrate the value of RDT evaluation under simulated field conditions.

▶ Over the last 2 decades, increasing regulations have decreased the risk of viral transfusion-transmitted infections (TTIs) caused by hepatitis C virus (HCV), hepatitis B virus, and human immunodeficiency virus. However, in settings in which time or resources are limited, the risk of TTIs is often higher. An example is in military deployment operations in which blood products are needed for emergency release before donors and products can be comprehensively screened. More than 250 000 units of blood products were transfused between 2003 and 2010, of which 6.2% were freshly collected products that were incompletely screened for TTI pathogens. Previous studies have found that the donors used for these blood products have a lower HCV seroprevalence than the general population. However, cases of HCV transmission have occurred, and the potential risk of an unscreened unit being infected is significantly higher than reported residual rates after HCV product testing in the United States. Therefore, there is a need for effective TTI risk mitigation, especially considering the mortality and morbidity related to HCV infection. In addition to careful donor selection, rapid device tests (RDTs) can be used for predonation screening before transfusion of urgent freshly collected blood products. The authors of this study assessed available HCV RDTs for use in urgent settings with a focus on test performance and ease-of-use determinations using a variety of specimen matrixes and experimental storage and test conditions. Regarding sensitivity, OraQuick HCV was the best performer and showed similar performance to previously published studies. Axiom HCV card sensitivity was lower than that of OraQuick but was not statistically inferior to OraQuick HCV. Hot storage or testing temperatures decreased sensitivity in all RDT methods compared, whereas cold storage had a more modest effect. These findings are important, as in many of the settings in which RDT testing is most relevant, adherence to storage and testing recommendations can be difficult. However, test specificity was not significantly affected by any of the temperature conditions tested except in the performance of the CORE HCV when stored under hot conditions. This article presented a nice comparison among RDTs that can be used to screen for TTIs in urgent or emergent predonation settings. The sample size for this study was small, and spiked plasma samples were used in lieu of fresh whole blood. The characteristics of the population used for these specimens are different than those of the military walking blood bank donors, and the sensitivity rates may not directly translate between groups. The results of this study have helped redefine current US military policies on predonation testing. These findings can also be used to develop policies and procedures in other settings in which mandated and regulated donor screening is not possible.

H. Signorelli, DO

The role of failure modes and effects analysis in showing the benefits of automation in the blood bank

Han TH, Kim MJ, Kim S, et al (Inje Univ, Seoul, Korea; Yonsei Univ, Seoul, Korea; Ewha Womans Univ, Seoul, Korea; et al)

Transfusion 53:1077-1082, 2013

Background.—Failure modes and effects analysis (FMEA) is a risk management tool used by the manufacturing industry but now being applied in laboratories.

Study Design and Methods.—Teams from six South Korean blood banks used this tool to map their manual and automated blood grouping processes and determine the risk priority numbers (RPNs) as a total measure of error risk.

Results.—The RPNs determined by each of the teams consistently showed that the use of automation dramatically reduced the RPN compared to manual processes. In addition, FMEA showed where the major risks occur in each of the manual processes and where attention should be prioritized to improve the process. Despite no previous experience with FMEA, the teams found the technique relatively easy to use and the subjectivity associated with assigning risk numbers did not affect the validity of the data.

Conclusion.—FMEA should become a routine technique for improving processes in laboratories.

▶ The current approach to error by most laboratories is to investigate them when they occur and change processes accordingly, but the continuing emphasis on reducing errors is leading to the adoption from other industries of so-called risk management tools. Failure modes and effects analysis (FMEA) is already an important part of good manufacturing processes and is associated with the manufacture of medical devices, where it is used to proactively assess processes for their error potential and their severity. A recent International Organization for Standardization (ISO) document (ISO/TS 22367) describes the use of FMEA in laboratories to find and characterize medical laboratory errors. However, to do this on a proactive basis, as recommended in the ISO document, requires a much more systematic approach to laboratory operations than is currently practiced. Such a systems approach is advocated through the discipline of process excellence or lean thinking. The latter includes tools such as value stream mapping, which is widely used to identify waste in processes, particularly the waiting periods, but can also be used to carefully identify all the steps in a process as a prerequisite to FMEA. The FMEA process consists of identifying errors and using scales to determine the severity of the error, the probability of occurrence, and the likelihood of detection. From these assessments, a risk priority number (RPN) can be determined. Error-free processes will have low RPNs while complex, multiple-step processes will have high RPNs. Given the myriad processes in any one laboratory, the proactive approach to risk analysis will first need to determine which processes are most at risk and prioritize these for examination. Blood grouping and related procedures, such as irregular antibody screening, are laboratory procedures in which obtaining the correct result is of critical importance and, therefore, are obvious targets for the use of FMEA techniques. Having identified processes that have high risk of errors, one approach to reducing that risk is the use of automation. However, although automation has been readily taken up in the clinical chemistry and hematology laboratory, many blood banks, including those with high volumes of testing, continue to use manual testing for various reasons, including cost. FMEA is one way to show the relative risks associated with manual techniques compared with automated techniques.

M. G. Bissell, MD, PhD, MPH

Establishment of a medium-throughput approach for the genotyping of *RHD* variants and report of nine novel rare alleles

Fichou Y, Le Maréchal C, Jamet D, et al (Etablissement Français du Sang (EFS)—Bretagne, Brest, France; Institut National de la Santé et de la Recherche Médicale (INSERM), Brest, France; Université de Bretagne Occidentale, Brest, France; et al)
Transfusion 53:1821-1828, 2013

Background.—The routinely used serologic methods are robust in accurately typing standard D− or D+ blood. However, they result in discrepancy in weak or partial D blood, which requires genetic analysis. We have previously used denaturing high-performance liquid chromatography (DHPLC) to screen the entire *RHD*-coding sequence. However, DHPLC is technically challenging, labor-intensive, and time-consuming. To overcome these inconveniences, we sought to develop a new two-step approach.

Study Design and Methods.—A total of 430 blood samples with D phenotype ambiguity were recruited for this study. The three most frequent weak *D* alleles (i.e., weak *D*, Type 1; weak *D*, Type 2; and weak *D*, Type 3), which altogether account for 60% to 90% of the atypical *RHD* alleles in the Caucasian population, were first identified by Tm-shift genotyping. The remaining unidentified samples were then subjected to a single-tube multiplex polymerase chain reaction (PCR) amplification of all 10 *RHD* exons followed by direct sequencing.

Results.—Optimal conditions for efficient and reliable identification of the three most common weak *D* variants by Tm-shift genotyping were established. All 10 *RHD* exons were successfully amplified in a single-multiplex PCR procedure. Employment of the two-step analysis identified *RHD* variants in 91.6% of the 430 studied samples. Two of the nine previously undescribed variants, c.335G>T and c.939G>A, were found to cause aberrant mRNA splicing by means of a splicing minigene assay.

Conclusion.—The new two-step analysis proved to be much easier and cheaper than the DHPLC method and therefore is convenient to be used as a routine, medium-throughput approach for *RHD* genotyping.

▶ Accidental transfusion of D+ blood has serious consequences including fatal hemolytic transfusion reactions for alloimmunized D− recipients and hemolytic disease of the fetus and newborn in D− mothers carrying a D+ fetus. Standard serologic methods for typing D− or D+ blood are accurate except in cases of weak or partial D blood. There is a lot of interest in developing a large-scale genotyping method for these atypical D phenotypes. The authors of this study used a denaturing high-performance liquid chromatography (DHPLC)-based method to screen subjects with D phenotype ambiguity and identified novel potential weak or partial D alleles. However, this method is not practical for high-throughput clinical use. Therefore, the authors sought to develop a new 2-step approach. The first step was to identify the most frequent weak D alleles through genotyping. For those unidentified samples, a single-tube multiplex polymerase chain reaction (PCR) amplification for all 10 *RHD* exons followed by direct sequencing would be used. This approach was compared with their previously adopted DHPLC-based strategy and showed many advantages logistically within the method's procedure. The first step identified the molecular basis of the D phenotype in more than 50% of the studied samples. The remaining samples were moved to a technically challenging second-step analysis where all 10 exons of the *RHD* gene were amplified successfully in a multiplex PCR procedure. Only approximately 8% of samples remained unidentified for the D phenotype, which is similar to other previously, published reports. This may be caused by a common founder variation located in the deep intronic regions or remote regulatory control regions of the *RHD* gene. Other methods like the SNaPshot method have been developed to identify 14 known *RHD* variants and have also been useful for these atypical D phenotypes. The authors also identified 9 novel rare RHD variants. Their 2-step approach could be used in a medium-throughput setting for rapid *RHD* genotyping to supplement serologic methods and was shown to be superior to the DHPLC method. Comparison of this 2-step method to the SNaPshot method would be useful.

H. Signorelli, DO

Evaluation of automated immunoassays in the diagnosis of heparin induced thrombocytopenia

Althaus K, Hron G, Strobel U, et al (Ernst-Moritz-Arndt Univ Greifswald, Germany; et al)

Thromb Res 131:e85-e90, 2013

Background.—Heparin-induced thrombocytopenia (HIT) is caused by platelet-activating antibodies that recognize platelet factor 4/heparin (PF4/hep) complexes. The *in vitro* demonstration of PF4/hep antibodies using functional and immunological methods is essential for optimal management of patients suspected to have HIT. Since functional assays are technically challenging and limited to specialized laboratories, antigen-binding assays are commonly used in routine laboratories.

Study Design.—Blood samples from 448 consecutive patients in whom HIT was suspected were investigated using a latex agglutination test HemosIL® HIT-Ab(PF4-H) (HemosIL-Ab), two chemiluminescence tests HemosIL AcuStar HIT-Ab(PF4-H) (HemosIL AcuStar-Ab) and AcuStar HIT-IgG(PF4-H) (HemosIL AcuStar-IgG), an in-house PF4/hep IgG enzyme immunoassay (EIA) and the heparin induced platelet aggregation (HIPA) test.

Results.—Antibodies against PF4/hep were detectable in 44 out of 119 samples using HemosIL-Ab among which 20 samples were also reactive in the HIPA; and in 122, 64 and 108 out of 448 sera using HemosIL AcuStar-Ab, HemosIL AcuStar-IgG and in-house PF4/hep IgG-EIA, respectively, among which 52 sera were also reactive in the HIPA. All assays had high sensitivities of >95% for platelet activating antibodies; however, they differed in their specificities. The highest specificity and positive predictive value was observed by HemosIL AcuStar-IgG (96% and 78%, respectively).

Conclusion.—Automated immunoassays are useful in the laboratory investigations of HIT and present a potential improvement toward standardization of laboratory investigations of HIT. The high positive predictive capability may justify treating the patient with alternative anticoagulants without waiting for the results of a functional assay.

▶ Heparin-induced thrombocytopenia (HIT) is a prothrombotic, immune-mediated adverse reaction that occurs after exposure to unfractionated heparin, low molecular heparin, or other polyanions such as hypersulfated chondroitin sulfate. HIT is usually caused by platelet-activating antibodies that recognize platelet factor 4 (PF4) heparin complexes. Typical clinical manifestations of HIT are a decrease in platelet count by more than 50%, beginning between days 4 and 10 of heparin therapy, often complicated by new thrombotic complications. However, the clinical diagnosis of HIT is often difficult, especially in patient populations with a high prevalence of thrombocytopenia, such as intensive care patients. Thus, the clinical diagnosis must be corroborated by in vitro demonstration of heparin-dependent antibodies, such as platelet-activating or anti-PF4/heparin IgG antibodies. Two different classes of assays are available: enzyme immunoassays (EIAs), which detect binding of antibodies to immobilized PF4/heparin complexes, and functional assays. Three automated PF4/heparin antigen assays, one based on the agglutination of latex particles and the 2 others with chemiluminescent detection, have recently been introduced. In the latex agglutination assay, agglutination of PF4/polyvinylsulfonate-coated beads by a monoclonal anti-PF4/heparin antibody is inhibited in the presence of human anti-PF4/heparin antibodies. This assay can only be performed with plasma, and it cannot differentiate between IgG, IgM, or IgA antibodies. The chemiluminescence assays are based on binding of anti-PF4/heparin antibodies to PF4/polyvinylsulfonate. They can be performed with serum or plasma and can differentiate between different immunoglobulin classes (IgG only or total antibody). They show a wide range of reactivity and might thus provide additional information compared with the EIAs. These automated assays might allow greater standardization and better comparability of results obtained in different laboratories. Furthermore, they allow single sample testing and provide a rapid turnaround time of results of approximately 13 minutes for the latex immunoassay and about 30 minutes on the chemiluminescent system. In this study, the authors assessed these 3 assays in comparison with an in-house PF4/heparin EIA and the HIPA test.

M. G. Bissell, MD, PhD, MPH

Effect of inositol hexaphosphate–loaded red blood cells (RBCs) on the rheology of sickle RBCs

Lamarre Y, Bourgeaux V, Pichon A, et al (UMR Inserm U665, Guadeloupe, France; ERYtech Pharma, Bâtiment Adénine, Lyon, France; Université Paris 13, Bobigny, France; et al)
Transfusion 53:627-636, 2013

Background.—The recent in vitro demonstration that inositol hexaphosphate–loaded red blood cells (IHP-RBCs) may reduce the risks of sickling of sickle RBCs (SS RBCs) exposed to hypoxia make these modified RBCs potentially useful in transfused sickle cell anemia (SCA) patients.

Study Design and Methods.—Hemorheologic properties of IHP-RBCs, normal RBCs (AA RBCs), SS RBCs, SS RBCs plus AA RBCs, and SS RBCs plus IHP-RBCs were compared under normoxia and/or after hypoxic challenges.

Results.—Although IHP-RBCs have reduced deformability compared with SS RBCs or AA RBCs, IHP-RBCs exhibited lower aggregability than AA RBCs and SS RBCs and, when mixed with SS RBCs, the aggregation level was below the one of SS RBCs alone or SS RBCs plus AA RBCs. Blood viscosity of SS RBC plus IHP-RBC suspension was lower than the viscosity of SS RBCs alone and greater than viscosity of SS RBCs plus AA RBCs. The hypoxic challenge was detrimental for deformability and viscosity of SS RBCs alone or SS plus AA RBC suspension but not for SS plus IHP-RBC suspension.

Conclusion.—Our results support the fact that IHP-RBCs could be useful in SCA by decreasing RBC aggregation and blunting the adverse effects of hypoxia on RBC deformability and blood viscosity.

► For patients with sickle cell disease (SCD), hypoxia is an important trigger for vascular occlusion events. Inositol hexaphosphate (IHP) has been shown to reduce the oxygen-hemoglobin affinity, thus improving the oxygen release in the blood stream and in the tissues, and may prevent sickling of red blood cells (RBCs) from sickle cell patients (SS RBCs) under physiologic conditions. Bourgeaux and colleagues showed that transfusion of IHP-loaded homologous red blood cells (IHP-RBCs) reduces SCD disorders in sickle transgenic mice and may be useful in transfused sickle cell anemia (SCA) patients.[1] IHP-RBCs may be able to decrease the transfusion volumes, thus reducing problems of blood availability and alloimmunization. The authors of this study compared the hemorheologic properties of different suspensions of IHP-RBCs, normal RBCs (AA RBCs), and SS RBCs. Hemorheologic variables were measured by looking at the RBC elongation indexes (EIs) at different shear stresses and osmotic gradients. The higher the index, the more deformable the RBCs are. They also compared the effects of adding either human IHP-RBCs or human AA RBCs on the rheology of human SS RBC suspension under normoxia and hypoxic conditions.

IHP-RBCs showed lower deformability than SS RBCs and AA RBCs. However, when IHP-RBCs are added to SS RBCs, the deformability was not improved and may not be adequate for massive transfusions. The effect of IHP-RBCs and AA RBCs on the membrane stability of the SS RBC suspensions was similar. Aggregation was decreased with IHP-RBCs mixed with SS RBCs when compared with the other suspensions, which may play an important role in improving blood flow hemodynamics in SCA patients. Blood viscosity of IHP-RBC suspension mixed with SS RBCs is lower than viscosity of SS RBCs alone and greater than viscosity of SS RBCs plus AA RBCs. One of the most important aspects of this study included their observations in hypoxic challenges. The authors showed that during the partial re-oxygenation state, IHP-RBCs release their oxygen to the adjacent SS RBCs, making them better oxygenated and less able to become sickle and rigid. This may play down the negative effects of IHP-RBCs on the SS RBC deformability. The diluting effect of AA RBCs did not counteract the increase of sickle and rigid SS RBCs caused by hypoxia. The positive hemorheologic effect of IHP-RBCs on SS RBC suspensions during hypoxia was observed for blood viscosity as well. At baseline, the deformability and blood viscosity was not improved for IHP-RBCs over AA RBCs. More importantly, however, during hypoxic conditions, SS plus IHP-RBC suspension showed superior beneficial hemorheologic effects than that of SS plus AA RBC suspension. These results, along with the findings in the recent study published by Bourgeaux and colleagues, give a strong foundation for future studies on the effects of IHP-RBCs in transfusion therapy in SCA.

H. Signorelli, DO

Reference

1. Bourgeaux V, Hequet O, Campion Y, et al. Inositol hexaphosphate-loaded red blood cells prevent in vitro sickling. *Transfusion*. 2010;50:2176-2184.

Assessment of the impact of rivaroxaban on coagulation assays: Laboratory recommendations for the monitoring of rivaroxaban and review of the literature

Douxfils J, Mullier F, Loosen C, et al (Namur Res Inst for Life Sciences (NARILIS), Mont-Godinne, Belgium)

Thromb Res 130:956-966, 2012

Introduction.—Rivaroxaban does not require monitoring nor frequent dose adjustment. However, searching for the optimal dose in the individual patient may be useful in some situations.

Aim.—To determine which coagulation assay could be used to assess the impact of rivaroxaban on haemostasis and provide guidelines for the interpretation of routine lab tests.

Materials.—Rivaroxaban was spiked at concentrations ranging from 11 to 1090 ng/mL in plateletpoor plasma. A large panel of coagulation assays was tested.

Results.—A concentration dependent prolongation of aPTT, PT, dPT, PiCT was observed. PT and dPT were the most sensitive chronometric assays but results varied depending on the reagent (Triniclot PT Excel S > Recombiplastin 2 G > Neoplastin R > Neoplastin CI + > Triniclot PT Excel > Triniclot PT HTF > Innovin). FXa chromogenic assays showed the highest sensitivity. In TGA, Cmax was the most sensitive parameter with the tissue factor induced pathway. Rivaroxaban interferes on haemostasis diagnostic tests such the measurement of clotting factors, fibrinogen, antithrombin, proteins C and S, activated protein-C resistance and Xa-based chomogenic assays.

Conclusions.—PT may be used as screening test to assess the risk of bleedings. A more specific and sensitive assay such as Biophen DiXaI using calibrators should be used to confirm the concentration of rivaroxaban. We also propose cut-off associated with a bleeding or thrombosis risk based on pharmacokinetic studies. Standardization of the time between the last intake of rivaroxaban and the sampling is mandatory.

► Rivaroxaban (Xarelto®) is a direct antithrombin-independent and orally active factor Xa (FXa) inhibitor that inhibits not only free FXa but also the prothrombinase complex and clot-bound FXa. The net clinical benefit of rivaroxaban, and other new oral anticoagulants, vs warfarin in patients with high risk of bleeding and stroke, suggests a wider use of these compounds in the near future. The absolute bioavailability of rivaroxaban is high (80% to 100%). Thanks to its predictable pharmacokinetic and pharmacodynamic profiles, monitoring is generally not recommended. However, clinical surveillance is recommended throughout the treatment period in several subgroups of patients. Thus, in patients with severe renal impairment (creatinine clearance < 30 mL/min) rivaroxaban plasma levels may be significantly increased, which may lead to a moderate increased bleeding risk. The use of rivaroxaban is not recommended in patients with creatinine clearance less than 15 mL/min and is to be used with caution in patients with creatinine clearance between 15 and 29 mL/min. In addition, Xarelto®

is a substrate of P-gp transporter and is partially metabolized by CYP3A4, resulting in some clinically relevant drug interactions. Moreover, it should be used with caution in cirrhotic patients with hepatic impairment (classified as Child Pugh B) and is contraindicated in patients with hepatic disease associated with a coagulopathy. Therefore, biological monitoring would be valuable in acute situations, such as recurrent thrombosis, bleedings, before urgent surgery, in case of bridging, and in case of at least 2 risk factors among the following: drug interactions with caution, moderate renal impairment, and moderate hepatic impairment. Monitoring may also be useful in infants, pregnant women, or in those with extreme body weights, although no relevant data on drug levels associated with approximate therapeutic and harmful ranges are currently available. The primary aim of this study is to assess which coagulation assay(s) could be proposed to measure the pharmacodynamic effects of rivaroxaban and to compare our results with those found in the literature. Secondly, the authors also provide laboratory recommendations for the accurate determination of plasma drug concentration in patients treated by rivaroxaban as well as a correct interpretation of routine laboratory tests influenced by the presence of rivaroxaban.

M. G. Bissell, MD, PhD, MPH

Does Rh immune globulin suppress HLA sensitization in pregnancy?

Kaufman RM, for the NHLBI Retrovirus Epidemiology Donor Study-II (REDS-II) (Brigham and Women's Hosp, Boston, MA; et al)

Transfusion 53:2069-2077, 2013

Background.—How Rh immune globulin (RhIG) prevents sensitization to D antigen is unclear. If RhIG Fc delivers a nonspecific immunosuppressive signal, then RhIG may inhibit sensitization to antigens other than D. HLA antibody prevalence was compared in previously pregnant D− versus D+ women to investigate whether RhIG suppresses HLA sensitization.

Study Design and Methods.—In the Leukocyte Antibody Prevalence Study (LAPS), 7920 volunteer blood donors were screened for anti-HLA and surveyed about prior pregnancies and transfusions. A secondary analysis of the LAPS database was performed.

Results.—D− women not more than 40 years old (presumed to have received antenatal with or without postpartum RhIG in all pregnancies) had a significantly lower HLA sensitization rate than D+ women (relative risk, 0.58; 95% confidence interval [CI], 0.40-0.83). When stratified by deliveries (one, two, three, or four or more), D− women not older than 40 were HLA sensitized less often than D+ women in every case. In contrast, a clear relationship between D type and HLA sensitization was not seen in older previously pregnant women whose childbearing years are presumed to have preceded the use of routine RhIG prophylaxis. In a multivariable logistic regression model, D− women not more than 40 years old remained significantly less likely to be HLA sensitized compared with D+ women after adjusting for parity, time from last pregnancy, lost pregnancies, and transfusions (odds ratio [OR], 0.55; 95% CI, 0.34-0.88).

Conclusion.—Consistent with a nonspecific immunosuppressive effect of RhIG, younger previously pregnant D– women were less likely than previously pregnant D+ women to be HLA sensitized.

▶ Human leukocyte antigen (HLA) sensitization occurs in more than 24% of previously pregnant women with a host of potential adverse consequences like transfusion-related acute lung injury, platelet refractoriness, and stem cell and solid organ transplant rejection. HLA sensitization occurs more often than D-negative women becoming sensitized to D antigen after a single pregnancy with a D-positive fetus. And since Rh immune globulin (RhIG) was introduced, that number has drastically decreased. Immunoglobulin therapies have been used successfully to prevent not only D sensitization in pregnancy but also HPA-1A sensitization. The authors of this study hypothesize that previously pregnant D-negative women (presumed to have received RhIG) would have a lower rate of HLA sensitization than previously pregnant D-positive women (presumed not to have received RhIG). The mechanism of RhIG in preventing D sensitization remains somewhat elusive, but the hope that the mechanisms may carry over to other antigens has been seen in prior studies. This retrospective study used a large data set that had been previously used and reanalyzed the data. For each subject, the age at enrollment was known as well as the D type, total number of pregnancies and deliveries, and the date of the last pregnancy. Previously pregnant female subjects were grouped into different age groups: not more than 40 years, 41 to 50, 51 to 60, 61 to 70, and 71 years and older. The authors then used the age groups to infer if the patients would have received antenatal or postpartum RhIG based on utilization data and standards of care at that time. They assumed that all younger—but not older—D-negative women would have received RhIG in essentially all pregnancies. This group had a significantly lower HLA sensitization rate than their D-positive counterparts, which remained significant after multivariable logistic regression analysis. In older previously pregnant women, men, and nulliparous women, there was no clear relationship between D type and HLA sensitization. This approach should be reasonably accurate for the youngest and the oldest subjects but is most likely less accurate for the subjects in the middle of the age spectrum. Overall, this study showed that there is evidence that RhIG may suppress HLA sensitization in pregnancy. A major limitation in this study is that no information on actual RhIG administration during pregnancy was available. Although the assumptions on RhIG administration based on the year when each of the women was pregnant may be fairly accurate, more prospective studies need to be done. Additionally, because the original data set was done in healthy blood donors it is possible that the older D-negative subjects who became sensitized to D antigen would have been excluded from the donor pool, therefore skewing the older D-negative group toward a lower rate of HLA sensitization. The possibility that RhIG administration or other immunoglobulin therapies may prevent HLA sensitization warrants further investigation in prospective studies.

H. Signorelli, DO

Evaluation of single-nucleotide polymorphisms as internal controls in prenatal diagnosis of fetal blood groups

Doescher A, Petershofen EK, Wagner FF, et al (Institut Bremen-Oldenburg, Germany; Institut Springe, Germany; St Josefs-Hosp, Wiesbaden, Germany)

Transfusion 53:353-362, 2013

Background.—Determination of fetal blood groups in maternal plasma samples critically depends on adequate amplification of fetal DNA. We evaluated the routine inclusion of 52 single-nucleotide polymorphisms (SNPs) as internal reference in our polymerase chain reaction (PCR) settings to obtain a positive internal control for fetal DNA.

Study Design and Methods.—DNA from 223 plasma samples of pregnant women was screened for *RHD* Exons 3, 4, 5, and 7 in a multiplex PCR including 52 SNPs divided into four primer pools. Amplicons were analyzed by single-base extension and the GeneScan method in a genetic analyzer. Results of D screening were compared to standard *RHD* genotyping of amniotic fluid or real-time PCR of fetal DNA from maternal plasma.

Results.—The vast majority of all samples (97.8%) demonstrated differences in maternal and fetal SNP patterns when tested with four primer pools. These differences were not observed in less than 2.2% of the samples most probably due to an extraction failure for adequate amounts of fetal DNA. Comparison of the fetal genotypes with independent results did not reveal a single false-negative case among samples (n = 42) with positive internal control and negative fetal *RHD* typing.

Conclusion.—Coamplification of 52 SNPs with *RHD*-specific sequences for fetal blood group determination introduces a valid positive control for the amplification of fetal DNA to avoid false-negative results. This new approach does not require a paternal blood sample. It may also be applicable to other assays for fetal genotyping in maternal blood samples.

▶ Determination of fetal *RHD* from maternal plasma is increasingly used as a tool for prenatal diagnosis. A remaining pitfall that hampers its use in situations of severe consequences is a limited reliability of negative results caused by difficulties in distinguishing negative results from false-negative results because of insufficient amounts of free fetal DNA (ffDNA). Large studies were performed in the last 10 years to investigate the reliability of noninvasive fetal *RHD* typing with real-time polymerase chain reaction (PCR). Most of the assays were performed without internal controls. A few studies included the *SRY* gene as proof for ffDNA. This approach is, however, limited to pregnancies with a male fetus. A valid control for ffDNA that neither depends on the sex of the fetus nor requires a paternal control sample is essential to fully exploit the potential of methods for noninvasive fetal genotyping. Detection of *RHD*+ ffDNA in D− mothers will trigger careful monitoring of the pregnancy and, if necessary, appropriate interventions. A negative result of fetal *RHD* genotyping in maternal blood samples is not conclusive. Insufficient amplification of fetal DNA could occur because of problems with the effectiveness of DNA extraction, especially if the ffDNA concentration in the maternal plasma is very low. Because most plasma DNA is of maternal origin, such false-negative results cannot be recognized by generic control amplifications. Low ffDNA concentrations are a special problem very early in pregnancy. A valid result in fetal genotyping may, however, be clinically meaningful for the diagnostic monitoring of pregnancies as early as 10 to 13 weeks of gestation, especially if antibodies are already detectable in the maternal serum. The authors, therefore, evaluated 52 single-nucleotide polymorphisms (SNPs) as internal positive controls for the amplification of fetal DNA in our PCR setting. A multiplex PCR for 4 *RHD* exons, including SNPs as the positive control, was established. The results of the new method were compared with those from genotyping by either real time PCR of the identical maternal blood samples or PCR of amniocentesis samples from the same pregnancy.

M. G. Bissell, MD, PhD, MPH

Fresh and Citrated Whole-Blood Specimens Can Produce Different Thromboelastography Results in Patients on Extracorporeal Membrane Oxygenation

Gilman EA, Koch CD, Santrach PJ, et al (Mayo Clinic, Rochester, MN)
Am J Clin Pathol 140:165-169, 2013

Objectives.—To compare thromboelastography (TEG) tracings obtained from fresh and citrated whole-blood samples in patients on extracorporeal membrane oxygenation (ECMO) or after cardiopulmonary bypass and in healthy volunteers.

Methods.—Samples of fresh and citrated whole blood were analyzed for 25 patients and 4 healthy volunteers. Thromboelastography analysis was performed in both plain and heparinase cups.

Results.—In 5 of 6 patients on ECMO, use of citrated samples resulted in apparent partial or complete heparin reversal. In TEG tracings from patients following cardiopulmonary bypass, there was a slight hypercoagulable appearance in the citrated sample. No differences were noted between fresh and citrated samples from healthy volunteers whose blood was spiked with heparin.

Conclusions.—In some patients on ECMO, use of samples collected in sodium citrate tubes for TEG analysis results in significant artifacts, which could lead to heparin overdosing in these patients.

▶ Thromboelastography (TEG) is a point-of-care viscoelastic assay that records the assembly of a clot in whole blood and provides an assessment of overall hemostasis. It evaluates the dynamics of clot formation and clot strength and, unlike standard tests of coagulation, it assesses the contribution of platelets as well as other cellular components. TEG was initially developed for use with fresh whole blood, but the test needs to be initiated within 4 minutes of sample collection, which is often impractical for many hospitals. The use of citrated whole blood has been published as an alternative, which allows for more time between the blood draw and initiation of the test. However, some studies have shown an effect of the citrate anticoagulated on the parameters of the assay. The use of TEG has been shown to decrease the transfusion of blood products for liver transplant and cardiovascular surgery, and this study validated the use of citrated whole blood for kaolin-activated TEG on patients on extracorporeal membrane oxygenation (ECMO) and for patients after cardiovascular surgery. Samples of fresh and citrated whole blood were collected nearly simultaneously from 6 patients on ECMO and 19 cardiovascular patients after protamine reversal of heparin and discontinuation of cardiopulmonary bypass. Whole blood samples from 4 healthy volunteers were also drawn and spiked with incremental levels of unfractionated heparin, which were either tested as whole blood within 4 minutes or aliquoted into 3.2% sodium citrate tubes and tested as citrated samples within 15 minutes. The fresh whole blood samples were collected and immediately transported within 4 minutes of the sample draw. TEG parameters measured included reaction time, angle, and maximum amplitude. See article for explanation of parameters. They found that in some patients on ECMO, the TEG tracings using citrated whole blood sample led to apparent heparin reversal in some patients with near-normal TEG results. In the fresh whole blood from these same patients, the TEG tracings showed profound coagulopathy, and because this assay is used to adjust heparin dose for these patients, the use of citrated whole blood samples could pose a serious risk of patient harm. Only moderate differences were seen in patients after cardiovascular surgery. The samples from healthy volunteers that were spiked with heparin showed that the presence of heparin alone is not sufficient to cause significant artifacts in TEG tracings with the use of citrated whole blood samples. While this study observed clinically significant differences between citrated whole blood and fresh whole blood samples on TEG tracings, the number of patients was extremely low. Additionally, the study did not look at the effect storage time had on the assays results. Many published studies looking at TEG parameters between samples collected in citrate and fresh whole blood have found varying results, making it difficult to generalize the effect citrated blood samples have on TEG testing in any specific patient population. This study emphasizes the need for institutions wishing to use citrated samples for TEG analysis to investigate the impact of citrated sample collection and storage time on the patient populations for which TEG testing will be utilized.

H. Signorelli, DO

Small deletions within the *RHD* coding sequence: a report of two novel mutational events and a survey of the underlying pathophysiologic mechanisms

Chen J-M, Fichou Y, Jamet D, et al (Institut National de la Santé et de la Recherche Médicale (INSERM), France; Université de Bretagne Occidentale, France; Hôpital Morvan, Brest, France; et al)
Transfusion 53:206-210, 2013

Background.—Some 270 variants in the *RHD* gene have so far been identified. Of these, approximately 6% (n = 17) are small (≤20 bp) deletions occurring within the gene's coding sequence. Fourteen of these small deletions disrupted the reading frame of the *RHD* gene, resulting almost invariably in a D−phenotype.

Study Design and Methods.—Two subjects who displayed D phenotype ambiguity or a genotype-phenotype discrepancy were referred to our laboratory for *RHD* genetic analysis. Hemizygosity for the most common 70-kb *RHD* deletion was first determined in both subjects by long-range polymerase chain reaction (PCR) followed by PCR amplification and sequencing of all 10 exons of the *RHD* gene in the nondeleted allele individually.

Results.—Two novel lesions in the *RHD* gene were identified on the nondeleted alleles, a 14-bp frameshifting deletion within Exon 1 (i.e., c.29-42delGGCGCTGCCTGCCC) and an 11-bp frameshifting deletion within Exon 3 (i.e., c.361-371delTTGTCGGTGCT), in Subjects 1 and 2, respectively.

Conclusion.—By reference to previously reported small deletions in the *RHD* gene, the 11-bp deletion in Exon 3 may be safely regarded as a bona fide D−variant. Although the association of the 14-bp deletion in Exon 1 with a weak D phenotype appears to be genuine, the underlying molecular mechanism still remains to be clarified. Evaluation of all known small *RHD* deletions points to slippage mutagenesis as the major underlying mutational mechanism. [Correction statement added after online publication 21-May2012: The spelling of bona has been updated.]

► The highly polymorphic and immunogenic RhD blood group system is of critical importance to the field of transfusion medicine. To date, some 270 variants in the *RHD* gene have been registered by the Rhesus website.[1] However, new variants continue to be discovered, as exemplified by multiple recent reports in this journal. Approximately 6% (n = 17) of currently reported *RHD* variants are small deletions (< 20 bp in accordance with the Human Gene Mutation Database) that have occurred within the *RHD* coding sequence. Here, the authors report on 2 further small deletions in the *RHD* gene and provide a brief overview of this particular category of variant with respect to their functional consequences and underlying mutational mechanisms.

M. G. Bissell, MD, PhD, MPH

Reference

1. http://www.uni-ulm.de/-wflegel/RH/. Accessed April 24, 2013.

Autologous stem cell transplant recipients tolerate haploidentical related-donor natural killer cell–enriched infusions

Klingemann H, Grodman C, Cutler E, et al (Tufts Med Ctr, Boston, MA; Lahey Clinic Med Ctr, Burlington, MA; American Red Cross Blood Services, Dedham, MA; et al)

Transfusion 53:412-418, 2013

Background.—In the setting of allogeneic stem cell transplantation (SCT), infusing natural killer (NK) cells from a major histocompatibility complex (MHC)- mismatched donor can mediate an antileukemic effect. The graft-versus-tumor effect after autologous stem cell transplantation (ASCT) may result in less disease relapse.

Study Design and Methods.—We performed a Phase I clinical trial to assess the safety and feasibility of infusing distantly processed donor NK-enriched mononuclear cell (NK-MNC) infusions from a MHC haplotype—mismatched (haploidentical) donor to patients who recently underwent ASCT for a hematologic malignancy. On Day 1, peripheral blood MNCs were obtained by steady-state leukapheresis and sent from Boston to the Production Assistance for Cellular Therapies (PACT) facility at the University of Minnesota, where immunomagnetic depletion of CD3 cells was performed on Day 2. NK-MNC products were then returned to Boston on Day 2 for infusion on Day 3. Toxicity, cellular product characteristics, and logistic events were monitored.

Results.—At a median of 90 days (range, 49-191 days) after ASCT, 13 patients were treated with escalating doses of NK-MNCs per kilogram from 10^5 to 2×10^7. Adverse effects included Grade 2 rigors and muscle aches, but no Grade 3 or 4 events and no graft-versus- host disease or marrow suppression. One air courier delay occurred. NK-MNC products were viable with cytotoxic activity after transport.

Conclusion.—CD3-depleted, MHC-mismatched allogeneic NK-MNC infusions can be safely and feasibly administered to patients after ASCT after distant processing and transport, justifying further development of this approach.

▶ Many patients with hematologic malignancies treated with autologous hematopoietic stem cell transplantation (ASCT) often relapse due to residual disease. High-dose radiation and chemotherapy are inadequate treatments for most of these patients; therefore, there is a need for innovative therapeutic modalities. Patients receiving ASCT lack the graft-versus-tumor (GVT) effect of allogeneic hematopoietic stem cell recipients. GVT is mediated by complex interactions in the allograft. The hypothesis is that MHC-mismatched allogeneic natural killer (NK) cellular therapy in ASCT patients may contribute to GVT effect with limited risk of graft-versus-host disease (GVHD). This has been shown in a few previously published reports, but safety data for NK cell infusion have not been published. Autologous NK cells would likely not have the same affect, as recognition of target antigens by NK cells requires that the target does not express self—major histocompatibility complex (MHC).

The authors in this study used a phase I design to determine if MHC-mismatched NK-cell—enriched mononuclear cell (NK-MNC) infusions from related donors can be safely administered. They wanted to also assess if distant processing of the units had an effect and what the maximum dose of the allogeneic NK-MNCs is given the limits in production. The apheresis MNC product was collected and shipped to a distant processing site where it was manipulated and returned to the originating site as an NK-MNC product. Thirteen patients who had received ASCT for hematologic malignancies were enrolled and divided into 4 escalating NK-MNC dose groups. All the donors shared only one MHC haplotype with their corresponding recipients to increase the probability of donor NK-cell alloreactivity against host tumor cells. The products had to have greater than 70% cell viability and fewer than 5×10^5/kg CD3+ lymphocytes, greater than 20% CD3-/CD56+ NK cells, negative Gram stain, and acceptable endotoxin level. The product was supplemented with interleukin-2 before transportation and washed on arrival. The NK-MNC infusion was administered as a one-time intravenous infusion along with diphenhydramine. The highest number of NK-MNCs obtainable by their method was 2×10^7 MNCs/kg and, therefore, was the highest dose given to their subjects. The first subject received fludarabine the day before the infusion, but all other subjects did not receive immunosuppression before infusion. Two patients received lower-than-intended cell dose because of a shipment issue and a clot issue with the product. Only one of the products had decreased viability less than 90%. The study showed that the infusions were well tolerated by all patients with a few transient minor side effects at higher dose levels, which resolved with supportive treatment. None of the patients had signs or symptoms of acute or chronic GVHD, marrow suppression, or graft rejection. Higher doses of NK-MNCs may be tolerated if larger-volume leukapheresis protocols are used. Chimerism analysis on the 3 patients who had received the highest allogeneic NK-MNC dose level did not detect donor-derived NK-MNCs in the recipients. This could be related to the sensitivity of the assay used or to the fact that the recipient's T rejected the infused cells. It is unclear if, based on current research, patients should be immunosuppressed before infusion. The authors showed that the logistics of collection, cell processing, and infusion at distant facilities was feasible with minor issues. Additional studies validating the processing and transportation would need to be done to minimize a loss in CD56+ cell recovery and also to assess the disease outcome effects for ASCT recipients. NK cell therapy holds great promise for treatment of not only patients with hematologic malignancies but also many other cancers. Although this study shows that NK cell—based immunotherapy is feasible and safe in a select population, progress in understanding NK cell function and ways to monitor NK cells during treatment is necessary to improve clinical success.

H. Signorelli, DO

Whole-Blood Thrombin Generation Monitored with a Calibrated Automated Thrombogram-Based Assay

Ninivaggi M, Apitz-Castro R, Dargaud Y, et al (Maastricht Univ Med Ctr, the Netherlands; Edouard Herriot, Lyon, France)
Clin Chem 58:1252-1259, 2012

Background.—The calibrated automated thrombogram (CAT) assay in plasma is a versatile tool to investigate patients with hypo- or hypercoagulable phenotypes. The objective was to make this method applicable for whole blood measurements.

Methods.—Thin-layer technology and the use of a rhodamine 110—based thrombin substrate appear to be essential for a reliable thrombin generation

(TG) assay in whole blood. Using this knowledge we developed a whole blood CAT-based assay.

Results.—We demonstrated that the whole blood CAT-based assay is a sensitive and rapid screening test to assess function of the hemostatic system under more nearly physiological conditions than the TG assay in plasma. Under conditions of low tissue factor concentration (0.5 pmol/L) and 50% diluted blood, the intraassay CV of the thrombogram parameters, endogenous thrombin potential and thrombin peak height, were 6.7% and 6.5%, respectively. The respective interassay CVs were 12% and 11%. The mean interindividual variation (SD) of 40 healthy volunteers was 633 (146) nmol·min/L for the endogenous thrombin potential and 128 (23) nmol/L for the thrombin peak. Surprisingly, erythrocytes contributed more than platelets to the procoagulant blood cell membranes necessary for optimal TG. Statistically significant ($P < 0.001$) and potentially clinically significant correlations were observed between circulating factor-VIII concentrations in blood of hemophilia A patients and endogenous thrombin potential ($r = 0.62$) and thrombin peak height ($r = 0.58$).

Conclusions.—We have developed a reliable method to measure TG in whole blood. The assay can be performed with a drop of blood and may provide a useful measurement of TG under more physiological conditions than plasma.

▶ The thrombin generation (TG) assay is increasingly being recognized as a versatile diagnostic tool in the field of thrombosis and hemostasis. It is well accepted that the transient TG profile in clotting plasma is a better determinant of the overall function of the hemostatic system than are clotting time—based assays, such as prothrombin time and activated partial thromboplastin time. TG in plasma is most accurately measured with the calibrated automated thrombogram (CAT) assay. This method has been designed for application with platelet-free and platelet-rich plasma as analytes. The method is, however, not applicable for measuring TG in whole blood. Variable quenching of the fluorescent signal by hemoglobin and red blood cells that sediment, cluster, and retract with the clot leads to highly erratic signals. A reliable whole blood TG assay is important because it enables us to go a step closer to physiological conditions than is possible in present practice. Apart from this conceptual advantage, there is the practical advantage that no centrifugation step is required, which opens the way to point-of-care TG measurements.

The authors of this article found that the problems caused by the presence of red blood cells can be overcome by dispersing the blood in a porous matrix, thereby creating a thin layer of blood, and by using rhodamine-110 as a signaling product. By these modifications of the plasma CAT assay, they acceptably reduced quenching and issues related to unequal distribution of red blood cells. Here, they report the technical validation of a whole blood CAT-based assay of acceptable imprecision that measures TG in a thin layer of whole blood. As proof of concept, they compared the whole blood thrombogram parameters with factor-VIII plasma concentrations in hemophilia A patients.

M. G. Bissell, MD, PhD, MPH

Routine use of a rapid test to detect bacteria at the time of issue for nonleukoreduced, whole blood–derived platelets

Harm SK, Delaney M, Charapata M, et al (Univ of Pittsburgh Med Ctr, PA; Univ of Washington, Seattle; The Inst for Transfusion Medicine, Pittsburgh, PA)

Transfusion 53:843-850, 2013

Background.—The Pan Genera detection (PGD) test is used to screen platelet (PLT) products for bacterial contamination. We report the experience of using the PGD test on whole blood–derived PLTs (WBPs) at two large centralized transfusion services (CTS).

Study Design and Methods.—Records of PGD test results were retrospectively reviewed. The PGD test was performed on individual WBP units or pools of WBPs ranging in size from 2 to 6 units at the time of issue. Bacterial culture was performed on PLT products with positive PGD tests, and at one CTS, the available cocomponents.

Results.—A total of 70,561 WBP pools were screened with the PGD test. There were seven true-positive PGD tests and 242 false-positive tests (positive predictive value of PGD test, 2.81%). The overall contamination rate was 99 per 10^6 WBP pools (1:10,080; 95% confidence interval [CI], 40-204), and the false-positive rate was 3430 per 10^6 WBP pools (1:292; 95% CI, 3011-3890). All seven bacterial isolates were Gram positive. The median age of the individual WBP units in the seven contaminated pools was 5 days (range, 3-5 days) compared to 4 days (range, 1-5 days) in the false-positive pools ($p = 0.0012$). The same bacteria isolated from a positive PLT pool also grew in one red blood cell cocomponent.

Conclusion.—After testing more than 70,000 WBP pools at two large CTSs, the rate of contaminated WBP pools detected by the PGD test was 99 per 10^6 pools (1:10,080).

▶ Bacterially contaminated platelet (PLT) products can cause serious morbidity and mortality. Between 2007 and 2011, septic reactions were the fourth leading cause of transfusion-related fatalities reported to the US Food and Drug Administration (FDA) with 4 of 24 fatalities caused by contaminated pooled whole blood–derived PLTs (SBPs) and 10 of 24 caused by contaminated apheresis PLTs. Prevention of transfusion-associated bacterial infection remains a major challenge. The reported bacterial contamination rate varies depending on the type of PLT component and method of detection. Blood centers and transfusion services that are accredited by the AABB must have a system in place to limit and detect or inactivate bacteria in all PLT components. These methods include culture of products close to the time of production and the use of near-issue test methods such as measurement of pH and glucose levels. While culturing remains the gold standard for detecting bacteria, there has been a lot of focus on the residual risk of bacterial contamination of PLTs despite negative cultures early in storage. Pan Genera Detection (PGD) test is an FDA-approved device for the detection of bacteria in both WBP and apheresis PLT products. It is a qualitative immunoassay that detects gram-negative–specific lipopolysaccharide antigens as well as gram-positive bacteria-specific lipoteichoic acid. The authors of this study published their experience with the PGD test across 2 large centralized transfusion centers serving a total of 35 hospitals with pooled WBPs. A total of 70 561 WBP pools (representing approximately 350 000 individual WBP units) were screened with the PGD test between the 2 transfusion centers. All of the PLT units reported here had been prepared via the PLT-rich plasma method and stored until the time of pooling and testing without leukoreduction. At both centers, positive reactions in the PGD test resulted in repeat PGD testing, test culture follow-up, bacterial identification, and product quarantine according to their algorithm. If the follow-up culture to a PGD-positive test result was negative after the 5-day incubation, then the PGD test result was considered to be a false-positive. A true-positive PGD result was defined as one in which the PGD test was positive and bacteria were isolated. There were 242 WBP pools with a false-positive PGD test result, and the study showed a positive predictive value of 2.81% for their centers. There were 7 true-positive PGD test results, which were all caused by gram-positive bacteria for an overall contamination rate of 99 per 106, which is lower than that of other published studies. The positive predictive value of the PGD test from this author was lower than other smaller published studies and was slightly but not significantly higher than that reported for the pH test for bacterial screening. Clearly, culture is a more sensitive method but has limitations because for practical reasons it must be performed early in the storage period of PLTs when bacteria levels are lower. False-positive PGD test results in this study were significantly lower than when this test was used to screen apheresis platelets. However, false-positive PGD results lead to an unnecessary waste of units, technologist time, and cartridge use with repeat PGD testing. The centers in this study had successful application of the PGD test. However, they did not evaluate the PGD-negative WBP pools with culture and, therefore, sensitivity could not be addressed. Some published studies have shown a large number of false-negatives with the PGD test. Improvements in the false-positive rate and sensitivity are necessary for this assay. Although culture remains the gold standard method of detecting bacterial contamination, the use of near-issue methods will play an important role in the future of transfusion medicine. Emerging appealing alternatives to the PGD method are flow cytometric and nucleic acid amplification techniques. For further reading, see reference list.[1]

H. Signorelli, DO

Reference

1. Brecher ME, Jacobs MR, Katz LM, et al. Survey of methods used to detect bacterial contamination of platelet products in the United States in 2011. *Transfusion.* 2013;53:911-918.

Routine use of a rapid test to detect bacteria at the time of issue for nonleukoreduced, whole blood–derived platelets

Harm SK, Delaney M, Charapata M, et al (Univ of Pittsburgh Med Ctr, PA; Univ of Washington, Seattle; The Inst for Transfusion Medicine, Pittsburgh, PA)

Transfusion 53:843-850, 2013

Background.—The Pan Genera detection (PGD) test is used to screen platelet (PLT) products for bacterial contamination. We report the experience of using the PGD test on whole blood–derived PLTs (WBPs) at two large centralized transfusion services (CTS).

Study Design and Methods.—Records of PGD test results were retrospectively reviewed. The PGD test was performed on individual WBP units or pools of WBPs ranging in size from 2 to 6 units at the time of issue. Bacterial culture was performed on PLT products with positive PGD tests, and at one CTS, the available cocomponents.

Results.—A total of 70,561 WBP pools were screened with the PGD test. There were seven true-positive PGD tests and 242 false-positive tests (positive predictive value of PGD test, 2.81%). The overall contamination rate was 99 per 10^6 WBP pools (1:10,080; 95% confidence interval [CI], 40-204), and the false-positive rate was 3430 per 10^6 WBP pools (1:292; 95% CI, 3011-3890). All seven bacterial isolates were Gram positive. The median age of the individual WBP units in the seven contaminated pools was 5 days (range, 3-5 days) compared to 4 days (range, 1-5 days) in the false-positive pools ($p = 0.0012$). The same bacteria isolated from a positive PLT pool also grew in one red blood cell cocomponent.

Conclusion.—After testing more than 70,000 WBP pools at two large CTSs, the rate of contaminated WBP pools detected by the PGD test was 99 per 10^6 pools (1:10,080).

▶ The reported rates of bacterial contamination in platelet (PLT) components vary by the type of PLT component, methods of bacterial detection, and study methods. These confounders make comparisons of the rate of observed bacterial contamination between and among PLT components challenging. Bacterially contaminated PLT products can lead to septic transfusion reactions and deaths. In the report of one large experience, the rate of transfusion-associated sepsis after the introduction of inlet-line sample diversion pouches and greater volumes of cultured product was approximately 1.2 septic reactions per 105 apheresis PLT collections. Between 2007 and 2011, septic reactions were the fourth leading cause of transfusion-related fatalities reported to the US Food and Drug Administration (FDA) with 4 of 24 fatalities caused by contaminated pooled WBPs and 10 of 24 due to contaminated apheresis PLTs. A device that has been FDA approved for the detection of bacteria in both whole blood–derived PLTs and apheresis PLT products is a Pan Genera Detection (PGD) test. This test is a qualitative immunoassay that uses lateral flow immunoprecipitation to detect gram-negative specific lipopolysaccharide antigens on one end of the cartridge and gram-positive bacteria-specific lipoteichoic acid on the opposite end of the cartridge. According to the manufacturer, the PGD has a sensitivity of 103 to 105 colony-forming units (CFUs) per milliliter. In practice, the lower limit of detection for gram-positive bacteria is on the order of 103 to 104 CFUs/mL, whereas for some strains of gram-negative bacteria, the lower limit of detection can be more than 106 CFUs/mL. The PGD test can be applied using various testing protocols immediately before the PLTs are issued to the patient. The initial results after implementing the PGD test to supplant pH testing at one of the author's centers has been previously reported. The PGD test had a superior positive predictive value compared with the pH test, and this resulted in significantly reduced wastage of what were ultimately found to be WBP pools that were tested negative in culture. The purpose of this study was to determine whether the initial experience with the PGD test was maintained after several years of use across 2 large centralized transfusion services that used slightly different testing protocols in serving a total of 35 hospitals with pooled WBPs.

M. G. Bissell, MD, PhD, MPH

Evaluation of single-nucleotide polymorphisms as internal controls in prenatal diagnosis of fetal blood groups

Doescher A, Petershofen EK, Wagner FF, et al (Institut Bremen-Oldenburg, Germany; Institut Springe, Germany; St Josefs-Hosp, Wiesbaden, Germany)
Transfusion 53:353-362, 2013

Background.—Determination of fetal blood groups in maternal plasma samples critically depends on adequate amplification of fetal DNA. We evaluated the routine inclusion of 52 single-nucleotide polymorphisms (SNPs) as internal reference in our polymerase chain reaction (PCR) settings to obtain a positive internal control for fetal DNA.

Study Design and Methods.—DNA from 223 plasma samples of pregnant women was screened for *RHD* Exons 3, 4, 5, and 7 in a multiplex PCR including 52 SNPs divided into four primer pools. Amplicons were analyzed by single-base extension and the GeneScan method in a genetic analyzer. Results of D screening were compared to standard *RHD* genotyping of amniotic fluid or real-time PCR of fetal DNA from maternal plasma.

Results.—The vast majority of all samples (97.8%) demonstrated differences in maternal and fetal SNP patterns when tested with four primer pools. These differences were not observed in less than 2.2% of the samples most probably due to an extraction failure for adequate amounts of fetal DNA. Comparison of the fetal genotypes with independent results did not reveal a single false-negative case among samples (n = 42) with positive internal control and negative fetal *RHD* typing.

Conclusion.—Coamplification of 52 SNPs with *RHD*-specific sequences for fetal blood group determination introduces a valid positive control for the amplification of fetal DNA to avoid false-negative results. This new approach does not require a paternal blood sample. It may also be

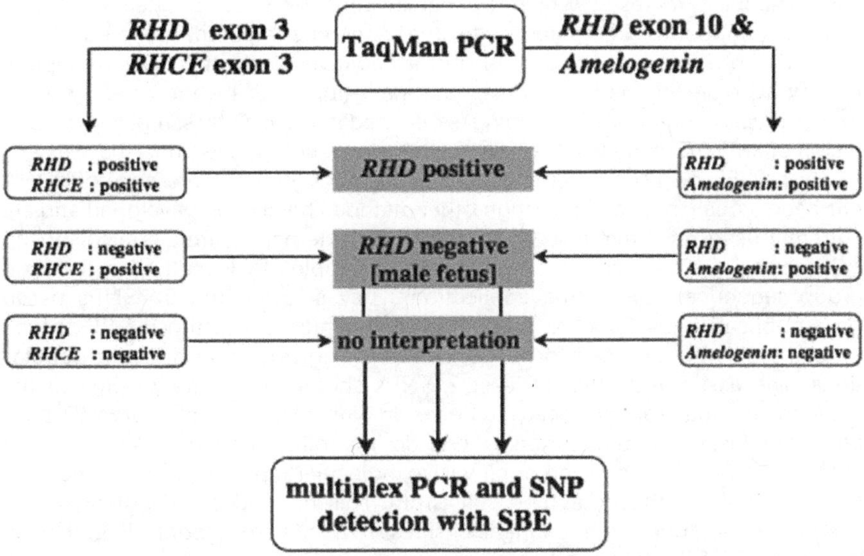

FIGURE 4.—Work flow for fetal *RHD* detection. Use of internal controls with SBE can be restricted to pregnancies with a female *RHD*− fetus. (Reprinted from Doescher A, Petershofen EK, Wagner FF, et al. Evaluation of single-nucleotide polymorphisms as internal controls in prenatal diagnosis of fetal blood groups. *Transfusion*. 2013;53:353-362 with permission from Transfusion and John Wiley and Sons, www.interscience.wiley.com.)

applicable to other assays for fetal genotyping in maternal blood samples (Fig 4).

▶ Despite widespread use of RH immune globulin prophylaxis, RH isoimmunization still occurs, which can lead to hemolytic disease of the newborn. Prenatal determination of *RHD* status is clinically useful because further testing and therapeutic procedures will not be necessary if the fetus is *RHD* negative. The ability to determine fetal *RHD* status noninvasively with maternal plasma avoids the risks associated with amniotic fluid or chorionic villi sampling. However, many real-time polymerase chain reaction (PCR) assays currently do not have an internal control limiting the reliability of the negative results. A negative result could represent a true negative or could be caused by insufficient amounts of free fetal DNA (ffDNA). Therefore, a negative result using ffDNA from maternal plasma is not currently conclusive, and those patients continue to need monitoring and therapeutic interventions. Some assays use the *SRY* gene as proof of ffDNA but are limited to pregnancies with a male fetus. This study evaluated single-nucleotide polymorphisms (SNPs) as internal positive controls for the amplification of fetal DNA in their PCR assay. The authors assumed that at least 2 or more SNPs should be different between fetal and maternal DNA for sufficient proof of the presence of fetal DNA. A total of 210 samples (94.2%) showed 2 or more SNPs to be different between fetal and maternal DNA. The remaining 13 samples were considered to not have proof of ffDNA or an unbalanced genotyping of some SNPs. This method had a very high sensitivity, and 7 samples had a false-positive *RHD* result, which is generally considered less problematic from a clinical standpoint. Compared with the reference method, no single case showed a positive internal control and a negative result in *RHD* genotyping. A flow scheme for the inclusion of this new approach in our routine setting for noninvasive prenatal *RHD* typing is depicted in Fig 4. Only samples with suspicion of an *RHD*- female fetus need further evaluation by the single-base extension assay. Finding sex-independent methods to confirm the presence of ffDNA has been a challenge, and although other methods have been developed and are currently used by some laboratories, they use external controls in a follow-up PCR setting. This study is the first to use a multiplex PCR method with blood group sequences for routine application. They selected the 52 SNPs based on a publication by Sanchez and colleagues, which chose those SNPs based on allele distribution used for identification of individuals in different populations. The assumption that at least 2 SNPs should be different between the maternal and fetal samples needs to be tested with a larger number of *RHD*-negative samples, which the authors plan to do in a follow-up study. Although this study shows a very promising noninvasive molecular typing procedure, the general limitations with genotyping still apply. This method could potentially be used for other blood group antigens besides *RHD* that are responsible for hemolytic disease of the fetus and newborn.

H. Signorelli, DO

Incomplete pretransfusion testing leads to surgical delays

McWilliams B, Yazer MH, Cramer J, et al (Univ of Pittsburgh, PA)

Transfusion 52:2139-2144, 2012

Background.—The Joint Commission has highlighted the importance of having appropriate and complete pretransfusion testing before surgery begins. The maximum surgical blood ordering schedule (MSBOS) indicates which patients require preoperative transfusion testing. We determined the number of times surgical delays were caused due to the lack of completed pretransfusion testing.

Study Design and Methods.—All transfusion events reported through the common medical event reporting system of eight networked hospitals over a 12-month period were evaluated to determine how often patients experienced surgical delays due to not having complete pretransfusion testing.

Results.—During this 12-month period 12 patients were identified who were either in or en route to the operating room with incomplete pretransfusion testing leading to a delay in providing crossmatched red blood cells (RBCs). In 6 of 12 cases a new antibody was discovered, which required extra time for the provision of crossmatched RBCs, while in 4 of 12 patients the samples were not sent or were lost on the way to the blood bank. In the remaining two patients other parts of the pretransfusion testing process were not followed according to hospital policy. The median surgery start time delay was approximately 12 hours (range, 1-168 hr) in 11 of 12 cases. One patient's case was not aborted when it was discovered that crossmatched RBCs were not immediately available due to newly detected alloantibodies.

Conclusions.—We identified three mechanisms by which delays in completing pretransfusion testing in surgical patients occurred. Adherence to the MSBOS and sample collection policies should reduce delays.

▶ Red blood cell (RBC) transfusion is an important support for modern surgical practice. In 2008, there were 5.8 million RBC recipients in the United States, and behind each of these transfusions was an elaborate process designed to identify and collect a sample from the intended recipient and to deliver the product that was ordered in a timely manner to that recipient. The sheer number of health care professionals involved in the process of transfusion creates many different sources of error. Perhaps the most egregious and life-threatening error involves a mistransfusion, whereby the patient receives the wrong unit of blood. The incidence of this type of error in the United States has been estimated between 1 in 19 000 and 1 in 12 000 per RBC unit transfused. Many other sources of error during the process of ordering, testing, and administering a transfusion have also been described generally in the context of analyzing the events submitted to a hospital's medical error reporting system. Avoidable delays in providing a necessary transfusion should be viewed as process errors. A particularly time-sensitive situation where delays in providing cross-matched RBCs can be especially problematic involves patients who are taken to the operating room (OR) before their pretransfusion testing has been completed. If RBCs are required during the surgery while the blood bank is performing the testing, then uncross-matched units, with their small but nonnegligible risk of hemolysis, would be issued. Even if RBCs are not required to begin the case, the surgical team might still decide to delay or defer its start while the specimen is collected and the testing is performed. To try to minimize the number of times when patients arrive in the OR without complete and appropriate pretransfusion testing, many hospitals employ a maximum surgical blood ordering schedule (MSBOS). The MSBOS lists all of the procedures that are performed at that site and the extent of blood bank testing that should be completed before the case begins based on local experience. Thus, ideally the MSBOS should be consulted and a specimen drawn days or weeks before the patient's scheduled OR date to allow the blood bank to perform the testing and locate antigen-negative units if necessary. Furthermore, if the surgical team has reason to believe that their patient has an underlying condition predisposing him or her to blood product replacement requirements in excess of the MSBOS recommendation, then it is appropriate to ensure that pretransfusion testing is complete before an elective case begins. The Joint Commission considers timely and accurate pretransfusion testing to be an important blood management performance measure, highlighting, in particular, the need to have appropriate testing completed before the start of anesthesia. This study sought to determine the number of times surgical patients were in or were en route to the OR without completed pretransfusion testing and to try to find ways to prevent this error from occurring in the future.

M. G. Bissell, MD, PhD, MPH

The Development of a Novel Molecular Assay Examining the Role of Aminopeptidase P Polymorphisms in Acute Hypotensive Transfusion Reactions

Hui Y, Wu YY, Tormey CA (Univ at Buffalo, NY; Yale Univ School of Medicine, New Haven, CT; et al)

Arch Pathol Lab Med 137:96-99, 2013

Context.—Acute hypotensive transfusion reactions are potentially harmful adverse effects of transfusion attributable to bradykinin generation. They are most often seen in patients taking angiotensin-converting enzyme (ACE) inhibitors (ACE-Is) because of the role ACE plays in metabolizing bradykinin. However, a number of acute hypotensive transfusion reactions occur in patients not taking ACE-Is. Aminopeptidase P (APP), another important enzyme responsible for bradykinin degradation, is encoded by the polymorphic *XPNPEP2* gene. Some polymorphisms in *XPNPEP2* have been associated with decreased APP activity. However, the role that APP polymorphisms play in acute hypotensive transfusion reactions has never been investigated.

Objective.—To develop a molecular assay to examine for the C-2399A single-nucleotide polymorphism (SNP) in the APP gene, *XPNPEP2*, in patients experiencing acute hypotensive transfusion reactions unassociated with ACEIs.

Design.—We developed an assay using polymerase chain reaction and DNA sequencing with primers targeted at *XPNPEP2* (59-GAGTATTATGTGGGACCATCC-3' and 5'-ATGCCTCGCAGAGACAAGAG-3'). Polymorphism zygosity was determined by comparing the sense/antisense sequencing results. This assay was then applied to patients with acute hypotensive transfusion reactions not taking ACE-Is (n = 4).

Results.—A C-2399A SNP assay was successfully developed and applied to patients with acute hypotensive transfusion reactions. In a pilot study, 2 patients (50%) were found to possess C-2399A polymorphisms. One was found to be homozygous, and the other was heterozygous.

Conclusions.—Our C-2399A SNP assay can be used to study acute hypotensive transfusion reactions in patients not taking ACE-Is. Initial data indicate that the C-2399A polymorphism may be a contributing factor in such reactions. However, further studies are necessary to better define the role of APP polymorphisms in relation to acute hypotensive transfusion reactions unassociated with ACEIs.

▶ Acute hypotensive transfusion reactions are relatively rare but potentially serious adverse events in which a transfusion recipient manifests a marked decrease in blood pressure with a virtual absence of other signs and symptoms. Much of the pathophysiology of acute hypotensive transfusion reactions has been linked to bradykinins and their metabolites, mediators that can induce substantial vasodilation and smooth muscle relaxation in vivo, with a resultant decrease in blood pressure. Some studies have also shown that bradykinin accumulation and hypotensive episodes may be exacerbated in transfused patients taking angiotensin-converting enzyme (ACE) inhibitors (ACE-Is), because ACE is a key enzyme in the degradation of bradykinin. However, based on reports of acute hypotensive transfusion reactions occurring in the absence of ACE-I use, it is possible that other pathways may contribute to the accumulation of bradykinin or its metabolites and result in hypotension in the setting of transfusion. With regard to alternative pathways of bradykinin metabolism, the enzyme aminopeptidase P (APP) is of particular interest. APP, present in cytosolic and membrane-bound forms, is estimated to be responsible for the degradation of about 20% to 25% of circulating bradykinin. More importantly, APP is the enzyme primarily responsible for the degradation of desArg9-bradykinin, the active metabolite of bradykinin. Notably, the *XPNPEP2* gene responsible for coding membrane-bound APP is polymorphic. The C-2399A single-nucleotide polymorphism (SNP) in *XPNPEP2* results in a substantially truncated APP protein that cannot adequately bind to the membrane of host epithelial cells, thereby reducing its ability to participate in bradykinin–bradykinin metabolite degradation. In fact, several studies have demonstrated that the C-2399A SNP in *XPNPEP2* is associated with decreased APP activity and angioedema in selected populations. To date, however, few studies have investigated the role of APP in acute hypotensive transfusion reactions, and no studies have determined whether the C-2399A SNP may be a contributing factor to acute hypotensive transfusion reactions in patients not taking ACE-Is. The primary aim of this study was to develop an assay for the C-2399A SNP, but further studies will be necessary to more deeply explore the possible relationship between acute hypotensive transfusion reactions and polymorphisms in the *APP* gene.

M. G. Bissell, MD, PhD, MPH

New direct and indirect methods for the detection of cyclooxygenase 1 acetylation by aspirin; the lack of aspirin resistance among healthy individuals

Kovács EG, Katona É, Bereczky Z, et al (Med and Health Science Ctr, Debrecen, Hungary; et al)

Thromb Res 131:320-324, 2013

Background.—Aspirin is widely used in the prevention of acute atherothrombotic complications. It acetylates Ser529 residue in cyclooxygenase-1 (COX-1) and prevents thromboxane A_2 (TXA_2) formation from arachidonic acid (AA) in platelets. Laboratory methods used for the detection of aspirin effect provide inconsistent results.

Methods.—Two new methods were developed for the direct and indirect detection of COX-1 acetylation by aspirin in 108 healthy volunteers treated daily with 100 mg enteric-coated aspirin for 7 days. Monoclonal antibodies were raised against acetylated and non-acetylated nonapeptides corresponding to the amino acid sequence of human COX-1 525–533 residues. Using Western blotting technique the antibodies clearly distinguished between acetylated and non-acetylated COX-1 in platelet lysate. The

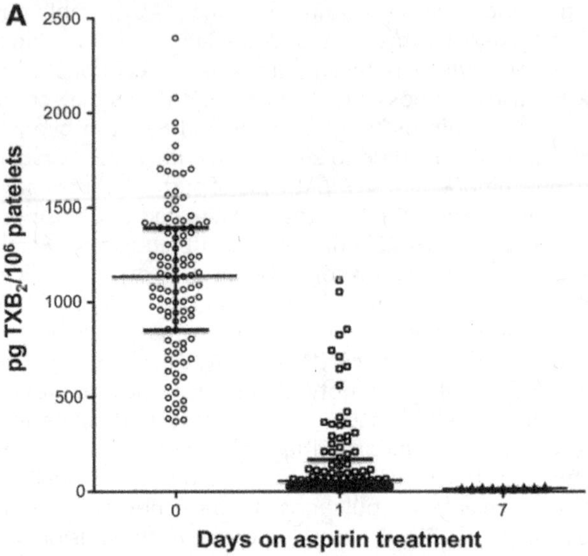

B

Arachidonic acid induced TXB_2 production of platelets ($pg\ TXB_2/10^6$ platelets)		
Day 0	Day 1	Day 7
1140 IQR: 854-1396 range 372-2394	**59** IQR: 28-171 range 7-1118	**16** IQR: 12-19 range 4-35

FIGURE 1.—The effect of aspirin treatment on arachidonic acid-induced TXB_2 production of platelets. Individual values on day 0 (○), day 1 (□) and day 7 (Δ) of aspirin treatment are demonstrated in the upper part (A) of the Figure. Long horizontal lines represent median values, while shorter horizontal lines correspond to the upper and lower limits of interquartile ranges (IQRs). As on day 7 very low TXB_2 production was observed in all cases, crowded individual values cannot be distinguished from each other and horizontal lines are hardly seen. In the lower part (B) the median values with IQRs and with total ranges are shown. The differences between day 0 and day1 or day7 values are highly significant ($p < 0.001$). (Reprinted from Thrombosis Research. Kovács EG, Katona É, Bereczky Z, et al. New direct and indirect methods for the detection of cyclooxygenase 1 acetylation by aspirin; the lack of aspirin resistance among healthy individuals. *Thromb Res*. 2013;131:320-324, Copyright 2013, with permission from Elsevier.)

second method measures AA-induced TXB_2 production of platelets in diluted platelet rich plasma.

Results.—No acetylated COX-1 was detected in platelets before aspirin treatment. At the same time antibodies raised against non-acetylated peptide gave intense reaction with COX-1 on the Western blot. In contrast, after 7 days of aspirin treatment, with a single exception, only acetylated COX-1 could be detected in the platelet lysate. The non-responding volunteer showed full response to aspirin after controlled drug intake. In parallel experiments aspirin treatment for 7 days practically completely inhibited AA-induced TXB_2 production by platelets.

Conclusions.—Chemical ("true") aspirin resistance, if it exists, must be a rarity among healthy individuals. The new methods could be used for detecting the acetylation of COX-1 by aspirin in patients on preventive aspirin therapy and for evaluating methods routinely used for such purpose (Fig 1).

► Low-dose aspirin (acetylsalicylic acid) treatment is a cornerstone in the prevention and treatment of acute atherothrombotic complications, like myocardial infarction and stroke. It reduces vascular death and nonfatal vascular events by approximately 15% and 30%, respectively. The antithrombotic action of aspirin is primarily based on its antiplatelet action. As an acetylating agent, it acetylates Ser529 residue in cyclooxygenase-1 (COX-1). COX-1 catalyzes the production of cyclic endoperoxides, prostaglandins G and H, from arachidonic acid (M). M is released from membrane phospholipids by phospholipase A_2 activated after the interaction of agonists with their platelet receptors. Prostaglandin H is then converted to thromboxane A_2 (TXA_2), a highly powerful platelet activator, by thromboxane synthase. The covalent modification of Ser529, sitting in the wall of the active site pocket of COX-1, prevents the access of M to the active site and blocks TXA_2 production by platelet throughout its lifespan. The fact that aspirin prevents acute vascular events only in some of the patients suggested that significant individual variations exist in the responsiveness to the drug. For this reason, the term "aspirin resistance" was introduced. Unfortunately, "aspirin resistance" has not been unequivocally defined, creating difficulties in the interpretation of results and also in setting up recommendations for the treatment of patients. The term covers 3 different, although not unrelated, definitions: (1) chemical (true) aspirin resistance—the lack of acetylation of platelet COX-I at Ser529 by aspirin; (2) laboratory resistance, or preferably, nonresponsiveness—diminished response to aspirin as measured by a laboratory test; (3) clinical resistance, or rather, ineffectiveness—aspirin does not protect the individual from acute vascular events. Clinical ineffectiveness could be established only retrospectively, as routinely used laboratory tests show high inter- and intraindividual variation, and there is considerable discrepancy between results obtained by different tests. Surprisingly, no laboratory test that directly detects chemical resistance, such as, the acetylation of COX-I, has been described. The aim of this study was 2-fold: (1) to develop 2 new methods, one for the direct detection of chemical aspirin resistance by using monoclonal antibodies specific to acetylated COX-I, or to nonacetylated COX-I, and another one that measures AA-induced production of TXB_2, the inactive metabolite of TXA_2 in platelet-rich plasma and (2) using the aforementioned methods to establish the frequency of true aspirin resistance among healthy individuals (Fig 1).

M. G. Bissell, MD, PhD, MPH

18 Cytogenetics and Molecular Pathology

Exome and Whole-Genome Sequencing as Clinical Tests: A Transformative Practice in Molecular Diagnostics

Yu Y, Wu B-L, Wu J, et al (Jiaotong Univ School of Medicine, Shanghai, China; Boston Children's Hosp, MA)

Clin Chem 58:1507-1509, 2012

Background.—Next-generation sequencing (NGS) has rapidly moved from revolutionizing how one interrogates the genetic causes of rare single-gene disorders into roles in clinical diagnostic areas. Molecular diagnostic testing reflects NGS principles, with many NGS-based tests for multigene panels not available. Exome sequencing is now emerging as a feasible way to conduct clinical tests. Few patients have been tested by whole-exome sequencing (WES) or whole-genome sequencing (WGS), but the results obtained to date have demonstrated the practicality of NGS testing. Some of the characteristics of NGS-based tests and issues related to analytic pursuits were outlined.

Validation.—Depending on the capture method used, exome areas can variably be resistant. Even the same exome-capturing kit can have different capture efficiency in different experiments and can demonstrate different total numbers of sequence reads generated by each run. Variant-calling algorithms can generate variant sets that overlap. As a result, the number of variants detected will differ. Validating NGS-based tests is difficult, but assays should become more standardized and consistent in the future.

Function.—WES/WGS tests assay all the genes or the whole genome. Both discovery and diagnostic functionalities are associated with WES/WGS tests. This dual functionality has direct implications for the selection of patients and family members and for the process of data analysis. After all the variants are filtered, the inheritance pattern, information on segregation, functional annotation of the variant, and correlation with a predicted disease mechanism are needed to identify the most likely candidate gene. Dominant disorder identifications are facilitated by parental samples to detect de novo variants. Having samples from additional family members helps in both dominant and recessive disorders, reducing considerably the number of candidate genes. It is then crucial to pinpoint the causal variant(s). Eventually gene expression profiling with high-throughput whole-transcriptome sequencing technologies and high-throughput functional assays will extend the clinical diagnostic step that will clarify causation.

Comparison.—Choosing WES or WGS is often based on pragmatic concerns such as cost, turnaround time, labor needed for data generation, and data storage requirements. WGS is anticipated to become more widely used in clinical situations, but current practice uses WES and gene panel-n-based tests. The full potential of WGS awaits a fuller understanding of how noncoding regions function. WES, WGS, and comprehensive gene panel tests offer options for different disease groups and specific conditions. A combined approach has the advantage of allowing the capture of all genomic variants.

Conclusions.—NGS-based molecular diagnostic tests have shown excellent clinical usefulness for single-gene disorders. Further developments and a better understanding of the potential of WES/WGS should greatly improve the practice of genomic medicine and the patient care associated with it.

▶ In the last few years, next-generation sequencing (NGS) has revolutionized the approaches by which we interrogate the genetic causes of rare single-gene disorders. More recently, NGS has been rapidly moving into the clinical diagnostics arena and transforming the practice of molecular diagnostics testing. Many NGS-based tests for multigene panels are available in clinical laboratories. Now, proof-of-principle studies are showing the feasibility of using exome sequencing for clinical testing. Conventional molecular diagnostics tests evaluate a defined number of exons for one or more genes, the selection of which is based on the best clinical judgment after thorough evaluation of the patient's clinical presentation. These tests, which are performed in Clinical Laboratory Improvement Amendments-certified laboratories, are mainly for Mendelian disorders with well-established causal relationships between genes and diseases. NGS-based comprehensive gene panels, whole exome sequencing–based tests, or whole genome sequencing–based tests, however, assay for a substantially larger number of genes and genomic regions, only a small proportion of which would potentially be associated with the patient's condition. NGS-based tests are performed mainly for patients without a clear clinical diagnosis or for patients who have negative test results for genes known to be associated with the disorder. Clinical diagnostics laboratories are actively engaged in implementing NGS-based tests. This article reviews some important characteristics of NGS-based tests and discusses a few outstanding analytical issues, with the hope of gaining a better understanding of the nature of this transformative diagnostic approach and achieving a glimpse into the future of NGS-based tests.

M. G. Bissell, MD, PhD, MPH

Development of a Genomic DNA Reference Material Panel for Myotonic Dystrophy Type 1 (DM1) Genetic Testing

Kalman L, Tarleton J, Hitch M, et al (Ctrs for Disease Control and Prevention, Atlanta, GA; Mission Hosp, Asheville, NC; et al)

J Mol Diagn 15:518-525, 2013

Myotonic dystrophy type 1 (DM1) is caused by expansion of a CTG triplet repeat in the 3′ untranslated region of the *DMPK* gene that encodes a serine-threonine kinase. Patients with larger repeats tend to have a more severe phenotype. Clinical laboratories require reference and quality control materials for DM1 diagnostic and carrier genetic testing. Well-characterized reference materials are not available. To address this need, the Centers for Disease Control and Prevention–based Genetic Testing Reference Material Coordination Program, in collaboration with members of the genetic testing community, the National Registry of Myotonic Dystrophy and Facioscapulohumeral Muscular Dystrophy Patients and Family Members, and the Coriell Cell Repositories, has established and characterized cell lines from patients with DM1 to create a reference material panel. The CTG repeats in genomic DNA samples from 10 DM1 cell lines were characterized in three clinical genetic testing laboratories using PCR and Southern blot analysis. *DMPK* alleles in the samples cover four of five DM1 clinical categories: normal (5 to 34 repeats), mild (50 to 100 repeats), classical (101 to 1000 repeats), and congenital (>1000 repeats). We did not identify or establish Coriell cell lines in the premutation range (35 to 49 repeats). These samples are publicly available for quality control, proficiency testing, test development, and research and should help improve the accuracy of DM1 testing.

▶ Myotonic dystrophy type 1 (DM1; Steinert disease), the most common form of adult muscular dystrophy, is a dominantly inherited, multisystem disorder that typically affects skeletal, smooth, and cardiac muscle; the eyes; the brain; and endocrine function. Although penetrance is approximately 100% by age 50 years, there is variable expressivity, and mild cases may be misdiagnosed or undiagnosed. DM1 results from an unstable CTG triplet expansion in the 3′ untranslated region of the *DMPK* gene (encodes a serine-threonine kinase) located on chromosome 19q13.3. Molecular genetic testing for DM1 relies primarily on measurement of the number of CTG repeats in the *DMPK* gene isolated from circulating leukocyte DNA. Polymerase chain reaction can be used to measure repeat length in *DMPK* alleles up to approximately 100 CTG repeats. Southern blot analysis is used to detect larger expansions. There are currently no US Food and Drug Administration–approved or cleared molecular genetic tests for DM1. All clinical testing is currently performed using tests developed in the individual laboratory. Clinical laboratories use characterized reference materials for several quality assurance purposes, including test development, test validation, quality control, and for alternative assessment. There are no commercial or other sources of characterized reference materials for molecular genetic testing of DM1. Laboratories that perform this test typically use characterized genomic

DNA from cell lines, such as those available from the National Institute of General Medical Sciences (NIGMS) repository at the Coriell Institute for Medical Research (Camden, NJ) or residual patient samples, as reference materials. Laboratories and proficiency testing programs have been unable to obtain many of the necessary reference materials because cell lines and patient samples with the complete range of CTG repeat lengths are not readily available. To address this need, the Centers for Disease Control and Prevention's Genetic Testing Reference Material Coordination Program collaborated with members of the genetic testing community, the NIGMS repository, and the National Institutes of Health–funded National Registry of Myotonic Dystrophy and Facioscapulohumeral Muscular Dystrophy Patients and Family Members. This report describes the characterization of new and preexisting cell lines in 3 clinical genetic testing laboratories and the development of a DM1 reference material panel for research and improved clinical testing.

M. G. Bissell, MD, PhD, MPH

Very Low PSA Concentrations and Deletions of the *KLK3* Gene

Rodriguez S, Al-Ghamdi OA, Burrows K, et al (Univ of Bristol, UK; et al)

Clin Chem 59:234-244, 2012

Background.—Prostate-specific antigen (PSA), a widely used biomarker for prostate cancer (PCa), is encoded by a kallikrein gene (*KLK3*, kallikrein-related peptidase 3). Serum PSA concentrations vary in the population, with PCa patients generally showing higher PSA concentrations than control individuals, although a small proportion of individuals in the population display very low PSA concentrations. We hypothesized that very low PSA concentrations might reflect gene-inactivating mutations in *KLK3* that lead to abnormally reduced gene expression.

Methods.—We have sequenced all *KLK3* exons and the promoter and searched for gross deletions or duplications in *KLK3* in the 30 individuals with the lowest observed PSA concentrations in a sample of approximately 85 000 men from the Prostate Testing for Cancer and Treatment (ProtecT) study. The ProtecT study examines a community-based population of men from across the UK with little prior PSA testing.

Results.—We observed no stop codons or frameshift mutations, but we did find 30 single-base genetic variants, including 3 variants not described previously. These variants included missense variants that could be functionally inactivating and splicing variants. At this stage, however, we cannot confidently conclude whether these variants markedly lower PSA concentration or activity. More importantly, we identified 3 individuals with different large heterozygous deletions that encompass all *KLK3* exons. The absence of a functional copy of *KLK3* in these individuals is consistent with their reduced serum PSA concentrations.

Conclusions.—The clinical interpretation of the PSA test for individuals with *KLK3* gene inactivation could lead to false-negative PSA findings used for screening, diagnosis, or monitoring of PCa.

▶ Prostate-specific antigen (PSA) is a serine protease produced specifically in the prostate. Although most PSA is found in semen, a small proportion is found in the bloodstream. The PSA test is used for diagnosis and disease monitoring and has been advocated for prostate cancer (PCa) screening. Serum PSA concentrations are generally increased in PCa, although this test lacks specificity, and the reference interval is quite wide. In addition, there is variation in the distribution of PSA concentrations in the general population, which is caused by differences in the volume of prostatic tissue and ethnicity. Drugs (eg, finasteride) and genetic variation also influence PSA concentrations. Intraindividual variations in PSA, PSA measurement error, and their implications for early detection of PCa have also been described. PSA is encoded by *KLK3* (kallikrein-related peptidase 3), a member of a family of 15 kallikrein genes located on human chromosome 19. Common single-nucleotide polymorphisms in *KLK3* have been associated with variation in PSA concentrations. The authors' hypothesis is that very low serum PSA concentrations may reflect inactivating gene mutations or gross genetic rearrangements involving *KLK3*. To test this hypothesis, they conducted a detailed genetic analysis of 30 individuals with the lowest observed PSA concentrations (<0.1 μg/L) in a cohort of approximately 85 000 men from the Prostate Testing for Cancer and Treatment Study.

M. G. Bissell, MD, PhD, MPH

Karyotype versus Microarray Testing for Genetic Abnormalities after Stillbirth

Reddy UM, for the NICHD Stillbirth Collaborative Research Network (Natl Insts of Health, Bethesda, MD; et al)
N Engl J Med 367:2185-2193, 2012

Background.—Genetic abnormalities have been associated with 6 to 13% of stillbirths, but the true prevalence may be higher. Unlike karyotype analysis, microarray analysis does not require live cells, and it detects small deletions and duplications called copy-number variants.

Methods.—The Stillbirth Collaborative Research Network conducted a population-based study of stillbirth in five geographic catchment areas. Standardized postmortem examinations and karyotype analyses were performed. A single-nucleotide polymorphism array was used to detect copy-number variants of at least 500 kb in placental or fetal tissue. Variants that were not identified in any of three databases of apparently unaffected persons were then classified into three groups: probably benign, clinical significance unknown, or pathogenic. We compared the results of karyotype and microarray analyses of samples obtained after delivery.

Results.—In our analysis of samples from 532 stillbirths, microarray analysis yielded results more often than did karyotype analysis (87.4% vs. 70.5%, $P < 0.001$) and provided better detection of genetic abnormalities (aneuploidy or pathogenic copy-number variants, 8.3% vs. 5.8%; $P = 0.007$). Microarray analysis also identified more genetic abnormalities among 443 antepartum stillbirths (8.8% vs. 6.5%, $P = 0.02$) and 67 stillbirths with congenital anomalies (29.9% vs. 19.4%, $P = 0.008$). As compared with karyotype analysis, microarray analysis provided a relative increase in the diagnosis of genetic abnormalities of 41.9% in all stillbirths, 34.5% in antepartum stillbirths, and 53.8% in stillbirths with anomalies.

Conclusions.—Microarray analysis is more likely than karyotype analysis to provide a genetic diagnosis, primarily because of its success with nonviable tissue, and is especially valuable in analyses of stillbirths with congenital anomalies or in cases in which karyotype results cannot be obtained. (Funded by the Eunice Kennedy Shriver National Institute of Child Health and Human Development.)

▶ Stillbirth, which is defined as fetal death at or after 20 weeks of gestation, occurs in one of every 160 births in the United States. Despite extensive evaluation, 25% to 60% of stillbirths remain unexplained. Karyotypic abnormalities are detected in 6% to 13% of stillbirths with a successful karyotype analysis. Some stillbirths may have chromosomal imbalances below the resolution of conventional cytogenetic analysis, which is typically 5 to 10 Mb. Single-nucleotide polymorphism oligonucleotide microarray analysis detects almost all genomic imbalances recognized by karyotyping, as well as smaller deletions and duplications in the kilobase range, termed *copy-number variants*. Microarray analysis can be performed on DNA from nonviable, or even macerated, tissue. The authors tested the hypothesis that microarray analysis detects abnormalities in stillbirth samples more often than karyotype analysis.

M. G. Bissell, MD, PhD, MPH

Chromosomal Microarray versus Karyotyping for Prenatal Diagnosis

Wapner RJ, Martin CL, Levy B, et al (Columbia Univ Med Ctr, NY; Emory Univ School of Medicine, Atlanta, GA; et al)

N Engl J Med 367:2175-2184, 2012

Background.—Chromosomal microarray analysis has emerged as a primary diagnostic tool for the evaluation of developmental delay and structural malformations in children. We aimed to evaluate the accuracy, efficacy, and incremental yield of chromosomal microarray analysis as compared with karyotyping for routine prenatal diagnosis.

Methods.—Samples from women undergoing prenatal diagnosis at 29 centers were sent to a central karyotyping laboratory. Each sample was split in two; standard karyotyping was performed on one portion and the other was sent to one of four laboratories for chromosomal microarray.

Results.—We enrolled a total of 4406 women. Indications for prenatal diagnosis were advanced maternal age (46.6%), abnormal result on Down's syndrome screening (18.8%), structural anomalies on ultrasonography (25.2%), and other indications (9.4%). In 4340 (98.8%) of the fetal samples, microarray analysis was successful; 87.9% of samples could be used without tissue culture. Microarray analysis of the 4282 nonmosaic samples identified all the aneuploidies and unbalanced rearrangements identified on karyotyping but did not identify balanced translocations and fetal triploidy. In samples with a normal karyotype, microarray analysis revealed clinically relevant deletions or duplications in 6.0% with a structural anomaly and in 1.7% of those whose indications were advanced maternal age or positive screening results.

Conclusions.—In the context of prenatal diagnostic testing, chromosomal microarray analysis identified additional, clinically significant cytogenetic information as compared with karyotyping and was equally efficacious in identifying aneuploidies and unbalanced rearrangements but did not identify balanced translocations and triploidies. (Funded by the Eunice Kennedy Shriver National Institute of Child Health and Human Development and others; ClinicalTrials.gov number, NCT01279733.)

▶ The development of array-based molecular cytogenetic techniques has improved the detection of small genomic deletions and duplications (called copy-number variants) that are not routinely seen on karyotyping, the standard cytogenetic analysis performed. Copy-number variants result in a variation from the expected number of copies of a segment of DNA (ie, the number in a normal genome). Copy-number variants can be either benign or pathogenic, depending on their location and genetic content. They are identified with the use of chromosomal microarray analysis in which a test sample of DNA from the patient is compared directly or indirectly with a reference (normal) genome. Identification of copy-number variants has been particularly helpful in the evaluation of children with congenital structural anomalies or altered neurocognitive development, including those diagnosed with autism spectrum disorders. Chromosomal microarray analysis identifies a genetic cause in an additional 12% to 15% of affected children, as compared with the current standard of karyotyping, leading to recommendations that microarray analysis should become the first-tier test for such children. The incremental value of chromosomal microarray in the analysis of stillborn pregnancies has been demonstrated. As compared with karyotyping, microarray analysis had a higher likelihood of obtaining a result and identified an increased incidence of genomic abnormalities among stillborn infants. Microarray analysis for prenatal diagnosis has been evaluated in small studies involving women whose fetus had a high probability of having chromosome abnormalities, such as those resulting in structural anomalies. These studies have shown the technical feasibility of microarray analysis. It remains uncertain, however, whether microarray analysis reliably detects all chromosome abnormalities diagnosed on standard karyotyping, and how often abnormal microarray results are not detected on karyotyping. The authors conducted a large, prospective study of prenatal diagnostic samples to assess, in blinded fashion, the ability of microarray analysis to diagnose common chromosome abnormalities and to gauge the extent of additional information provided by microarray analysis as compared with standard karyotyping.

M. G. Bissell, MD, PhD, MPH

Comparative Analytical Utility of DNA Derived from Alternative Human Specimens for Molecular Autopsy and Diagnostics

Klassen TL, von Rüden E-L, Drabek J, et al (Baylor College of Medicine, Houston, TX)

J Mol Diagn 14:451-457, 2012

Genetic testing and research have increased the demand for high-quality DNA that has traditionally been obtained by venipuncture. However, venous blood collection may prove difficult in special populations and when large-scale specimen collection or exchange is prerequisite for international collaborative investigations. Guthrie/FTA card–based blood spots, buccal scrapes, and finger nail clippings are DNA-containing specimens that are uniquely accessible and thus attractive as alternative tissue sources (ATS). The literature details a variety of protocols for extraction of nucleic acids from a singular ATS type, but their utility has not been systematically analyzed in comparison with conventional sources such as venous blood. Additionally, the efficacy of each protocol is often equated with the overall nucleic acid yield but not with the analytical performance of the DNA during mutation detection. Together with a critical in-depth literature review of published extraction methods, we developed and evaluated an all-inclusive approach for serial, systematic, and direct comparison of DNA utility from multiple biological samples. Our results point to the often underappreciated value of these alternative tissue sources and highlight ways to maximize the ATS-derived DNA for optimal quantity, quality, and utility as a function of extraction method. Our comparative analysis clarifies the value of ATS in genomic analysis projects for population-based screening, diagnostics, molecular autopsy, medico-legal investigations, or multi-organ surveys of suspected mosaicisms.

▶ The demand for genetic diagnosis is rising steeply, including preemptive screening, diagnostics, adverse reaction risk assessment, familial and population genetic profiling, and molecular autopsy. This dramatically increases the need for optimal collection and processing so that samples are amenable to a wide range of research and diagnostic applications and often to the establishment of a renewable tissue source such as perpetual cell lines. Blood and organ-derived specimens possess many of these attributes; however, their procurement often encounters logistical and ethical obstacles. DNA-containing specimens, such as saliva, buccal specimens, nail clippings, and blood spots, are alternative tissue sources (ATS) that offer cost-effective, practical, and minimally or noninvasive options that are appealing to medical professionals and candidate research participants. They are easy to collect, store, and ship, which is especially important in large-scale national and international familial or population screening programs and in molecular autopsy. There are numerous published reports on processing individual alternative samples using resulting DNA quantity or genotyping success as a surrogate measure of optimal methodology or sample utility. Unfortunately, this extensive technical knowledge base is inconsistent, lacking a rationale for the chosen processing steps and rigorous, systematic, comparative data on multiple ATS vs conventional blood samples as to their performance in downstream applications. This has hampered broader acceptance of alternative specimens as valuable research and diagnostic material.

The objectives of this study were to analyze the common processing steps and develop an informed extraction approach for the most commonly and easily available alternative samples, such as blood spots, buccal scrapes, and nail clippings, and to perform a parallel comparison of ATS vs conventional samples as to DNA quality, quantity, and genomic diagnostic ability. The authors have placed the results of this analysis in both a scientific and educational context that can be readily used by all personnel involved in translational genomic research and diagnostics.

M. G. Bissell, MD, PhD, MPH

Inherited Cardiomyopathies: Molecular Genetics and Clinical Genetic Testing in the Postgenomic Era

Teekakirikul P, Kelly MA, Rehm HL, et al (Harvard Med School, Boston, MA; Partners HealthCare Ctr for Personalized Genetic Medicine, Cambridge, MA; et al)

J Mol Diagn 15:158-170, 2013

Inherited cardiomyopathies include hypertrophic cardiomyopathy, dilated cardiomyopathy, arrhythmogenic right ventricular cardiomyopathy, left ventricular noncompaction, and restrictive cardiomyopathy. These diseases have a substantial genetic component and predispose to sudden cardiac death, which provides a high incentive to identify and sequence disease genes in affected individuals to identify pathogenic variants. Clinical genetic testing, which is now widely available, can be a powerful tool for identifying presymptomatic individuals. However, locus and allelic heterogeneity are the rule, as are clinical variability and reduced penetrance of disease in carriers of pathogenic variants. These factors, combined with genetic and phenotypic overlap between different cardiomyopathies, have made clinical genetic testing a lengthy and costly process. Next-generation sequencing technologies have removed many limitations such that comprehensive testing is now feasible, shortening diagnostic odysseys for clinically complex cases. Remaining challenges include the incomplete understanding of the spectrum of benign and pathogenic variants in the cardiomyopathy genes, which is a source of inconclusive results. This review provides an overview of inherited cardiomyopathies with a focus on their genetic etiology and diagnostic testing in the postgenomic era.

► Inherited cardiomyopathies are cardiovascular disorders classified based on ventricular morphology and function and include hypertrophic cardiomyopathy (HCM), dilated cardiomyopathy (DCM), arrhythmogenic right ventricular cardiomyopathy (ARVC), left ventricular noncompaction (LVNC), and restrictive cardiomyopathy (RCM). Of these, HCM is the most common, with an estimated prevalence of 1 in 500 individuals. Common complications can include heart failure and sudden cardiac death (SCD), and undiagnosed disease (particularly in HCM and ARVC) accounts for a significant proportion of SCD in young adults and athletes. Since the discovery that pathogenic variants in the sarcomere genes cause HCM, many advancements have been made to define the genetic etiology of inherited cardiomyopathies. The increased risk of SCD in individuals with disease encouraged interest in clinical genetic testing, which began approximately a decade ago and is now widely available through genetic testing laboratories in the United States and worldwide. However, the high degree of locus and allelic heterogeneity that is characteristic of all cardiomyopathies necessitates sequence analysis of the entire coding region of multiple genes, which has been a costly and lengthy process using traditional technologies. Growing genetic and phenotypic overlap among different cardiomyopathies adds further complexity, often resulting in stepwise testing of multiple disease-specific gene panels when the diagnosis is not entirely clear. Next-generation sequencing (NGS) technologies have removed these barriers and enabled testing of a large number of genes simultaneously. NGS-based test panels are now offered by a growing number of diagnostic laboratories worldwide, which is beginning to change the landscape of medical genetic testing. However, an unwelcome effect of this unprecedented ability to sequence any gene is an increased likelihood of detecting variants of unclear clinical significance (VUSs). This effect necessitates a stringent review of the evidence supporting claims of disease association as variants in insufficiently studied genes can be difficult to interpret. However, because genetic testing for inherited cardiomyopathies is a relatively young discipline, the spectrum of pathogenic variants present in the population is incompletely characterized, even in well-established disease genes. This leaves a high probability of detecting a novel sequence VUS, which can create substantial emotional difficulties for patients. This review summarizes the clinical features of inherited cardiomyopathies, current knowledge on the genetic etiologies, and clinical genetic testing in the postgenomic era (Fig 1 in the original article).

M. G. Bissell, MD, PhD, MPH

Bacterial Genomics in Infectious Disease and the Clinical Pathology Laboratory

Olsen RJ, Long SW, Musser JM (The Methodist Hosp System, Houston, TX; The Methodist Hosp Res Inst, Houston, TX)

Arch Pathol Lab Med 136:1414-1422, 2012

Context.—Throughout history, technologic advancements have fueled the engine of innovation, which, in turn, has driven discovery. Accordingly, recent advancements in DNA sequencing technology are revolutionizing bacterial genomics.

Objective.—To review important developments from the literature. The current state of bacterial genomics, with an emphasis on human pathogens and the clinical pathology laboratory, will be discussed.

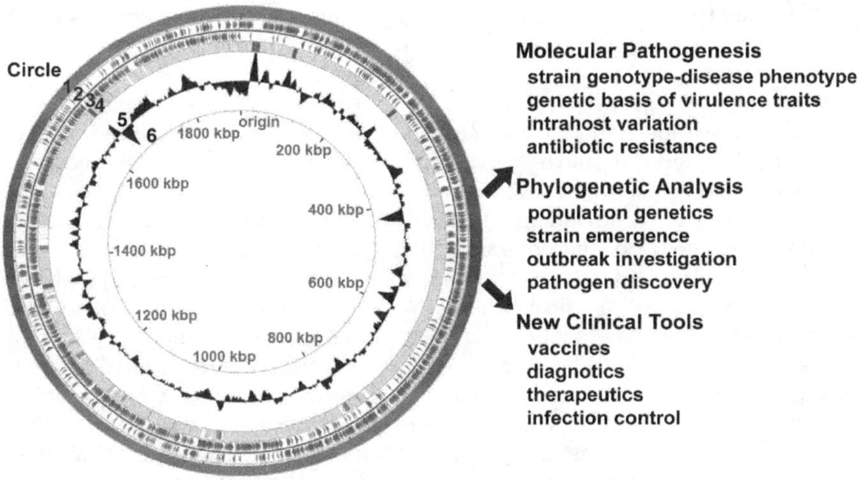

FIGURE 1.—Whole-genome sequence data for bacteria may be graphically displayed as a circular map. Each concentric circle confers a different piece of information. Shown here is a circular map comparing the whole-genome sequences of 2 hypothetical strains. The outermost circle depicts predicted gene function (color-coded to represent basic functions, such as carbohydrate metabolism or immune evasion). Moving inward, the second and third circles show the predicted coding sequences (arrows) on the forward and reverse strands of the chromosome, respectively. The fourth circle compares gene content between the 2 strains being analyzed. Sequences present in both genomes (the core genome) are shown as pink bars. In comparison, sequences that are unique to the reference genome (absent in the comparator strain) are shown as white bars, and sequences that are unique to the comparator genome (absent in the reference strain) are shown as red bars. In many bacterial species, mobile genetic elements, such as prophages, are the primary mechanism for strains to acquire new gene content. Prophages frequently encode virulence factors and antibiotic resistance genes responsible for the emergence of new subclonal lineages and lead to outbreaks. Alternatively, subtle genetic changes, such as single-nucleotide polymorphisms, may also significantly affect strain genotype—disease phenotype relationships. The fifth circle shows G + C nucleic acid content, a predictor of gene-encoding sequences. Finally, the innermost circle (circle 6) shows landmarks, such as the origin of replication, around the circular chromosome. Whole-genome sequencing and comparative genomics are powerful tools for infectious disease researchers and laboratory physicians, enabling them to gain insight into molecular pathogenesis and to perform fine-structure phylogenetic analyses. These data sets can then be used to create new clinical tools, such as vaccines, therapies, and diagnostics. For Interpretation of the references to color in this figure legend, the reader is referred to web version of this article. (Reproduced with permission of College of American Pathologists from Olsen RJ, Long SW, Musser JM. Bacterial genomics in infectious disease and the clinical pathology laboratory. *Arch Pathol Lab Med.* 2012;136:1414-1422, permission conveyed through Copyright Clearance Center, Inc.)

Data Sources.—A comprehensive review was performed of the relevant literature indexed in PubMed (National Library of Medicine) and referenced medical texts.

Conclusions.—Many important discoveries bearing on infectious disease research and pathology laboratory practice have been achieved through whole-genome sequencing strategies. Bacterial genomics has improved our understanding of molecular pathogenesis, host-pathogen interactions, and antibiotic-resistance mechanisms. Bacterial genomics has also facilitated the study of population structures, epidemics and outbreaks, and newly identified pathogens. Many opportunities now exist for clinical

pathologists to contribute to bacterial genomics, including in the design of new diagnostic tests, therapeutic agents, and vaccines (Fig 1).

▶ Microbial pathogenesis researchers and infectious disease specialists have long sought to understand the molecular basis of human disease caused by bacteria. Although new data can be generated with current methodologies, and paradigm shifts can occur with re-evaluation of current knowledge, the most historic advancements have followed an introduction of new technologies. Today, next-generation sequencing platforms and bioinformatics tools are opening a new chapter in the history of infectious disease research and clinical pathology laboratory practice. The authors review clinically relevant discoveries generated from bacterial whole-genome sequencing, with an emphasis on human pathogens and laboratory medicine. The studies discussed in this article represent illustrative examples and are not intended to be a comprehensive review. The first complete bacterial genome, *Haemophilus influenzae* strain Rd, was sequenced in 1995. Although the *H influenzae* genome was relatively small (only 1 830 137 base pairs), the project took more than 1 year to complete and cost an estimated $1 million. Two years later, DNA sequencing technology was advancing at a rate similar to Moore's law. Moore's law predicts a doubling of computational microprocessor power every 24 months. Importantly, the cost for generating sequence data has also steadily decreased. It is now possible, depending on the instrument used, to sequence the complete genome of a bacterial strain in 1 day for much less than $1000. Similarly, a single instrument can generate 100 or more bacterial genome sequences in less than 1 week. Assuming this trend continues, a $10 bacterial genome will be realistically obtained in the near future. The coupling of increased DNA sequencing capacity with decreased instrument and reagent cost and newly developed computational expertise has driven the intensive interrogation of the bacterial genomes into the forefront of modern infectious disease research. These advances are not projections for the future, but rather, they are mature technologies on the verge of routine clinical laboratory implementation. Importantly, recent achievements in bacterial genomics have transformed our understanding of virulence factors, host-pathogen interactions, and population genetics. Furthermore, they have opened new opportunities for the rational design of diagnostics, therapeutics, and vaccines that may significantly improve patient care (Fig 1).

M. G. Bissell, MD, PhD, MPH

Data Submission and Quality in Microarray-Based MicroRNA Profiling

Witwer KW (Johns Hopkins Univ School of Medicine, Baltimore, MD)

Clin Chem 59:392-400, 2013

Background.—Public sharing of scientific data has assumed greater importance in the omics era. Transparency is necessary for confirmation and validation, and multiple examiners aid in extracting maximal value from large data sets. Accordingly, database submission and provision of the Minimum Information About a Microarray Experiment

(MIAME)[3] are required by most journals as a prerequisite for review or acceptance.

Methods.—In this study, the level of data submission and MIAME compliance was reviewed for 127 articles that included microarray-based microRNA (miRNA) profiling and were published from July 2011 through April 2012 in the journals that published the largest number of such articles—*PLOS ONE*, the *Journal of Biological Chemistry, Blood*, and *Oncogene*—along with articles from 9 other journals, including *Clinical Chemistry*, that published smaller numbers of array-based articles.

Results.—Overall, data submission was reported at publication for <40% of all articles, and almost 75% of articles were MIAME noncompliant. On average, articles that included full data submission scored significantly higher on a quality metric than articles with limited or no data submission, and studies with adequate description of methods disproportionately included larger numbers of experimental repeats. Finally, for several articles that were not MIAME compliant, data reanalysis revealed less than complete support for the published conclusions, in 1 case leading to retraction.

Conclusions.—These findings buttress the hypothesis that reluctance to share data is associated with low study quality and suggest that most miRNA array investigations are underpowered and/or potentially compromised by a lack of appropriate reporting and data submission.

▶ Irreproducibility of scientific findings is a cause for ongoing concern. The authors of a recent analysis presented a parsimonious surrogate for poor quality: a "reluctance to share published research data," presumably stemming from investigators' "fear that reanalysis may expose errors in their work or may produce conclusions that contradict their own." For publication of research that involves array technology, mandatory full data deposition is already the norm, based on the Minimum Information About a Microarray Experiment (MIAME) standard. First published in 2001 and rapidly adopted by most journals, MIAME describes the minimum information that is needed to interpret "the results of the experiment unambiguously and potentially to reproduce the experiment." Only 10 of 18 *Nature Genetics* microarray studies that were examined in a 2009 study were found to link to MIAME-compliant data. The author noticed recently that many microRNA (miRNA) micro array profiling publications do not reference public data, suggesting that the miRNA field may be a special area of concern. Interest in miRNAs as regulators and biomarkers of clinical conditions has led to a rapid increase of miRNA profiling studies and funding opportunities. The influx of new investigators has been facilitated by the relatively small number of canonical miRNAs in comparison with, for example, protein-coding transcripts, combined with the availability of off-the-shelf profiling systems and mail-in services. Even experience with analysis of large data sets may appear to be an unnecessary prerequisite to miRNA profiling, because data analysis is offered by service companies, and vendors provide largely automated analysis workflows, obviating direct data manipulation by the investigator. Although access to research options is positive, black box services and software also present potential pitfalls and may contribute to irreproducible results and confusion in the miRNA-profiling field, as in any work that involves large data sets. To assess the current level of MIAME compliance in miRNA array studies, the author reviewed articles that reported array-based miRNA profiling in the 4 journals that published the largest number of such studies during a 10-month period from 2011 to 2012. To provide a sampling of the wider literature as well, he examined all such articles published during a 2-week period within these 10 months.

M. G. Bissell, MD, PhD, MPH

Diagnosing fetal alcohol syndrome: new insights from newer genetic technologies

Douzgou S, Breen C, Crow Y, et al (Univ of Manchester, UK)
Arch Dis Child 97:812-817, 2012

Objective.—A genetic opinion is frequently requested in the assessment of a child with suspected fetal alcohol spectrum disorders (FASD). We studied the outcome of genetic assessment of 80 children referred to a regional genetics centre between 2004 and 2010 to identify the value of the genetic assessment in cases of suspected FASD.

Design.—Retrospective case series.

Patients.—80 patients, aged between 1 month and 26 years.

Methods.—Data from the medical records was abstracted, entered onto a standard study pro forma, recorded in an Excel spreadsheet and analysed using simple frequency analysis.

Results.—In 20% of cases fetal alcohol syndrome was confirmed at the genetic consultation. The most common facial features were thin upper lip (86.6%) and short palpebral fissures (82%). A lip–philtrum score of 4 or 5 was identified in two-thirds of cases. The most common alternative diagnosis was a chromosome disorder, representing 8.75% of the FASD referrals.

Setting.—A regional genetics service in the North West of England.

Conclusions.—Genetic assessment was of particular value in excluding other diagnoses and providing information to carers. Two-thirds of the children referred were subject to a care order increasing the difficulty to obtain a family and alcohol exposure history. Classification of FASD was difficult in children under a year old when data on growth and development were limited. Structural malformations were not common in the group overall and some previously reported diagnostic signs were not found to be reliable markers of FASD. Chromosome disorders showed phenotypic overlap with FASD and are an important differential diagnosis.

▶ In 1973, a landmark report on birth defects in children of alcoholic mothers was published, which correlated prenatal alcohol exposure with a pattern of major and minor malformations, growth failure, and cognitive and behavioral problems. Although this condition was initially designated "fetal alcohol syndrome" (FAS), the term "fetal alcohol spectrum disorders" (FASD) has been proposed more recently to describe a broader range of adverse outcomes of prenatal alcohol exposure. The incidence of FASD is thought to range from 0.2 to 2.0 per 1000 live births. Diagnostic criteria for FASD were defined in 1996, and 5 diagnostic categories were proposed: FAS with confirmed maternal alcohol exposure, FAS without confirmed maternal alcohol exposure, partial FAS with confirmed alcohol exposure, alcohol-related birth defects, and alcohol-related neurodevelopmental disorder. These criteria were subsequently updated in 2005, and further comprehensive guidelines have been published subsequently. Despite this guidance and the introduction of more objective scoring systems for FASD, it can still be difficult to confirm or refute this diagnosis in an individual child. Biomarkers for prenatal alcohol exposure exist, most notably the levels of fatty acid ethyl esters in meconium and hair, but utilizing these in routine clinical practice has proven difficult. Obtaining an accurate history of alcohol exposure can be problematic, as mothers may not be willing to disclose their true alcohol intake during pregnancy. Several prenatal screening tools exist for identification of mothers at an increased risk of having a child with FASD, including T-ACE, TWEAK, and AUDIT-C. Many children presenting for diagnosis of FASD do not live with their mothers, making the use of these tools difficult. British Medical Association guidelines recommend referral of all children with suspected FASD to a clinical geneticist. A genetic assessment is similar to other consultations involving the processes of history taking, clinical examination and investigation, and tying all these together to arrive at a diagnosis. However, more attention is paid to the family and perinatal history, and a detailed examination for morphologic differences is carried out. The geneticist may order specific investigations, such as chromosomal microarray analysis and single gene tests. When searching for a diagnosis, the clinical geneticist uses a variety of resources, including specialized literature, databases, and opinions from other colleagues. Some clinical geneticists question the value of their input to the diagnosis of FASD, an environmental disorder in which there is often limited maternal and family information available. The authors, therefore, sought to explore the value of genetic assessment of children with suspected FASD in the setting of a regional genetics center.

M. G. Bissell, MD, PhD, MPH

Importance of the Efficiency of Double-Stranded DNA Formation in cDNA Synthesis for the Imprecision of Microarray Expression Analysis

Thormar HG, Gudmundsson B, Eiriksdottir F, et al (Univ of Iceland, Reykjavik; Lifeind ehf, Reykjavik, Iceland; et al)
Clin Chem 59:667-674, 2013

Background.—The causes of imprecision in microarray expression analysis are poorly understood, limiting the use of this technology in molecular diagnostics. Two-dimensional strandness-dependent electrophoresis (2D-SDE) separates nucleic acid molecules on the basis of length and strandness, i.e., double-stranded DNA (dsDNA), single-stranded DNA (ssDNA), and RNA·DNA hybrids.

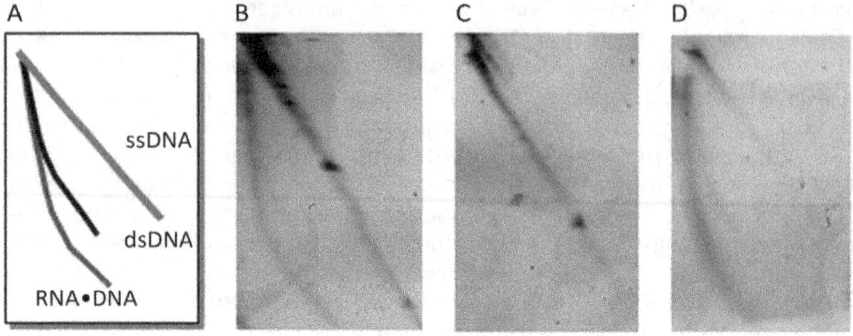

FIGURE 1.—Analysis of cDNA synthesis with 2D-SDE. (A), Schematic representation of analysis of cDNA synthesis with 2D-SDE. The RNA and ssDNA fragments in the original sample form a diagonal line in front of an arc of dsDNA. RNA·DNA hybrids form an arc lying behind the dsDNA arc. Separation of the fractions allows measurements of the percentage and length distribution of each fraction. (B), Products of cDNA synthesis showing ssRNA template, RNA·DNA hybrids, and only a small amount of dsDNA. (C), Products of a cDNA synthesis reaction without deoxynucleoside triphosphates, showing only RNA from the original template. (D), Products of a cDNA synthesis reaction treated with RNase A. Treatment decreased the ssRNA/ssDNA fraction from 80% to 12%, indicating that most of this fraction was RNA. (Reprinted from Thormar HG, Gudmundsson B, Eiriksdottir F, et al. Importance of the efficiency of double-stranded DNA formation in cDNA synthesis for the imprecision of microarray expression analysis. *Clin Chem.* 2013;59:667-674, used with permission from the American Association for Clinical Chemistry.)

Methods.—We used 2D-SDE to measure the efficiency of cDNA synthesis and its importance for the imprecision of an in vitro transcription–based microarray expression analysis.

Results.—The relative amount of double-stranded cDNA formed in replicate experiments that used the same RNA sample template was highly variable, ranging between 0% and 72% of the total DNA. Microarray experiments showed an inverse relationship between the difference between sample pairs in probe variance and the relative amount of dsDNA. Approximately 15% of probes showed between sample variation ($P < 0.05$) when the dsDNA percentage was between 12% and 35%. In contrast, only 3% of probes showed between-sample variation when the dsDNA percentage was 69% and 72%. Replication experiments of the 35% dsDNA and 72% dsDNA samples were used to separate sample variation from probe replication variation. The estimated SD of the sample-to-sample variation and of the probe replicates was lower in 72% dsDNA samples than in 35% dsDNA samples.

Conclusions.—Variation in the relative amount of double-stranded cDNA synthesized can be an important component of the imprecision in T7 RNA polymerase–based microarray expression analysis (Fig 1).

► Analysis of gene expression with microarrays is a major application in functional genomics. This technology is also becoming important in clinical diagnostics, such as the monitoring of gene expression profiles in breast cancer. Despite new technologies for sample preparation, array treatment, and data analysis, concerns have been raised regarding the quality of the experimental results.

The steps in sample processing, including cDNA synthesis and antisense RNA (aRNA) transcription (if used), are critical and have direct implications for the quality of the analytical phase. These steps have received less attention than factors affecting reproducibility, most likely because of a lack of methods to characterize the composition of complex nucleic acid samples and how composition affects quality. Measurements of the amounts and length distributions of single-stranded DNA (ssDNA), RNA-DNA hybrids, and double-stranded DNA (dsDNA), in particular, might provide useful information about the sample. Such measurements could be used to estimate the effects of these variables on sample quality. One of the most commonly used methods in microarray expression analysis is in vitro transcription (IVT) that uses T7 RNA polymerase to transcribe double-stranded cDNA to aRNA. Experiments have found that IVT and RNA-labeling procedures are a large source of technical variation. The T7 RNA polymerase can initiate transcription only if the promoter-binding site in the cDNA is double stranded. This fact suggests that the composition and strandness of the cDNA sample is an important parameter affecting the quality of gene expression analysis based on IVT. The authors previously described 2-dimensional strandness-dependent electrophoresis (2D-SDE), a method for relative quantification and length analysis of the ssDNA, ssRNA, dsDNA, and RNA-DNA hybrid fractions in complex nucleic acid samples. In the first dimension of the electrophoresis, molecules in the sample are separated on the basis of both length and strandness, that is, whether they are ssDNA/ssRNA, dsDNA (B-form helix), or RNA-DNA hybrids (A-form helix). Of these 3 fractions, ssDNA/ssRNA migrates slowest, dsDNA has an intermediate mobility, and RNA-DNA hybrids have the fastest mobility (A-form helices are shorter than B-form helices per base pair). In the second dimension of the electrophoresis, all the molecules are single stranded and are separated only according to length. The method of 2D-SDE, therefore, separates these 3 different fractions present in the original sample (Fig 1). In this study, the authors used 2D-SDE to analyze the efficiency of cDNA synthesis. Their hypothesis was that cDNA synthesis is a major factor affecting imprecision in microarray expression analysis. Identifying such factors might allow modifications in sample preparation procedures that could improve precision and facilitate the use of microarrays in molecular diagnostics.

M. G. Bissell, MD, PhD, MPH

Article Index

Chapter 1: Outcomes Analysis

Chapter 2: Breast

Chapter 3: Gastrointestinal System

Chapter 4: Hepatobiliary System and Pancreas

Chapter 5: Lung and Mediastinum

Chapter 6: Soft Tissue and Bone

Chapter 7: Female Genital Tract

Chapter 8: Kidney

Chapter 9: Head and Neck

Chapter 10: Cytopathology

Chapter 11: Hematolymphoid

Chapter 12: Techniques/Molecular

Chapter 13: Laboratory Management and Outcomes

Chapter 14: Clinical Chemistry

Chapter 15: Clinical Microbiology

Chapter 16: Hematology and Immunology

Chapter 17: Transfusion Medicine and Coagulation

Chapter 18: Cytogenetics and Molecular Pathology

Author Index

H

I

J

K

L

M

N

O

P

Q

R

S

T

Sheridan
Hanover, PA USA
October 16, 2018